753.50

D1088044

Essential Hypertension as an Endocrine Disease

Butterworths International Medical Reviews

Clinical Endocrinology

Published volumes

1   The Pituitary
Edited by Colin Beardwell and Gary L. Robertson

2   Calcium Disorders
Edited by David A. Heath and Stephen J. Marx

Next title

Adrenal Cortex
Edited by David C. Anderson and Jeremy S. D. Winter

Essential Hypertension as an Endocrine Disease

Edited by

Christopher R. W. Edwards, MD, FRCP, FRCP(Edin.)
Professor of Clinical Medicine, University of Edinburgh Department of Medicine, Western General Hospital, Edinburgh, UK

and

Robert M. Carey, MD
Professor of Internal Medicine; Head, Division of Endocrinology and Metabolism, University of Virginia Medical Center, Charlottesville, Virginia, USA

Butterworths
London Boston Durban Singapore Sydney Toronto Wellington

First published 1985

© Butterworth & Co. (Publishers) Ltd. 1985

British Library Cataloguing in Publication Data

Essential hypertension as an endocrine disease
  –(Butterworth's international medical reviews
  Clinical endocrinology, ISSN 0260-0072; 3)
  1. Hypertension
  I. Edwards, C.R.W.   II. Carey, R.M.
  616.1'32071   RC685.H8

  ISBN 0-407-02274-0

Photoset by Butterworths Litho Preparation Department
Printed and bound in England by Robert Hartnoll Ltd., Bodmin, Cornwall

Contributors

Karen L. Barnes, PhD
Staff, Research Division, Section of Cardiovascular Neurobiology, Department of Cardiovascular Research, Cleveland Clinic Foundation, Cleveland, Ohio, USA

K. Bridget Brosnihan, PhD
Staff, Research Division, Section of Cardiovascular Neurobiology, Department of Cardiovascular Research, Cleveland Clinic Foundation, Cleveland, Ohio, USA

Morris J. Brown, MSc, MRCP
Senior Lecturer in Clinical Pharmacology, Royal Postgraduate Medical School, London, UK

Paul L. Drury, MA, MRCP
Lecturer in Medicine, Department of Medicine, Medical College of St Bartholomew's Hospital, London, UK

Fernando Elijovich, MD
Internal Medicine Associate, Hypertension Division, Mount Sinai Medical Center, New York, New York, USA

Carlos M. Ferrario, MD
Acting Chairman, Section of Cardiovascular Neurobiology, Department of Cardiovascular Research, Cleveland Clinic Foundation, Cleveland, Ohio, USA

R. Fraser, MSc, PhD, FRSE
Medical Research Council Blood Research Unit, Glasgow, UK

Norman K. Hollenberg, MD, PhD
Professor of Radiology, Harvard Medical School and Brigham Women's Hospital, Boston, Massachusetts, USA

Lawrence R. Krakoff, MD
Professor of Medicine; Chief, Hypertension Division, Mount Sinai Medical Center, New York, New York, USA

A. F. Lever, MB BS, FRCP, FRSE
Director, Medical Research Council Blood Pressure Unit, Glasgow, UK

Graham A. MacGregor, MA, FRCP
Senior Lecturer; Honorary Consultant Physician, Department of Medicine, Charing Cross Hospital Medical School, London, UK

E. E. Muirhead, MD
Director, Department of Pathology, Baptist Memorial Hospital; Professor and Chairman, Department of Pathology, University of Tennessee Center for the Health Sciences, Memphis, Tennessee, USA

Henry W. Overbeck, MD, PhD
Departments of Medicine and Physiology/Biophysics, Cardiovascular Research and Training Center, University of Alabama School of Medicine, Birmingham, Alabama, USA

P. L. Padfield, MB, BCh, MRCP
Consultant Physician/Senior Lecturer, Department of Medicine, Western General Hospital, Edinburgh, UK

Michael J. Peach, BS, MS, PhD
Professor of Pharmacology, Department of Pharmacology, University of Virginia School of Medicine, Charlottesville, USA

Peter C. Rubin, MA, DM, FRCP
Wellcome Senior Fellow in Clinical Science, University Department of Materia Medica, Stobhill General Hospital, Glasgow, UK

Marc T. Schiavone, PhD
Research Fellow, Section of Cardiovascular Neurobiology, Department of Cardiovascular Research, Cleveland Clinic Foundation, Cleveland, Ohio, USA

Harold A. Singer, BS, PhD
Research Fellow in Physiology, Department of Pharmacology, University of Virginia School of Medicine, Charlottesville, Virginia, USA

Robert C. Speth, PhD
Associate Staff, Research Division, Section of Cardiovascular Neurobiology, Department of Cardiovascular Research, Cleveland Clinic Foundation, Cleveland, Ohio, USA

Michael L. Tuck, MD
Professor of Medicine, UCLA School of Medicine; Chief of Endocrinology/
Metabolism, UCLA San Fernando Valley Program, Sepulveda, California, USA

H. E. de Wardener, MD, FRCP
Emeritus Professor of Medicine, Research Laboratories, Charing Cross Hospital,
London, UK

Michael L. Watson, MB, ChB, MRCP
Consultant Physician, Royal Infirmary, Edinburgh, UK

Gordon H. Williams, MD
Professor of Medicine, Harvard Medical School, Brigham and Women's Hospital,
Boston, Massachusetts, USA

Contents

Introduction

Christopher R. W. Edwards and Robert M. Carey

There have been several excellent reviews and monographs on endocrine hypertension but these have largely concentrated on the classical endocrine conditions such as Cushing's and Conn's syndromes, phaeochromocytoma, hypertensive types of congenital adrenal hyperplasia, angiotensin II-dependent hypertension, acromegaly and primary hypothyroidism. Although these conditions are of particular interest in that they highlight different endocrine mechanisms leading to hypertension, they appear to have little relevance to the majority of patients with high blood pressure. This book was prompted by our feeling that there was a need to gather together in one volume a selection of the pieces of evidence suggesting that there are significant endocrine abnormalities in patients with essential hypertension. While we believe that many of these abnormalities are likely to be primary contributing factors in the pathophysiology and/or maintenance of essential hypertension, it also is possible that some of these abnormalities may be secondary to the hypertensive process.

Any consideration of the aetiology of hypertension, be it hormonal or otherwise, must include a definition of hypertension. This has proved to be difficult because frequency distribution curves for blood pressure in a population have shown that there is no subpopulation with high blood pressure that can be distinguished from those with normal pressure. Hence, Pickering proposed that hypertension is not a qualitative entity, and thus any distinction between normal and high blood pressure must of necessity be arbitrary. If then blood pressure itself is a graded phenomenon with no clear distinction between normal and abnormal, it may well be that factors leading to high blood pressure are related to those that modulate normal pressure, and hence the fault lies in their homeostatic control. On the other hand, factors leading to high blood pressure may be unrelated to normal control mechanisms and these putatively inherited causal agent(s) would presumably have such variable penetrance and be so common as to make hypertensives indistinguishable as a separate subpopulation.

Teleologically, it would seem appropriate that the endocrine system, which is based on the release of products of specialized cells into an aqueous compartment

1

to have an effect on cells at a distance from the site of secretion, should control the transport of hormones to their target sites of action. Thus, hormonal regulation of volume and pressure of the aqueous compartment would be critical for effective delivery of the message.

The role that hormones play in the control of normal and high blood pressure has been made much easier to determine by the introduction of specific pharmacological agents that block the effects or decrease the production of different hormones. For example, the competitive antagonists of angiotensin II and captopril, the first orally active angiotensin converting enzyme (ACE) inhibitor, have given new insight into the role of the renin-angiotensin system in blood pressure homeostasis. Thus, in idiopathic hyperaldosteronism we now know that the zona glomerulosa has a markedly enhanced sensitivity to angiotensin II and that treatment with an ACE inhibitor will lower aldosterone secretion, elevate plasma potassium and lower blood pressure to normal. However, not surprisingly such responses in patients with low renin essential hypertension have focused attention on the possibility that angiotensin converting enzyme inhibitors might be lowering blood pressure by means other than a reduction of angiotensin II. These include effects on the degradation of kinins, production of prostaglandins, and the sympathetic nervous system. In addition, the fact that almost all hypertensive patients can be controlled on the combination of an angiotensin converting enzyme inhibitor with a diuretic or sodium restriction has given emphasis to the role that sodium intake may play. Similarly, in normal subjects a low sodium intake markedly increases the hypotensive effect of angiotensin converting enzyme inhibitors.

Useful though these drugs have been in treating hypertension, caution is necessary in interpreting the response in terms of the aetiology of the problem. Are angiotensin converting enzyme inhibitors lowering blood pressure by interfering with a normal or a pathological control mechanism? In the case of calcium antagonists some authors have claimed that their effect is greater in hypertensive than in normotensive subjects and have suggested that such drugs are treating a specific cause for the high blood pressure. However, other authors have clearly shown that alternative pharmacological agents with a specific mechanism of action also are more effective in lowering blood pressure in hypertensive than in normotensive patients. For example, the specific dopamine-1 (DA-1) receptor stimulating agent, SKF 82526-J, normalizes blood pressure in hypertensive subjects but is ineffective in normal subjects. Thus, reduction of blood pressure to normal by a pharmacological agent does not necessarily imply that the mechanism altered by that agent is responsible for the underlying hypertensive process.

If then the endocrine system is important in the control of blood pressure, what hormones could play a role in either the genesis or maintenance of essential hypertension? In this book we have selected some of the areas of hypertension research in which there is evidence for a hormonal mechanism. The various authors look at the possible involvement of the peripheral and the brain renin–angiotensin system, vasopressin, epinephrine, the natriuretic hormone, mineralocorticoids, prostanoids and the renomedullary interstitial cell antihypertensive hormone, Hormones, however, cannot be considered in isolation. Hence the chapters on the role of salt and the endothelium in hypertension, and reviews of high blood pressure associated with pregnancy, diabetes and obesity.

Hypertension research has been likened to the man who lost his car keys in a poorly lighted car park. A passing stranger offered to help and spent some minutes searching in vain before asking the hapless motorist 'Are you sure you lost your keys in this part of the car park?' 'No', replied the man, 'I am not sure, but the light is much brighter here.'

Our hope is that this book, which is the first to our knowledge to concentrate on the endocrinology of essential hypertension rather than the more esoteric causes of endocrine hypertension, will shed some light on this exciting and critical field.

1

Role of central mechanisms in the development of endocrine hypertension

Carlos M. Ferrario, Marc T. Schiavone,
Karen L. Barnes, K. Bridget Brosnihan and
Robert C. Speth

INTRODUCTION

Not very long ago the task of outlining this chapter would have been a straightforward undertaking, since the hypertension literature provided us with a clear cut classification of those diastolic and systolic hypertensions that are either produced by or associated with disturbances in endocrine function. In current textbooks of medicine (such as Conn and Conn, 1980) the involvement of the endocrine system as a cause of high blood pressure is limited to a discussion of adrenal hypertension, pheochromocytoma, Cushing's disease and the adreno-genital syndrome; a more complete survey of the subject would include the 'secondary' association of hypertension with myxedema, hyperparathyroidism and acromegaly. Restriction of the topic to the diseases listed above is no longer tenable since we now know that the nervous and endocrine systems serve a variety of integrative functions. With the consideration that blood, tissue and brain hormones modify the activity of the peripheral and central aspects of the sympathetic control mechanism, the involvement of endocrine factors in the regulation of cardiac output and tissue perfusion pressure must be re-evaluated.

To begin with, hormonal factors may have a direct influence upon vascular contractility, as in the case of angiotensin II (Ang II) and pituitary vasopressin (Cowley, 1982; Westfall, 1980). However, in other situations the action of endocrine substances upon the regulation of blood pressure may either result from, or be masked by, accompanying disorders of the neurogenic control mechanism. For example, the adrenal cortex is linked strongly to blood pressure regulation through its major effects on the extracellular fluid and sodium balance (Reid and Ganong, 1977; Vecsei, Hackenthal and Ganten, 1978). However, steroid hormones can also act at presynaptic and postsynaptic sites to alter uptake and release of neurotransmitters, as well as affect the synthesis of neuronal proteins which, following either axonal or dendritic transport, may participate in neurojunctional events (McEwen *et al.*, 1979; Westfall, 1980). Adrenal steroids can

4

therefore exert an effect at several points in the blood pressure regulatory mechanism; identification of the site or sites at which an endocrine product exerts a major effect will require a parallel and precise understanding of the array of functions and their relative hierarchy.

Another factor must be considered in evaluating the role of the nervous and endocrine systems in blood pressure regulation. Although these systems are most clearly defined in vertebrates, recent evidence suggests that they may have their origins in the most primitive of eukaryotic and prokaryotic organisms (LeRoith *et al.*, 1983; Rosenzweig *et al.*, 1983). According to LeRoith *et al.* (1983) a peptide very similar to insulin exists in two strains of protozoa, two species of fungi and four strains of *Escherichia coli*. Somatostatin, ACTH(1-39) and beta-endorphin may also be present in protozoa (LeRoith *et al.*, 1983). These observations suggest that some of the pre-existing messenger molecules in microbes were incorporated by evolutionary forces into the nervous system to act as neurotransmitters, and into the endocrine system to act as hormones. Tracing the evolutionary origin of peptide hormones may provide a clue to the possible unity of the nervous and endocrine systems and thus establish the need to consider these two systems together in the understanding of blood pressure regulation.

The striking evidence that is emerging from the use of genetic probes and studies of comparative structure–activity relationships (Cooper and Martin, 1982; Rosenzweig *et al.*, 1983) raises an important question: *Are neurogenic and hormonal (endocrine) mechanisms unrelated expressions of the autonomic control of cardiovascular function, or are these two systems intertwined so intimately as to constitute parts of a more basic cellular regulatory control mechanism dealing with the constancy of the 'milieu interieur' and the adaptation of the organism to fluctuations in the surrounding environment?* This possibility has not been generally recognized by hypertensinologists, in part because the majority of the new and challenging information originates from basic neurobiology studies. Because we no longer believe that there are firm boundaries (other than anatomical ones) separating the endocrine system and the nervous system, the material reviewed in this chapter will be integrated by considering the facets of endocrine-based hypertensions as an aspect of a more generalized disturbance in the neuroendocrine control of the circulatory system.

BASIC FUNCTIONS OF THE AUTONOMIC NERVOUS SYSTEM

It is agreed that the central nervous system (CNS) plays a fundamental role in controlling arterial perfusion pressure by regulating the amount and pattern of the discharge of sympathetic and parasympathetic neurons to the heart and blood vessels, integrating reflexes, controlling the release of vasoactive hormones such as the output of renin by the kidneys and secretion of vasopressin by the neurohypophysis, and coupling the cardiovascular system to behavior (Abboud *et al.*, 1976; Abboud, 1982).

The peripheral autonomic nervous system is integrated with the CNS into a functional unit by both afferent and efferent pathways (Hilton, 1975). The afferent pathways transmit sensory information to the central controller from receptors which act as mechanochemical transducers converting the energy derived from cardiac and vascular wall stresses into nerve action potentials (Katchalsky and Rehovoth, 1971). Sensory receptors and afferent pathways that may be involved in hypertension include arterial and cardiopulmonary receptors and possibly somatic endings in skeletal muscle and skin (Abboud, 1982; Ferrario and Takishita, 1983; Tarazi, Fouad and Ferrario, 1983). Efforts to demonstrate a primary disturbance in the reflex regulation of arterial pressure as a cause of arterial hypertension have met with failure, inasmuch as sustained hypertension has not yet been produced by the removal of the carotid sinus and aortic nerves (Cowley, Monos and Guyton, 1974; Ferrario and Takishita, 1983). However, these observations do not negate an important role of pressor and possibly depressor reflexes in the pathogenesis of arterial hypertension since a change in their normal function could contribute to the evolution and/or maintenance of high blood pressure. A well-known example is the resetting of the carotid sinus baroreceptor, particularly important in the pathogenesis of renal hypertension (Krieger, Salgado and Michelini, 1982; McCubbin, Green and Page, 1956; McCubbin and Page, 1963; Page and McCubbin, 1965). Recent studies indicate that pressor reflexes originating from the myocardium, coronary vessels and aorta may be a cause of paroxysmal hypertension associated with coronary insufficiency, dissecting aneurysms, Lewis's angina and hypertension after coronary bypass surgery (Tarazi, Fouad and Ferrario, 1983). Because cardiopulmonary receptors are important in the regulation of renin release, renal function and the secretion of vasopressin (VP), they may also participate in the pathogenesis of high blood pressure. Esler, Julius and Randall (1976) suggest that low pressure intrathoracic receptors may be active in the expression of low renin hypertension. Sympathetic afferents have occasionally been considered as a source for disturbances in blood pressure regulation. Recent studies (Katholi *et al.,* 1982; Winternitz, Katholi and Oparil, 1982; Zanchetti, 1979) indicate that renal afferents may be involved causally in the pathogenesis of experimental hypertension.

The efferent pathways involved in the maintenance of arterial pressure include brain cardiovascular centers and sympathetic and parasympathetic effector pathways. The sympathetic and parasympathetic neuroeffector mechanisms in the heart are of major importance in the regulation of cardiac rate and output, whereas the sympathetic neuroeffector system in the blood vessels has been shown to be the dominant pathway by which autonomic neural activity is reflected in vasomotor tone. Although these efferent autonomic effects are predominantly vasoconstrictor, there is strong evidence for the existence of neurogenic vasodilator mechanisms including sympathetic cholinergic, histaminergic, dopaminergic and beta-adrenergic dilator systems (Abboud, 1982; Folkow, 1982). Each of these systems, or all combined, may have an important role in hypertension since they tend both to oppose as well as facilitate the adrenergic vasoconstrictor actions of the sympathetic nervous system (SNS).

There are other important ways by which the autonomic nervous system participates in the regulation of arterial pressure and, hence, hypertension. Both adrenergic and dopaminergic systems have been shown to influence the urinary excretion of sodium (Edwards *et al.*, 1982; Reid and Ganong, 1977). In addition, neurogenic factors interact with the renin–angiotensin system (RAS), in part via the blood-borne effects of angiotensin II upon neuroreceptors located in, or within the vicinity of, the brain circumventricular organs (CVOs) (Ferrario and McCubbin, 1974; Knigge *et al.*, 1980). Through its effects on the circulation, the excretory function of the kidneys and certain hormonal mechanisms (angiotensin II and vasopressin), the autonomic nervous system also plays an important role in the regulation of extracellular fluid and the distribution of the 'effective blood volume' between the peripheral and cardiopulmonary compartments (Berecek and Bohr, 1976; Brennan *et al.*, 1971; Cowley, Monos and Guyton, 1974; Ericsson, 1971; Esler, Julius and Randall, 1976; Folkow, 1960; Gavras *et al.*, 1982; Heyndrickx, Boettcher and Vatner, 1976; Hilton, 1975; Mark *et al.*, 1977; Share, 1976; Tarazi, Fouad and Ferrario, 1983). Thus neurogenic mechanisms influence arterial pressure in multiple ways by effects on cardiac function, vasomotor tone, humoral and hormonal mechanisms, renal function and sodium excretion, and the distribution of blood and extracellular fluid volumes. Neurogenic mechanisms of blood pressure regulation are also closely linked to behavioral and environmental influences. For example, stress and excessive intake of sodium are behavioral and environmental factors that are known to modify blood pressure. It is conceivable that they contribute to hypertension by affecting neurogenic control (Elliott and Eisdorfer, 1982). Lastly, these same mechanisms may trigger an increased contribution of renal, endocrine or vascular responses which might then sustain the elevated blood pressure (Ferrario and McCubbin, 1974; Ferrario *et al.*, 1981; Tobian, 1977).

It is therefore conceivable that disturbances in autonomic nervous system function may act as initiating, reinforcing and/or stabilizing elements of the disease process. An increase in sympathetic nerve activity due to the action of angiotensin II upon the intrinsic activity of bulbospinal vasomotor neurons (Ferrario and McCubbin, 1974), together with the effect of the peptide acting at presynaptic sites to release norepinephrine (NE) (McCubbin, 1974; Peach, Bumpus and Khairallah, 1969; Westfall, 1980), is one of the possible ways by which autonomic mechanisms can participate in the development of high blood pressure in experimental situations such as renovascular hypertension (Page and McCubbin, 1965, 1968). Adjustments in adrenergic activity to cardiac muscle may be associated with both the development and maintenance of left ventricular hypertrophy, a structural process which allows the heart muscle to cope with progressive increases in afterload (Folkow, 1982; Tarazi, Fouad and Ferrario, 1983).

Because the autonomic nervous system is endowed with such a variety of actions upon the cardiovascular system, apparent heterogeneities in the characteristics of various hypertensions may not necessarily imply the existence of several independent causes, but may instead represent a spectrum of variants with dominance shifting among neurogenic, hormonal and renal primary elements (Ferrario and Page, 1978; Folkow, 1982). The coexistence of aggravating factors such as stress, dietary imbalances or secondary disease may determine the predominant involvement of any one factor. There are thus no strict borders between primary and secondary elements; the initiation of hypertension should therefore be considered to originate from the interaction of neurogenic, hormonal and humoral mechanisms and their modulation by the environment. This does not deny, however, that predisposing factors may be common to either the human or animal species, or that the interplay between genetic and environmental influences will affect the disease process.

THE CONNECTION BETWEEN AUTONOMIC MECHANISMS AND NEUROENDOCRINE FACTORS

The discovery not too long ago that synapses both within and outside the CNS represented chemical switches led to the birth of a biochemical approach to the understanding of brain functions (Cooper and Martin, 1982; Frohman, 1980; Guillemin, 1980; McKelvy, Glasel and Foreman, 1980; Rotsztejn, 1980). At the synapse not only drugs but genetic factors, dietary constituents, hormones, metabolic products and immune and infectious processes could all be seen to act, altering the pattern of transynaptic activity to affect behavior, mental processes and organ system functions. At almost the same time it became increasingly evident that peripheral peptide hormones were not only able to gain access to the fluid environment of the brain (Cooper and Martin, 1982; Oldendorf, 1981; Rodriguez, 1976) but moreover were produced within the CNS itself. To date many (if not all) of the classically known peripheral peptide hormones such as insulin, kinins and angiotensin II, as well as the gut hormones gastrin, cholecystokinin and vasoactive intestinal peptide (VIP), have been localized in brain tissue, principally by employing immunohistochemical procedures (Cooper and Martin, 1982; Ganten and Speck, 1978; Guillemin, 1980; McKelvy, Glasel and Foreman, 1980). Although some questions exist regarding the chemical structure of some of these peptides (McKelvy, Glasel and Foreman, 1980; Rosenzweig *et al.*, 1983) it is likely that forthcoming information will verify their identity.

According to Charrer (1977) brain peptides acting as non-conventional chemical mediators represent a mode of information transfer that digresses from standard synaptic transmission. The discovery of these peptides (endorphins, brain–gut hormones, calcitonin, angiotensins, etc.) in the brain of mammals including man (Cooper and Martin, 1982) and the increasing progress that is being made in understanding their function have added another dimension to hypertension research. Although both peptide and steroid hormones convey a variety of messages at each receptor site, their possible mode of action at a synapse may not be vastly different. In a recent review of the subject Cooper and Martin (1982) indicated that peptidergic neurons are cells which manufacture and secrete peptides in a fashion similar or even identical to that of peripheral hormone-producing tissue. This principle is best exemplified by neurons of the supraoptic and paraventricular nuclei, the source of the posterior pituitary hormones vasopressin and oxytocin, and the hypophysiotropic neurons of the hypothalamus which secrete the pituitary releasing factors. At first the gland-like characteristics of these hypothalamic neurons may seem incongruous, yet all neurotransmission, even at the neuromuscular junction, is basically a form of neurosecretion (Cooper and

Martin, 1982). Indeed, it would appear that there is a *continuum* from neurons such as the anterior horn cell at one extreme to glandular cells such as the pancreatic beta-cell at the other, with hypothalamic neurons and certain peptide-secreting cells in the gastrointestinal tract occupying an intermediate position. The application of these concepts to the understanding of cardiovascular regulation has not been realized fully, even though today neuropeptides are the object of such intense research interest that it is hard to remember a time when they were not being actively studied.

According to Rotsztejn (1980), peptides can act as 'transmitters', 'neuro-hormones' or 'neuromodulators' depending upon the site at which the action takes place. An example of how a peptide can act as a *transmitter* is illustrated by the inhibitory effect of VIP on the release of somatostatin from medial basal hypothalamic fragments. The same peptide, however, can also behave as a *neurohormone*, as illustrated by the stimulatory effects of VIP upon prolactin (PRL) secretion by pituitary cells (Rotsztejn, 1980). In addition a peptide can also act as a *neuromodulator*. For example, methionine enkephalin, which has no effect by itself on the release of luteinizing hormone releasing hormone (LHRH), inhibits the dopamine (DA)-induced release of the hormone from LHRH terminals (Rotsztejn, 1980). In other words, neuromodulation by peptides appears to involve a long-lasting effect induced by a substance which then changes the capacity of the cell to respond to a given stimulus. Neuromodulation is not only a property of peptides but can also be extended to classic neurotransmitters (that is, involvement of serotonin with the suckling-induced PRL release) as well as certain steroid hormones (McEwen *et al.*, 1979). This observation points to further sites at which the action of the sympathetic and parasympathetic branches of autonomic function intertwines with the activity of peripheral and central endocrine products. As reviewed by McEwen *et al.* (1979), steroid hormones have both genomic and non-genomic effects in presynaptic and postsynaptic events. Non-genomic effects may involve the action of the hormone on the presynaptic or postsynaptic membrane to alter permeability (uptake, release) to neurotransmitters or their precursors and/or functioning of neurotransmitter receptors. Genomic actions of steroids lead to altered synthesis of proteins which, after axonal or dendritic transport, may participate in presynaptic or postsynaptic events. With the consideration that both glucocorticoid (Chatelain *et al.*, 1983; Krakoff, Nicolis and Amsel, 1975; Krakoff, Selvadura and Sutter, 1975) and mineralocorticoid (Edwards *et al.*, 1982; Vecsei, Hackenthal and Ganten, 1978) hormones participate in the pathogenesis of hypertension, a further understanding of both the molecular and biological events regulating the interaction of steroids with autonomic function is likely to offer new and important insights into the mechanisms of hypertension.

HYPERTENSION AND CENTRAL NERVOUS SYSTEM MECHANISMS

Under ordinary circumstances the arterial blood pressure, and hence the distribution of blood flow through various organs, is maintained within a normal range by the activity of neural systems largely contained within or relaying through the medulla oblongata. These centers drive preganglionic sympathetic neurons in the spinal cord, creating a background vasoconstrictor outflow that can alter peripheral resistance and thereby change arterial pressure. Moreover, this influence upon precapillary resistance vessels may be the product of an interaction between neural systems which exert opposite actions on sympathetic neurons. Reis (1981) suggests that the neuronal vasopressor system within the CNS may increase sympathetic discharges and hence arterial pressure; on the other hand, a counteracting neuronal vasodepressor system (such as the baroreceptors) may inhibit sympathetic activity and lower arterial pressure. The anatomical localization and physiology of these two systems have been investigated by a variety of techniques; these have demonstrated that pressor and depressor areas are anatomically segregated, driven in response to different behaviors, and excited reflexly by different stimuli (Reis, 1981).

Monoaminergic mechanisms

Many of the brain regions known to participate in cardiovascular regulation are densely supplied with bioamine-producing and/or releasing neurons. It is now known that the CNS contains three types of catecholamines: dopamine, norepinephrine and epinephrine (EPI). Although our understanding of the structure and function of the catecholamine-containing cells of the CNS is still incomplete, the progress that has been made thus far indicates that catecholaminergic neurons play an active role in the regulation of arterial pressure in both normotensive and hypertensive states. For a review of the anatomy and physiology of the central catecholaminergic system we recommend those published by Moore and Bloom (1978, 1979). For the purpose of this presentation it suffices to say that the norepinephrine neuron system contrasts with the dopamine and epinephrine neurons in having a remarkably extensive distribution throughout the neuroaxis. Dahlstrom and Fuxe (1964, 1965) numbered the norepinephrine-containing cell groups of the brain stem from A1 caudally to A12 rostrally; those containing serotonin have been classified as B1 to B9. Of particular importance is the demonstration of norepinephrine-containing neurons in the ventrolateral medulla (Loewy and McKellar, 1980); it has been suggested that these neurons may function as a part of the elusive 'brain stem vasomotor centers' (Bousquet *et al.*, 1979). Another important cell group (A2) lies within the complex of the nucleus tractus solitarius (nTS) and dorsal motor nucleus of the vagus (dmnX) and may also send fibers into the area postrema. Although the A1 and A2 groups were thought to innervate the spinal sympathetic preganglionic neurons (Dahlstrom and Fuxe, 1965), recent studies in rat (Loewy, McKellar and Saper, 1979) and rabbit (Chalmers *et al.*, 1981) reveal that the A5 and A7 cell groups innervate the intermediolateral cell column (IML), with minimal input from A1 to A2. On the other hand, Fleetwood-Walker and Coote (1981) reported that the major norepinephrine innervation of the intermediolateral cell column in the cat derives from A1, with little from A2 and none from A5. Whether the discrepancies result from *species or methodological differences* remains to be determined. Although the major norepinephrine innervation of hypothalamic regions appears to derive from A1, there may be small contributions from all the brainstem catecholaminergic cell groups. Epinephrine cell bodies have been reported in two cell groups in the rat (C1,C2) just rostral to the A1 and A2 norepinephrine cell groups (Ross *et al.*, 1981). Howe *et al.* (1980) have now found a third epinephrine-containing neuron cluster (C3) in the midline of the medulla just rostral to C2. In addition to confirming the nine serotonin (5-HT) cell groups reported by Dahlstrom and Fuxe (1965) in the rat midline raphe region, Steinbusch (1981) found five additional serotonergic cell clusters, including one in the area postrema. These new groups and the B1 and B3 groups in the medullary raphe are the most likely to have cardiovascular relevance. Loewy and McKellar (1980, 1981) have reported that B1 and B3 neurons project to the intermediolateral cell column of the thoracic spinal cord.

Some of the strongest evidence for central catecholaminergic involvement in regulation of arterial pressure derives from studies of centrally acting antihypertensive drugs (DeJong and Nijkamp, 1976; Gordon *et al.*, 1979; Korner and Head, 1983; Nashold, Mannarino and Wunderlich, 1961; Sowers, Nyby and Jasberg, 1982) which appear to operate by mimicking CNS catecholamines. Microinjection of norepinephrine or epinephrine into the rat nucleus tractus solitarius produces a rapid decrease in arterial pressure and heart rate. The effect can be blocked by prior microinjection of phentolamine (DeJong and Nijkamp, 1976); on the other hand, a microinjection of serotonin into the nucleus tractus solitarius produces increases in arterial pressure that are blocked by 5-HT antagonists (Coote *et al.*, 1981). Electrolytic and neurochemical lesion studies also support the importance of catecholamines in cardiovascular control. In the rabbit, Blessing, West and Chalmers (1981) have shown that destruction of the A1 norepinephrine region results in hypertension and profound bradycardia. On the other hand, destruction of A2 cells in the rat produces only lability of arterial pressure with unchanged mean pressure (Reis *et al.*, 1979). Recent studies by Ferrario and Barnes (unpublished observations) suggest that the initial hypertension due to central baroreceptor denervation (nucleus tractus solitarius hypertension) is accounted for by increased quantities of circulating vasopressin (*Figures 1.1* and *1.2*). These observations are of considerable interest since others (Sawchenko and Swanson, 1982; Sofroniew, 1980; Sofroniew and Schrell, 1981; Swanson and Sawchenko, 1980) have shown that vasopressin and oxytocin-containing neurons in the supraoptic and paraventricular nuclei are innervated by noradrenergic terminals in part arising from the A1 region.

There have been a number of studies emphasizing the importance of the role of central adrenergic and dopaminergic systems in the pathogenesis of steroid and renal hypertension. Reid, Zivin and Kopin (1975) have shown that in the rat destruction of noradrenergic neurons by the injection of 6-hydroxydopamine (6-OHDA) into the CSF prevents the development of deoxycorticosterone (DOC) salt hypertension. Activity of the enzyme phenylethanolamine *N*-methyltransferase (PNMT) which converts norepinephrine to epinephrine is increased in the brain stem of deoxycorticosterone and salt-treated rats (Saavedra, Grobecker and Axelrod, 1976; Saavedra, 1979; Saavedra, Kvetnansky and Kopin, 1979; Saavedra,

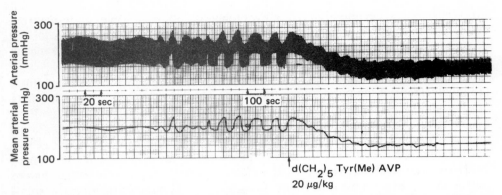

Figure 1.1 Within 1 hour after bilateral destruction of the solitary tracts and recovery from halothane anesthesia, the dog has become markedly hypertensive; the elevations in mean arterial pressure (MAP: 196 mmHg) are associated with great lability due to the presence of a complete atrioventricular block demonstrated electrocardiographically. At the *arrow* an intravenous injection of a competitive antagonist of the vasculotropic actions of arginine vasopressin [d(CH$_2$)$_5$Tyr(Me)AVP] causes a significant fall of the elevated pressure and restores the cardiac rhythm to normal. Experiment performed utilizing procedures as described by Ferrario, Barnes and Bohonek (1981)

Correa and Iwai, 1980). Moreover, central or peripheral administration of an active inhibitor of PNMT (SK & F 64139) reduces blood pressure in these rats to normal values (Black *et al.*, 1981). Mineralocorticoid hypertension also causes an increase in adrenoceptor binding sites in both brainstem and hypothalamus (Yamada, Yamamura and Roeske, 1980). Although Van Ameringen, deChamplain and Imbeault (1977) showed that the turnover of norepinephrine in the brainstem and

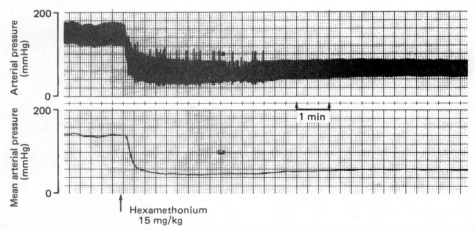

Figure 1.2 The further injection of a ganglion blocker causes a further fall of the arterial blood pressure to hypotensive values. The findings shown in this and the preceding figure indicate that the onset of nucleus tractus solitarius hypertension is predominantly due to increased quantities of circulating vasopressin

hypothalamus is decreased, and that transection of the spinal cord reverses deoxycorticosterone-salt hypertension, CSF injection of the neurotoxin 6-OHDA does not produce the same effects after the hypertension is established (Haeusler, Finch and Thoenen, 1972).

As reviewed by Scoggins *et al.* (1982b), there is considerable evidence regarding the involvement of the peripheral sympathetic nervous system in the pathogenesis of deoxycorticosterone-salt hypertension. Several investigators have provided evidence for enhanced activity of sympathetic efferent pathways to the adrenal medulla, the heart and the blood vessels (Chalmers, 1975; deChamplain, 1977; deChamplain, Krakoff and Axelrod, 1967; deChamplain and Van Ameringen, 1972). In deoxycorticosterone-salt hypertension plasma norepinephrine levels are augmented while peripheral norepinephrine turnover is increased. Majewski, Rand and Tung (1981) have proposed that epinephrine, via activation of prejunctional beta-adrenoreceptors, may act to facilitate release of neuronal norepinephrine and hence elevate blood pressure. On the other hand, plasma epinephrine is not always elevated following either steroid or ACTH administration (Scoggins *et al.*, 1982b). In a dog model of steroid hypertension, Bravo, Tarazi and Dustan (1977) found no evidence of sympathetic nervous system involvement; they suggested instead that the hypertension may be related to an intrinsic increase in vascular smooth muscle contractility (Onoyama, Bravo and Tarazi, 1979). Pharmacological maneuvers that interrupt sympathetic nerve activity have been reported to prevent the development of deoxycorticosterone-salt hypertension (Scoggins *et al.*, 1982b). Although the increases in sympathetic activity may have a cause within the brain, it has also been suggested that hypertension induced by steroid hyperactivity is due to changes in epinephrine production by the adrenal gland (Scoggins *et al.*, 1982b).

To recapitulate, steroid hormones have a profound effect upon neuronal function and there is reason to believe that the status of the sodium (Na^+) balance can act to modulate the activity of both the CNS and peripheral divisions of the SNS (Abboud, 1982; Chobanian *et al.*, 1978; Ferrario *et al.*, 1981; Liard and Silenzio, 1982; Mark *et al.*, 1977). Studies performed by us (Brosnihan, Szilagyi and Ferrario, 1981; Brosnihan, Smeby and Ferrario, 1982; Szilagyi *et al.*, 1981; Takishita and Ferrario, 1982) and Tanaka, Seki and Fujii (1982) indicate that changes in sodium balance have an important influence upon the activity of CNS adrenergic mechanisms. It is therefore not surprising that mineralocorticoid-induced hypertension may be associated with disturbances in sympathetic nervous system function. However, further studies are needed to determine whether adrenergic abnormalities are causally associated with the initiation of the hypertension, reflect a compensatory response to the blood pressure elevation, or are due to changes in either plasma or CSF–Na^+ concentrations (Ferrario *et al.*, 1981). With the exception of vasopressin and adrenocorticotropic hormones (*see below,* page 17) there is a considerable lack of information regarding the effect of steroid hypertension upon the activity of hypothalamic-pituitary hormones other than ACTH. Inasmuch as hypothalamic neurosecretory cells are heavily innervated by nerve terminals projecting from dopaminergic and noradrenergic cell bodies located elsewhere (Frohman, 1980), it is likely that alterations in adrenergic function will produce changes in the activity of these peptidergic neurons.

Hypertension of renal origin is another example of the involvement of CNS adrenergic mechanisms in the evolution of the disease process. Sympathetic overactivity has been regarded as a strong candidate for the maintenance of renal hypertension in its chronic form, but controversy exists with regard to the site and mechanism at which the defect may originate (Folkow, 1982). Pertinent literature regarding neurogenic influences in renal hypertension can be found in the following references: Buckley and Ferrario, 1981; Ferrario and McCubbin, 1974; Ferrario and Page, 1978; Krieger, Salgado and Michelini, 1982; Mark *et al.*, 1977; McCubbin and Page, 1963; Overbeck and Grissette, 1982; Page and McCubbin, 1965, 1968; Tobian, 1977; Waeber *et al.*, 1982. Here we will summarize only current evidence about central adrenergic involvement in this kind of experimental hypertension. In general, the procedures employed to evaluate the role of CNS adrenergic factors in the evolution of renal hypertension consisted of either the application of a neurotoxin (6-OHDA) or the assessment of changes in brain catecholamine turnover and content (Chalmers *et al.*, 1974; Chalmers, 1975; Petty and Reid, 1979). It has been shown that intraventricular administration of 6-OHDA prevents the development of cellophane wrap hypertension in the rabbit (Chalmers *et al.*, 1974) and that due to clipping of one renal artery and contralateral nephrectomy in rabbits (Chalmers *et al.*, 1974). The development of hypertension of the high renin type (two-kidney, one clip) was found not to be affected by intraventricular administration of 6-OHDA in rabbits (Chalmers *et al.*, 1974). Acute administration of the PNMT inhibitor SK & F 64139, which blocks the conversion of norepinephrine to epinephrine, had a small hypotensive effect upon the elevated blood pressure of rats with two-kidney, one-clip hypertension, whereas the same maneuver reversed the hypertension due to deoxycorticosterone-salt administration (Black *et al.*, 1981). Fuxe *et al.* (1981) have shown an increase in norepinephrine and epinephrine turnover in rats with two-kidney, two-clip hypertension compared to the two-kidney, one-clip type. According to Fuxe *et al.* (1981) the findings suggest the participation of central adrenergic mechanisms in the pathogenesis of *low* but not *high* renin hypertension. Tanaka *et al.* (1982) have shown that norepinephrine turnover in the aorta, mesenteric artery and left ventricle is increased in rabbits 14 days after onset of one-kidney, one-clip hypertension. On the other hand, the turnover of the transmitter from the same region was not changed in rabbits with two-kidney, one-clip hypertension. As to the brainstem, neither norepinephrine concentration nor its turnover were altered in either type of hypertension (Tanaka *et al.*, 1982). Further work will be required, however, to resolve this issue. It is difficult to accept that central noradrenergic pathways are not involved in the production of two-kidney, one-clip hypertension since there is evidence of decreased content of brainstem catecholamines in this model of renovascular hypertension (Fuxe *et al.*, 1981). As indicated above, central noradrenergic pathways participate in the CNS integration of the low and high pressure baroreceptor reflexes. Recently, Suzuki *et al.* (1983) and Krieger, Salgado and Michelini (1982) provided additional evidence for a central disturbance of noradrenergic mechanisms in the pathogenesis of two-kidney, one-clip hypertension in the dog and rat respectively. As shown in *Figures 1.3* and *1.4* from data obtained by Suzuki *et al.* (1983) the elevations in arterial pressure and heart rate

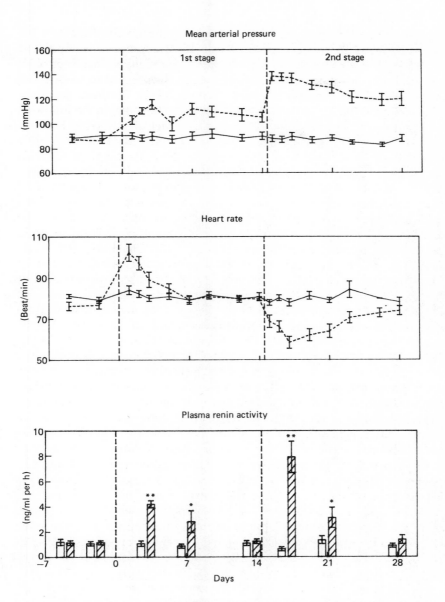

Figure 1.3 Time course of the changes in mean arterial pressure, heart rate, and plasma renin activity (PRA) for 14 days after clipping of the renal artery (first stage) and two 2 weeks following occlusion of the previously constricted vessel (second stage). Values are means ± 1 SE from eight dogs developing two-kidney, one-clip hypertension (broken lines and hatched bars) and nine sham-operated controls (solid lines and clear bars). Prior to constriction of the renal artery (RA), baseline values for MAP, HR, and PRA averaged 88 ± 3 mmHg, 76 ± 2 beats/min, and 1.1 ± 0.2 ng/ml/hr respectively. Corresponding values for nine sham-operated controls are: MAP: 87 ± 2 mmHg; HR: 81 ± 1 beats/min; PRA: 1.2 ± 0.2 ng/ml/hr. ** = $P < 0.01$; * = $P = 0.05$. (Reprinted from Suzuki *et al.* (1983) by kind permission)

associated with the production of two-kidney, one-clip hypertension in the conscious dog were accompanied by significant increases in the concentration of norepinephrine in both the plasma and the CSF obtained from the cisterna magna.

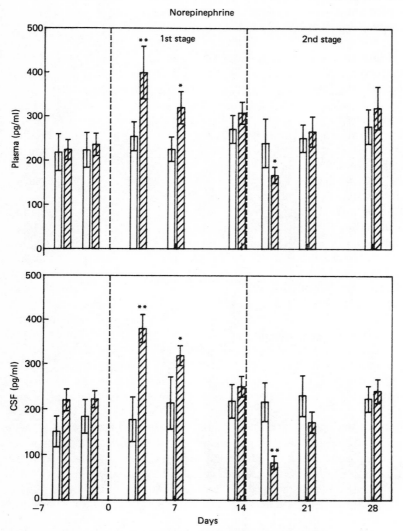

Figure 1.4 Development of two-kidney one-clip hypertension was associated with transient changes in the concentration of norepinephrine in both the plasma and cerebrospinal fluid compartments. Clear bars are means ± 1 SE of values determined in the sham-operated group; hatched bars are values for the group of dogs developing renovascular hypertension. For the group subjected to renal hypertension, control values for plasma and CSF norepinephrine averaged 223 ± 23 and 220 ± 24 pg/ml respectively. In the sham group, baseline plasma and CSF norepinephrine were 219 ± 42 and 151 ± 34 pg/ml respectively. Comparisons of control baseline values between the two groups of dogs showed no significant differences at $P > 0.05$. Other P values as in *Figure 1.3*. (From Suzuki *et al.*, 1983)

Role of vasopressin

Vasopressin is usually considered primarily in terms of its antidiuretic properties (Kleeman and Berl, 1979; Reichlin, 1981) because the concentrations of the peptide required for antidiuresis are much less than those needed to elevate blood pressure in the intact organism (Bisset and Lewis, 1962; Cowley, 1982; Mohring, 1978).

Vasopressin originates in cell bodies of hypothalamic nuclei, primarily the supraoptic and paraventricular nuclei (Scharrer and Scharrer, 1954). Axons from these nuclei extend via the median eminence to the neurohypophysis, with terminals immediately adjacent to a capillary bed (Bodian, 1963; Palay, 1957). Recent immunocytochemical studies indicate that vasopressin fibers may also extend from the paraventricular nucleus to the zona externa of the median eminence (Zimmerman *et al.*, 1977). Vasopressinergic fibers also project from the paraventricular and suprachiasmatic nuclei to the dorsal motor nucleus and nucleus tractus solitarius, thus suggesting that vasopressin may also play some modulatory role in the cardiovascular reflex pathway (Sofroniew, 1980).

Osmoregulation is the most extensively studied of the factors modulating vasopressin release (Bie, 1980). The observation that water diuresis in a dog was inhibited by injection of an hyperosmolar solution into the carotid artery led Verney (1947) to propose that osmoreceptors may regulate vasopressin release. Later studies by Jewell and Verney (1957) suggested that these osmoreceptors may be located in the anterior hypothalamus. Osmosensitive cells in the hypothalamus have since been demonstrated electrophysiologically (Cross and Green, 1959; Hayward and Vincent, 1970), and vasopressin secretion has been enhanced by hyperosmotic solutions in hypothalamo-neurohypophysial (HNS) explants of the rat (Sladek and Knigge, 1977). Osmoreceptor cells in the rat hypothalamus may be located in the anteroventral third ventricle (AV3V) region, inasmuch as it has been observed that HNS explants from rats subjected to anteroventral third ventricle lesions do not secrete vasopressin in response to osmotic stimuli (Sladek and Johnson, 1983).

Afferent fibers from cardiopulmonary and sinoaortic baroreceptors also modulate vasopressin release (Share, 1976). Henry, Gauer and Reeves (1956) first demonstrated that balloon distension of the left atrium of the dog was associated with diuresis. The afferent limb of this reflex is mediated by the vagus nerve (Henry and Pearce, 1956), and the diuresis results from inhibition of vasopressin release (Brennan *et al.*, 1971; Koizumi and Yamashita, 1978). Stimulation of carotid baroreceptors also inhibits vasopressin release, as seen by the observation that carotid occlusion is associated with augmented activity of neurons in the supraoptic nucleus and increased vasopressin release (Chien, Peric and Usami, 1962; Share and Levy, 1962; Yamashita and Koizumi, 1979). The relative importance of plasma osmolality and left atrial pressure (LAP) has also been evaluated in the regulation of vasopressin release. Quillen and Cowley (1983) have studied the relation between plasma osmolality and plasma vasopressin in hypovolemic, normovolemic and hypervolemic dogs. Vasopressin release in response to a rise in plasma osmolality was enhanced in the hypovolemic state and depressed in the hypervolemic state. Inasmuch as these changes in plasma volume were associated with changes in LAP within the normal range, it appears that atrial receptors play a significant modulatory role in the normal regulation of plasma vasopressin.

The antidiuretic hormone promotes vasoconstriction both directly (Altura and Altura, 1977) and indirectly by augmentation of pressor responses to sympatho-mimetic amines (Bartelstone and Nasmyth, 1965). The vasoconstrictor actions of vasopressin are primarily seen in the resistance vessels of the mesentery and the skeletal muscles; vasopressin does not cause significant vasoconstriction in the kidneys, heart or brain (Ericsson, 1971; Heyndrickx, Boettcher and Vatner, 1976). Thus it appears that vasopressin acts to optimize the distribution of body water during hemorrhage or dehydration.

Although the *in vitro* vasoconstrictor action of vasopressin is observed at concentrations similar to those observed in plasma, the physiological significance of this vasoconstrictor action has been questioned on the grounds that large concentrations of vasopressin are required to elevate blood pressure *in vivo* (Johnston, Newman and Wood, 1981). This does not rule out, however, a role for vasopressin in cardiovascular regulation. Montani *et al.* (1980) have shown that in dogs intravenous vasopressin infusion within a physiological range caused no elevations in arterial pressure since the increases in vascular resistance are offset by a proportional fall in cardiac output. That these effects of vasopressin may be related to an effect of the hormone upon the CNS control of the baroreceptor reflex was demonstrated by repeating the study in baroreceptor denervated and headless dogs. Removal of either the baroreceptor nerves or decapitation (Cowley, Monos and Guyton, 1974) unmasked the hypertensive effects of the hormone. These data suggest that the baroreceptor reflex may normally compensate for the vasopressin-induced vasoconstriction. The locus of this action is presumed to be a CNS site in the baroreceptor feedback loop (Liard *et al.*, 1981). Intraventricular injection of vasopressin is associated with bradycardia (Varma, Bhuwaneshwar and Bhargava, 1969) and a fall in arterial pressure (Nashold, Mannarino and Wunderlich, 1961). It has also been reported that microinjection of vasopressin into the nucleus tractus solitarius region triggers a marked increased in blood pressure and heart rate (Matsuguchi *et al.*, 1982); the significance of this observation has been questioned, inasmuch as it appears likely that the tissue was exposed to high concentrations of vasopressin (Cowley, 1982). Cowley, Monos and Guyton (1974) showed that the marked pressor response to vasopressin in headless dogs exceeds by two to three orders of magnitude the changes that would be predicted by merely removing the opposing effects of baroreceptor reflexes. This suggests that vasopressin normally enhances the ability of the baroreceptor reflex to offset changes in peripheral resistance, either by amplifying baroreceptor inhibition of sympathetic tone or baroreceptor enhancement of vagal tone (Liard *et al.*, 1981). Recently, Michelini, Barnes and Ferrario (1983) observed that the centrally mediated pressor response due to intravertebral infusion of angiotensin II can be abolished after pretreatment with an inhibitor of the vasculotropic actions of vasopressin given into the cisterna magna. These data suggest the existence of a CNS interaction between vasopressin and angiotensin II in the control of bulbospinal vasomotor outflow and cardiovascular reflexes.

It seems unlikely that vasopressin alone may be a causative agent in hypertension. Although chronic elevation of plasma vasopressin is associated with an increase in peripheral resistance (Montani *et al.*, 1980), the vasoconstriction is not associated with a sustained rise in blood pressure (Padfield *et al.*, 1981; Smith *et al.*, 1979). The fluid retention associated with vasopressin's antidiuretic action is transient, and urine osmolality returns to control level (Smith *et al.*, 1979). However, the urine osmolality remains greater than that appropriate for the concomitant plasma osmolality (Bartter and Schwartz, 1967).

Nevertheless, speculation persists that vasopressin could play a role in the onset and maintenance of some forms of hypertension. Vasopressin is elevated in many different hypertensive states (Mohring *et al.*, 1978). In addition, fluid retention is sustained during a prolonged elevation of vasopressin when kidney function is compromised (Manning *et al.*, 1979). The vasopressor action of vasopressin in hypertension may also be enhanced by decreased baroreceptor sensitivity, which is also seen in some types of hypertension (Takeshita *et al.*, 1975). Cowley (1982) has postulated that the sustained vasoconstrictive action of vasopressin could significantly influence the distribution of body fluid volume, vascular compliance, vascular segmental filling pressures, and extracellular sodium and potassium concentrations. These factors are considered to play a role in the pathogenesis of arterial hypertension.

In the deoxycorticosterone-salt model of hypertension, the severity of hypertension seems to be correlated with the plasma level of vasopressin. In the benign hypertensive phase plasma vasopressin is elevated three-fold greater than normal, while in the malignant phase plasma vasopressin increases ten-fold over the normal level (Mohring *et al.*, 1977). A role for vasopressin in the onset of deoxycorticosterone-salt hypertension is suggested by the observation that the rat with hereditary diabetes insipidus (Brattleboro rat) does not develop deoxycortico-sterone-salt hypertension (Crofton *et al.*, 1979; Berecek *et al.*, 1982a, 1982b). Replacement of vasopressin in these rats restored not only the ability of the steroid treatment to cause hypertension, but also returned the increased vascular reactivity to norepinephrine, angiotensin II, and vasopressin (Berecek *et al.*, 1982b). However, the role of vasopressin in the onset of deoxycorticosterone-salt hypertension may not be related to its direct pressor effect since administration of a selectively antidiuretic analog of vasopressin causes a rise in blood pressure in Brattleboro rats during deoxycorticosterone-salt treatment (Saito, Yajima and Watanabe, 1981). However, it is important to note that Rabito, Carretero and Scicli (1981) found no evidence of a role of vasopressin in the maintenance of high blood pressure in rats with either mineralocorticoid or renovascular hypertension.

Elevation of plasma vasopressin has also been reported in the rat with spontaneous hypertension (SHR) (Crofton *et al.*, 1978; Mohring, Kintz and Schoun, 1979). As with the deoxycorticosterone-salt rat, the increase of vasopressin in the spontaneous hypertension paralleled the progression of the disease, and injection of vasopressin antiserum brought about a significant reduction in the blood pressure (Mohring, Kintz and Schoun, 1979). Brain levels of vasopressin have been compared in the hypertension-prone (SBH) and hyperten-sion-resistant (SBR) strains of the Sabra rat (Feuerstein *et al.*, 1981). Vasopressin was more markedly elevated in the hypothalamus and pituitary of the SBH rat, but the SBR rat also demonstrated elevated levels of hypothalamic and pituitary vasopressin as compared with the control strain of the Sabra rat. It remains to be determined, however, whether these increased levels of central vasopressin are causative or adaptive phenomena in the pathogenesis of hypertension-susceptibility or resistance in the Sabra rat.

Vasopressin appears less likely to play a direct role in experimental renal hypertension. In two-kidney Goldblatt hypertensive rats renal artery clamping was associated with a variable rise in plasma vasopressin after 3–5 weeks, and the effect of vasopressin antiserum on blood pressure was also variable (Mohring *et al.*, 1978). Moreover, Woods and Johnston (1982) reported that two-kidney, one-clip Brattleboro rats develop malignant hypertension at the same rate and to the same degree as two-kidney, one-clip Long-Evans rats.

In summary, there is no compelling evidence that vasopressin plays a primary role in the pathogenesis of hypertension. On the other hand, plasma vasopressin is elevated in many hypertensive states. Moderate increases in plasma vasopressin do not bring about a rise in systemic blood pressure, in spite of vasopressin's vasoconstrictive action. This may be explained by vasopressin's enhancement of the baroreceptor reflex mechanism. However, in the hypertensive state, where factors such as vascular compliance and renal function are already compromised, then the vasoconstrictive and/or antidiuretic properties of vasopressin may serve to further aggravate the disease (the role of vasopressin in hypertension is further discussed in Chapter 3).

The brain and kidney renin–angiotensin systems

The importance of the kidney renin–angiotensin system (RAS) in blood pressure regulation and the control of extracellular fluid volume is firmly established. More recently, however, low concentrations of angiotensin II have been shown to activate the sympathetic nervous system centrally as well as to induce thirst, natriuresis and the secretion of vasopressin, ACTH and other pituitary hormones (Buckley and Ferrario, 1981; Buckley *et al.*, 1981; Di Nicolantonio *et al.*, 1982; Epstein, Fitzsimmons and Ralls, 1969; Ferrario, Dickinson and McCubbin, 1970; Ferrario, Gildenberg and McCubbin, 1972; Ferrario, 1983b; Fink, Bryan and Mokler, 1982; Maran and Yates, 1977; Phillips *et al.*, 1977; Reid *et al.*, 1982; Szilagyi and Ferrario, 1981). It is accepted that a part of the complex neurogenic, hemodynamic, behavioral and hormonal effects produced by angiotensin II are conveyed via receptors situated outside the blood–brain barrier. At these sites the parenchyma of the brain is in communication with the plasmatic environment because of the presence of fenestrated capillaries and lack of tight endothelial junctions (Knigge *et al.*, 1980). These anatomical features are characteristics of the so-called brain circumventricular organs, structures which are generally juxtaposed to the ventricular spaces with neuronal elements functioning as neurotransducers (Ferrario, 1983b). Blood-borne polypeptides can reach neuronal elements contained either within, or in the near proximity of, these structures to exert far-reaching neurotransmitter and neurohormonal effects. The available data indicate that angiotensin II may act at several circumventricular organs, namely, the subfornical organ (SFO), the organum vasculosum of the lamina terminalis (OVLT), the median eminence (ME) and the area postrema (AP). The predominant action of angiotensin II upon the circumventricular organs of the forebrain is to elicit thirst and sodium appetite as well as to alter the secretory activity of hypothalamic-hypophysial neurons (Phillips *et al.*, 1977). The area postrema of the medulla oblongata has been shown instead to augment the activity of bulbospinal vasomotor neurons leading to increased release of adrenomedullary epinephrine and neurogenic vasoconstriction in the splanchnic but not the renal vasculature (Ferrario, Dickinson and McCubbin, 1970; Ferrario, 1983a). The decrease in sympathetic activity to the kidneys may account for the absence of any neurogenically mediated release of renin during area postrema stimulation by angiotensin II (Reid *et al.*, 1982). Studies by Ferrario and colleagues (*see* Ferrario, 1983a; Ferrario *et al.*, 1979) indicate that the sympathoexcitatory actions of the area postrema pathway are involved in the regulation of the cardiovascular function in the dog. Preliminary observations also suggest that in the dog this structure may play a part in the evolution of one-kidney, one-clip hypertension (Ferrario, 1983a).

There is also growing evidence that angiotensin II is formed in the brain (Quinlan and Phillips, 1981). The existence of angiotensin-like bioactivity and immuno-reactivity was first reported in CSF by Finkielman *et al.* (1972) and in brain by Fischer-Ferraro *et al.* (1971). Hutchinson *et al.* (1978) reported that the immunoreactive angiotensin II (Ang II-ir) in canine cerebrospinal fluid was des-Asp[1] angiotensin II. Their proof was based upon comparison of angiotensin II-like activity of CSF to that of authentic heptapeptide by polyacrylamide-slab gel electrophoresis using Tris/borate buffers at pH 8.87. Later, a surprising report was made by Semple, McCrae and Morton (1980) suggesting that the detection of immunoreactive angiotensin II in CSF arises from an immunoassay artifact. Employing a paper chromatographic method, they observed that CSF–immunoreactive angiotensin II migrated differently from the plasma peptide. According to Bumpus and Ferrario (1984) they did not take into account the previous report of Hutchinson *et al.* (1978) nor the possibility that there may be a sequence difference between plasma and brain angiotensin. The latter possibility has been substantiated by recent studies of Husain *et al.* (1983). They showed that incubation of CSF with purified dog kidney renin yielded a number of angiotensin I isopeptides with molecular weights ranging between 1300 and 3000.

The occurrence of angiotensinogen in brain tissue and CSF is also well established but questions remain as to the source of its biosynthesis. Printz and Gregory (1981) injected rabbit plasma [^{125}I]-angiotensinogen intravenously into rabbits and measured its uptake in brain and CSF. Although they detected radioactivity in these areas, they were unable to show that the labeled protein crossed the blood brain barrier. Printz, Printz and Gregory (1978) demonstrated that CSF and plasma angiotensinogen had different microheterogeneity. However, most of these differences disappeared after removal of sialic acid by neuroamini-dase. Experiments entailing either adrenalectomy, nephrectomy or chronic treatment with reserpine revealed a clear dissociation between changes in plasma and brain renin substrates (Gregory, Wallis and Printz, 1982; Wallis and Printz,

1980). Ito *et al.* (1980) determined that in man CSF angiotensinogen was immunogenically different from that in plasma and that removal of the sialic acid residue by treatment with neuroaminidase did not abolish this immunological difference. These data provide additional support for the possibility that the angiotensin(s) synthesized in the brain may be structurally different from that of plasma (Husain *et al.,* 1983). On the other hand, leakage of plasma substrate into CSF has not been ruled out completely because of the similar electrophoretic protein patterns between CSF and plasma after neuroaminidase treatment (Ito *et al.,* 1980).

A renin-like activity in brain extracts was first reported by Ganten (*see* Ganten and Speck, 1978) but their assay procedure did not exclude the fact that acid proteases (such as cathepsin D) were responsible for the formation of the active peptide. Hirose, Yokosawa and Inagami (1978) and Osman, Smeby and Sen (1979) later separated cathepsin D from brain isorenin by using immunocytochemical techniques, Slater (1981) demonstrated a widespread distribution of renin in human brain. Angiotensin-converting enzyme has also been demonstrated by radiochemical assay in rat brain, with the highest concentration in the subfornical organ and the area postrema (Chevillard and Saavedra, 1982).

Angiotensin II has been identified immunocytochemically in cells of para-ventricular and supraoptic nuclei in rat, monkey and man by several investigators (Changaris, Severs and Keil, 1978; Fuxe *et al.,* 1976). Fibers immunoreactive to angiotensin II were seen in anterior and middle hypothalamus, locus coeruleus, nucleus tractus solitarius, dorsal motor nucleus and in the spinal cord substantia gelatinosa. The widespread distribution of angiotensin immunoreactivity in brain correlates with the distribution of angiotensin-binding sites. Bennett and Snyder (1976) studied angiotensin-binding sites in bovine and rat brain membranes. In calf brain, [^{125}I] angiotensin II binding was restricted to the cerebellum while in rat brain the binding was highest in thalamus–hypothalamus, midbrain and brain stem. Speth and colleagues (1983) have shown the existence of specific binding sites in the organum vasculosum of the lamina terminalis, subfornical organ and the nucleus tractus solitarius and dorsal motor nucleus region of the dog brain. These recent studies suggest a role for endogenous angiotensin II in the modulation of the baroreceptor reflex within the CNS. The mechanism by which angiotensin II may act to regulate cardiovascular function has not yet been established. It is accepted that acute and chronic administration of angiotensin II into the brain via either the cerebral blood supply (Ferrario, Dickinson and McCubbin, 1970; Reid *et al.,* 1982) or cerebral ventricles (Buckley *et al.,* 1981; Gordon *et al.,* 1979) produces a sustained rise in arterial pressure, in part due to activation of sympathetic nerve activity. The effect of the peptide, administered centrally, upon the release of hypothalamic pituitary hormones may also contribute to the elevation in arterial pressure, even though Fink, Bryan and Mokler (1982) showed that in rabbits increased release of vasopressin cannot account for the hypertension due to intraventricularly administered (IVT) angiotensin II. Angiotensin II is a potent stimulus for the secretion of ACTH (Scholkens *et al.,* 1982). Lohmeier and Carroll (1982) and Lohmeier and Kastner (1982) have shown that in dogs chronic administration of ACTH produced a marked potentiation of the hypertension due to norepinephrine infusion. It is thus possible that the stimulatory action of IVT angiotensin II upon ACTH and the secretion of corticosterone by the adrenal cortex could facilitate an increase in vascular reactivity since the steroid is known to decrease extraneuronal uptake of norepinephrine, inhibit the synthesis of prostacycline and stimulate the sodium–potassium (Na–K) ATPase pump (Scholkens *et al.*, 1982). Since corticosterone also stimulates hepatic synthesis of angiotensinogen (Wallis and Printz, 1980) a feedback relationship may exist between adrenal steroids and the brain renin–angiotensin system. With the consideration that chronic cerebroventricular administration of angiotensin II in conscious rabbits leads to an augmented pressor response to intravenous norepinephrine (Fink, Bryan and Mokler, 1982) an interplay among ACTH, angiotensin and sympathetic nerve activity also appears likely.

To recapitulate, the local formation of angiotensin II in the brain alone or in conjunction with the effects of the blood-borne peptide upon circumventricular organs may act to modulate the activity of CNS pathways involved in the expression of thirst, sodium conservation, overall volume control and blood pressure regulation (*Figure 1.5*). The widespread localization of the peptide in the brain of

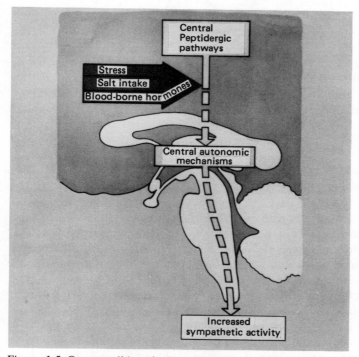

Figure 1.5 One possible way by which the brain may participate in the pathogenesis of arterial hypertension is by becoming a target organ for risk factors such as stress, changes in dietary sodium intake or increased production of blood-borne vasoactive and steroid hormones. These factors may activate brain peptidergic pathways having a neuromodulatory function upon central adrenergic mechanisms. (From Ferrario, 1983b)

mammals, its presence in the CSF and the possible occurrence of isopeptides suggest that the angiotensins may fulfil unique and unrelated roles at different sites of the neuroaxis. It is also possible that angiotensin II may function as a releasing factor for hypophysial hormones or the releasing peptides themselves (Aguilera, Hyde and Catt, 1982).

There is evidence that brain angiotensin II may participate in the pathogenesis of certain forms of arterial hypertension (Unger *et al.*, 1981), if one accepts the premise that the hypotensive effects resulting from the central administration of renin–angiotensin blockers are not related to the passage of the compound from the CSF into peripheral blood. Pitfalls regarding this interpretation have been outlined by Ferrario (1983b) recently.

Although adrenocortical steroids affect the activity of the renin–angiotensin system, there is still equivocal evidence regarding a role of angiotensin II in either the initiation or maintenance of either deoxycorticosteroid-salt or ACTH-mediated hypertension (Scoggins *et al.*, 1982b). The infusion of an angiotensin II antagonist into rats made hypertensive by 6-alpha-methylprednisolone has been reported to reduce the elevated blood pressure (Krakoff, Selvadura and Sutter, 1975). However, the same effects were not observed in patients with Cushing's syndrome (Swartz *et al.*, 1980) or in deoxycorticosteroid-salt hypertensive rats treated with captopril (Vetter *et al.*, 1976). Saralasin given into the ventricular system of deoxycorticosteroid-salt hypertensive rats produced a further elevation of the arterial pressure (Mann *et al.*, 1978). These data suggest that angiotensin II is not directly involved in the genesis of this form of hypertension. On the other hand, there is reason to believe that brain angiotensin II may be involved in the pathogenesis of renal and SHR hypertension; these findings are reviewed by Rubin, Antonaccio and Horovitz (1981), Scholkens *et al.* (1982) and Ganten and Speck (1978).

THE ROLE OF BRAIN MECHANISMS IN HYPERTENSION AS INDICATED BY LESION EXPERIMENTS

Ablation techniques are used with increasing frequency to evaluate the participation of brain mechanisms in the pathogenesis of arterial hypertension. The studies entailing the placement of an electrolytic lesion in the anteroventral aspects of the third ventricle have provided a significant impetus to the understanding of this aspect of hypertension research (Brody *et al.*, 1978; Brody and Johnson, 1980). The history, the characteristics of the brain structures removed by the procedure, and the results obtained in various models of experimental hypertension are reviewed by Brody *et al.* (1978). In general, these studies indicate that AV3V lesioned rats are refractory to the development of either renal hypertension or that due to central baroreceptor denervation. Studies of Fink and Bryan (1982) in renal hypertensive rabbits, Scoggins *et al.* (1982a) in ACTH induced hypertension in the sheep and Ferrario (1983a) in renovascular hypertensive dogs indicate that species differences must be considered when assessing the role of the AV3V region in the pathogenesis of hypertension.

Lesions in the AV3V region of the rat prevent the occurrence of deoxycortico-sterone-salt hypertension (Bryan and Fink, 1981). The same effects were not obtained when the subfornical organ was removed instead (Bryan and Fink, 1981). On the other hand, removal of the subfornical organ was effective in preventing the renal form. Berecek *et al.* (1982a) suggest that prevention of DOC-salt hypertension following AV3V lesion may in part result from the inhibition of vasopressin release (*see also* Sladek and Johnson, 1983). On the other hand, Pamnani *et al.* (1981) have proposed an alternative mechanism to explain the effect of AV3V lesions. They suggest that the surgical procedure prevents the release of a natriuretic hormone which acts in the periphery to inhibit the Na–K ATPase pump function in both the kidney and the blood vessels. Additional proof for this mechanism has been provided by Singu-Mize, Bealer and Caldwell (1982). Intriguing evidence supporting this contention has been described superbly by Haddy (1982). Studies by Scoggins *et al.* (1982a) raise some questions regarding the role of the AV3V region in mineralocorticoid hypertension in species other than the rat. In the sheep, ACTH administration causes hypertension and increases in plasma and CSF Na^+ and osmolarity. Although AV3V lesions abolished the dipsogenic response to hyperosmolarity in this species, the hypertensive response is not diminished (Scoggins *et al.*, 1982a). In another model of steroid hypertension Marson *et al.* (1981) showed that destruction of the AV3V region reduced the severity of the hypertension due to administration of methylprednisolone to rats. When the same procedure was performed during the chronic phase, the elevated blood pressure returned toward control values. Thus, in the glucocorticoid model of hypertension the AV3V region of the rat contributes to, but is not essential for, the expression of the hypertension.

Current research indicates that the AV3V region contains structures that mediate the pressor response to IVT angiotensin II, carbachol and hypertonic saline in the rat and also in the dog (Brody and Johnson, 1980; Ferrario, 1983b). Hartle *et al.* (1982) have identified two anatomically and functionally distinct vasoconstrictor pathways taking different routes through the anterior hypothalamus. The integrity of the more medial pathway appears to be required for the expression of the angiotensin II effect; a pathway lateral to the periventricular one might be involved in the central control of the baroreceptor reflex.

SUMMARY

The basic hemodynamic abnormality in chronic stable hypertension is an increase in vascular resistance and a multitude of factors may account for this change. Enhanced sympathetic nerve activity together with altered neuroendocrine function may contribute directly to the development of the hypertension and the associated hypertrophic vascular changes. Although abnormalities in the set point of arterial pressure may be due to a genetic, metabolic or structural alteration of brain cardiovascular centers, the biochemical basis of the disorder should be sought in the factors linking the relationship between neurotransmitters and neuropeptides, the chemical messengers favoring a neuroendocrine response which signals a greater vascular contraction, and hence increased blood pressure.

References

ABBOUD, F. M. (1982) The sympathetic system in hypertension. *Hypertension,* **4** (Suppl II), II-208–II-225

ABBOUD, F. M., HEISTAD, D. D., MARK, A. Z. and SCHMID, P. G. (1976) Reflex control of the peripheral circulation. *Progress of Cardiovascular Disease,* **18,** 371–403

AGUILERA, G., HYDE, C. L. and CATT, K. J. (1982) Angiotensin II receptors and prolactin release in pituitary lactotrophs. *Endocrinology,* **111,** 1045

ALTURA, B. M. and ALTURA, B. T. (1977) Vascular smooth muscle and neurohypophysial hormones. *Federation Proceedings,* **36,** 1853–1860

BARTELSTONE, H. J. and NASMYTH, P. A. (1965) Vasopressin potentiation of catecholamine action in dog, cat and rat aortic strip. *American Journal of Physiology,* **208,** 754–762

BARTTER, F. C. and SCHWARTZ, W. B. (1967) The syndrome of inappropriate secretion of antidiuretic hormone. *American Journal of Medicine,* **42,** 790–806

BENNETT, J. P. JR and SNYDER, S. H. (1976) Angiotensin II binding to mammalian brain membranes. *Journal of Biological Chemistry,* **251,** 7423–7430

BERECEK, K. H., BARRON, K. W., WEBB, R. L. and BRODY, M. J. (1982a) Vasopressin-central nervous system interactions in the development of DOCA hypertension. *Hypertension,* **4,** *(Suppl II),* II-131–II-137

BERECEK, K. H. and BOHR, D. F. (1976) Bases for increased vascular reactivity in experimental hypertension. In *Vascular Neuroeffector Mechanisms,* edited by J. A. Bevan, G. Burnstock, B. Johansson and O. A. Nedergaard, pp. 198–204. Basel: Karger

BERECEK, K. H., MURRAY, R. D., GROSS, F. and BRODY, M. J. (1982b) Vasopressin and vascular reactivity in the development of DOCA hypertension in rats with hereditary diabetes insipidus. *Hypertension,* **4,** 3–12

BIE, P. (1980) Osmoreceptors, vasopressin, and control of renal water excretion. *Physiological Reviews,* **60,** 961–1048

BISSET, G. W. and LEWIS, G. P. (1962) A spectrum of pharmacological activity in some biologically active peptides. *British Journal of Pharmacology,* **19,** 168–182

BLACK, J., WAEBER, B., BRESNAHAN, M. R., GAVRAS, I. and GAVRAS, H. (1981) Blood pressure response to central and/or peripheral inhibition of phenylethanolamine *N*-methyltransferase in normotensive and hypertensive rats. *Circulation Research,* **49,** 518–524

BLESSING, W. W., WEST, M. J. and CHALMERS, J. (1981) Hypertension, bradycardia and pulmonary edema in the conscious rabbit after brainstem lesions coinciding with the A1 group of catecholamine neurons. *Circulation Research,* **49,** 949–958

BODIAN, D. (1963) Cytological aspects of neurosecretion in opossum neurohypophysis. *Bulletin of Johns Hopkins Hospital,* **113,** 57–93

BOUSQUET, P., BLOCH, R., FELDMAN, J. and SCHWARTZ, J. (1979) The ventromedullary vasomotor centre. In *Nervous System and Hypertension,* edited by P. Meyer and H. Schmitt, pp. 363–370. New York: John Wiley Inc.

BRAVO, E. L., TARAZI, R. C. and DUSTAN, H. P. (1977) Multifactorial analysis of chronic hypertension induced by electrolyte-active steroids in trained, unanesthetized dogs. *Circulation Research,* **40** (Suppl. I), I-140–145

BRENNAN, L. A. JR, MALVIN, R. L., JOCHIM, K. E. and ROBERTS, D. E. (1971) Influence of right and left atrial receptors on plasma concentrations of ADH and renin. *American Journal of Physiology,* **221,** 273–278

BRODY, M. J., FINK, G. D., BUGGY, J., HAYWOOD, J. R., GORDON, F. J. and JOHNSON, A. K. (1978) The role of the anteroventral third ventricle (AV3V) region in experimental hypertension. *Circulation Research,* **43** (Suppl. I), I-2–I-13

BRODY, M. J. and JOHNSON, A. K. (1980) Role of the anteroventral third ventricle region in fluid and electrolyte balance, arterial pressure regulation, and hypertension. In *Frontiers in Endocrinology,* edited by L. Martini and W. F. Ganong, pp. 249–292. New York: Raven Press

BROSNIHAN, K. B., SMEBY, R. R. and FERRARIO, C. M. (1982) Effects of chronic sodium depletion on canine brain renin and cathepsin D activities. *Hypertension,* **4,** 604–608

BROSNIHAN, K. B., SZILAGYI, J. E. and FERRARIO, C. M. (1981) Effect of chronic sodium depletion on cerebrospinal fluid and plasma catecholamines. *Hypertension,* **3,** 233–239

BRYAN, W. F. and FINK, G. D. (1981) The effect of periventricular (AV3V) brain lesions on the development of renal hypertension in the rabbit. *Federation Proceedings,* **40,** 390

BUCKLEY, J. P. and FERRARIO, C. M. (Eds.) (1981) *Central Nervous System Mechanisms in Hypertension.* New York: Raven Press

BUCKLEY, J. P., LOKHANDWALA, M. F., JANDHYALA, B. S., FRANCIS, J. S. and TADEPALLI, A. (1981) Circulatory effects of chronic intraventricular administration of angiotensin II in dogs. In *Central Nervous System Mechanisms in Hypertension,* edited by J. P. Buckley and C. M. Ferrario, pp. 363–376. New York: Raven Press

BUMPUS, F. M. and FERRARIO, C. M. (1984) Extrarenal renin angiotensin system: comments on its occurrence and cardiovascular role. In *Topics in Pathophysiology of Hypertension,* edited by H. Villarreal and M. Sambhi, pp. 407–416. Boston: Martinus Nijhoff

CHALMERS, J. P. (1975) Brain amines and models of experimental hypertension. *Circulation Research,* **36,** 469–480

CHALMERS, J. P., BLESSING, W. W., WEST, M. J., HOWE, P. R. C., COSTA, M. and FURNESS, J. B. (1981) Importance of new catecholamine pathways in control of blood pressure. *Clinical and Experimental Hypertension,* **3,** 393–416

CHALMERS, J. P., DOLLERY, C. T., LEWIS, P. J. and REID, J. L. (1974) The importance of central adrenergic neurons in renal hypertension in rabbits. *Journal of Physiology,* **233,** 403–411

CHANGARIS, D. G., SEVERS, W. B. and KEIL, L. C. (1978) Localization of angiotensin in rat brain. *Journal of Histochemistry and Cytochemistry,* **26,** 593–607

CHARRER, B. (1977) Peptides in neurobiology: historical introduction. In *Peptides in Neurobiology,* edited by H. Gainer, pp. 1–8. New York: Plenum Press

CHATELAIN, R., BUMPUS, F. M., CHERNICKY, C. L. and FERRARIO, C. M. (1983) Different patterns of altered glucocorticoid secretion in experimental malignant and benign hypertension. *Journal of Pathology,* **139,** 69–88

CHEVILLARD, C. and SAAVEDRA, J. M. (1982) Distribution of angiotensin-converting enzyme activity in specific areas of the rat brain stem. *Journal of Neurochemistry,* **38,** 281–284

CHIEN, S., PERIC, B. and USAMI, S. (1962) The reflex nature of release of antidiuretic hormone upon common carotid occlusion in vagotomized dogs. *Proceedings of the Society of Experimental and Biological Medicine,* **111,** 193–196

CHOBANIAN, A. V., GAVRAS, H., GAVRAS, I., BRESNAHAN, M., SULLIVAN, P. and MELBY, J. C. (1978) Studies on the activity of the sympathetic nervous system in essential hypertension. *Journal of Human Stress,* **4,** 22–28

CONN, H. F. and CONN, R. B. JR (Eds.) (1980) *Current Diagnosis.* Philadelphia: W. B. Saunders Co.

COOPER, P. E. and MARTIN, J. B. (1982) Neuroendocrinology and brain peptides. *Trends in Neuroscience,* **5,** 186–189

COOTE, J. H., MACLEOD, V. H., FLEETWOOD-WALKER, S. M. and GILBEY, M. P. (1981) The response of individual sympathetic preganglionic neurons to microelectrophoretically applied endogenous monoamines. *Brain Research,* **215,** 135–145

COWLEY, A. W. JR (1982) Vasopressin and cardiovascular regulation. In *International Review of Physiology, Vol. 26, Cardiovascular Physiology IV,* edited by A. C. Guyton and J. E. Hall, pp. 189–242. Baltimore: University Park Press

COWLEY, A. W. JR, MONOS, E. and GUYTON, A. C. (1974) Interaction of vasopressin and the baroreceptor reflex system in the regulation of arterial blood pressure in the dog. *Circulation Research,* **34,** 505–514

CROFTON, J. T., SHARE, L., SHADE, R. E., ALLEN, C. and TARNOWSKI, D. (1978) Vasopressin in the rat with spontaneous hypertension. *American Journal of Physiology,* **235,** H361–H366

CROFTON, J. T., SHARE, L., SHADE, R. E., LEE-KWON, W. J., MANNING, M. and SAWYER, W. H. (1979) The importance of vasopressin in the development and maintenance of DOC-salt hypertension in the rat. *Hypertension,* **1,** 31–38

CROSS, B. A. and GREEN, J. B. (1959) Activity of single neurons in the hypothalamus. Effect of osmotic and other stimuli. *Journal of Physiology (London),* **148,** 554–569

DAHLSTROM, A. and FUXE, K. (1964) Evidence for the existence of monoamine-containing neurons in the central nervous system. I. Demonstration of monoamines in the cell bodies of brain stem neurons. *Acta Physiologica Scandinavia,* **62** (Suppl. 232), 1–55

DAHLSTROM, A. and FUXE, K. (1965) Evidence for the existence of monoamine-containing neurons in the central nervous system. II. Experimentally induced changes in the intraneuronal amine levels of bulbospinal neuron system. *Acta Physiologica Scandinavica,* **64** (Suppl. 247), 5–36

deCHAMPLAIN, J. (1977) The sympathetic system in hypertension. *Clinical Endocrinology and Metabolism,* **6,** 633–655

deCHAMPLAIN, J., KRAKOFF, L. R. and AXELROD, J. (1967) Catecholamine metabolism in experimental hypertension in the rat. *Circulation Research,* **20,** 136–145

deCHAMPLAIN, J. and VAN AMERINGEN, M. R. (1972) Regulation of blood pressure by sympathetic nerve fibers and adrenal medulla in normotensive and hypertensive rats. *Circulation Research,* **31,** 617–628

DE JONG, W. and NIJKAMP, F. P. (1976) Centrally induced hypotension and bradycardia after administration of alpha-methylnoradrenaline into the area of the nucleus tractus solitarii of the rat. *British Journal of Pharmacology,* **58,** 593–598

DI NICOLANTONIO, R., MENDELSOHN, F. A. O., HUTCHINSON, J. S., TAKATA, Y. and DOYLE, A. E. (1982) Dissociation of dipsogenic and pressor responses to chronic central angiotensin II in rats. *American Journal of Physiology,* **242,** R498–R504

EDWARDS, C. R. W., AL-DUJAILI, E. A. S., BOSCARO, M., GOW, I. and WILLIAMS, B. C. (1982) Peptidergic and monoaminergic regulation of aldosterone secretion. In *Endocrinology of Hypertension,* edited by F. Mantero, E. G. Biglieri and C. R. W. Edwards, pp. 11–18. London and New York: Academic Press

ELLIOTT, G. R. and EISDORFER, C. (Eds.) (1982) *Stress and Human Health: Analysis and Implications of Research.* A study by the Institute of Medicine, National Academy of Sciences. Springer Series on Psychiatry, New York: Springer Publishing Company

EPSTEIN, A. N., FITZSIMMONS, J. T. and RALLS, B. J. (1969) Drinking caused by the intracranial injection of angiotensin into the rat. *Journal of Physiology (London),* **200,** 98–100

ERICSSON, B. F. (1971) Effect of vasopressin on the distribution of cardiac output and organ blood flow in the anesthetized dog. *Acta Chirurgica Scandinavica,* **137,** 729–738

ESLER, M., JULIUS, S. and RANDALL, O. (1976) Relationship of volume factors, renin and neurogenic vascular resistance in borderline hypertension. In *The Arterial Hypertensive Disease, A Symposium,* edited by G. Rorive and H. van Cauwenberge, pp. 231–249. New York: Masson

FERRARIO, C. M. (1983a) Central nervous system mechanisms of blood pressure control in normotensive and hypertensive states. *Chest,* **83** (Suppl), 331S–335S

FERRARIO, C. M. (1983b) The neurogenic actions of angiotensin II. *Hypertension,* **5,** (Suppl. V) V-73–V-79

FERRARIO, C. M., BARNES, K. L., BOHONEK, S. (1981) Neurogenic hypertension produced by lesions of the nucleus tractus solitarii alone or with sinoaortic denervation in the dog. *Hypertension,* **3** (Suppl. II), 112–118

FERRARIO, C. M., BARNES, K. L., BROSNIHAN, K. B. and McCUBBIN, J. W. (1981) An analytical description of the role of neurogenic factors in the control of arterial pressure. In *Hypertension,* edited by H. Villarreal, pp. 185–194. New York: Wiley and Sons, Inc.

FERRARIO, C. M., BARNES, K. L., SZILAGYI, J. E. and BROSNIHAN, K. B. (1979) Physiological and pharmacological characterization of the area postrema pressor pathways in the normal dog. *Hypertension,* **1,** 235–245

FERRARIO, C. M., DICKINSON, C. J. and McCUBBIN, J. W. (1970) Central vasomotor stimulation by angiotensin. *Clinical Science,* **39,** 239–245

FERRARIO, C. M., GILDENBERG, P. L. and McCUBBIN, J. W. (1972) Cardiovascular effects of angiotensin mediated by the central nervous system. *Circulation Research,* **30,** 257–262

FERRARIO, C. M. and McCUBBIN, J. W. (1974) Neurogenic factors in hypertension. *Hospital Practice,* **9,** 71–81

FERRARIO, C. M. and PAGE, I. H. (1978) Current views concerning cardiac output in the genesis of experimental hypertension. *Circulation Research,* **43,** 821–831

FERRARIO, C. M. and TAKISHITA, S. (1983) Baroreceptor reflexes and hypertension. In *Hypertension: Physiopathology and Treatment,* edited by J. Genest, O. Kuchel, P. Hamet and M. Cantin, pp. 161–170. New York: McGraw-Hill Book Co.

FEUERSTEIN, G., ZERBE, R. L., BEN-ISHAY, D., KOPIN, I. J. and JACOBOWITZ, D. M. (1981) Catecholamines and vasopressin in forebrain nuclei of hypertension prone and resistant rats. *Brain Research Bulletin,* **7,** 671–676

FINK, G. D. and BRYAN, W. J. (1982) Influence of forebrain periventricular lesions on the development of renal hypertension in rabbits. *Hypertension,* **4,** 155–160

FINK, G. D., BRYAN, W. J. and MOKLER, D. J. (1982) Effects of chronic intracerebroventricular infusion of angiotensin II on arterial pressure and fluid homeostasis. *Hypertension,* **4,** 312–319

FINKIELMAN, S., FISCHER-FERRARO, C., DIAZ, A., GOLDSTEIN, D. J. and NAHMOD, V. E. (1972) A pressor substance in the cerebrospinal fluid of normotensive and hypertensive patients. *Proceedings of the National Academy of Sciences of the USA,* **69,** 3341–3344

FISCHER-FERRARO, C., NAHMOD, V. E., GOLDSTEIN, D. J. and FINKIELMAN, S. (1971) Angiotensin and renin in rat and dog brain. *Journal of Experimental Medicine,* **133,** 353–361

FLEETWOOD-WALKER, S. M. and COOTE, J. H. (1981) The contribution of brainstem catecholamine cell groups to the innervation of the sympathetic lateral cell column. *Brain Research,* **205,** 141–155

FOLKOW, B. (1960) Range of control of the cardiovascular system by the central nervous system. *Physiological Reviews,* **40** (Suppl. 4), 93–99

FOLKOW, B. (1982) Physiological aspects of primary hypertension. *Physiological Reviews,* **62,** 347–504

FROHMAN, L. A. (1980) Neurotransmitters as regulators of endocrine function. In *Neuroendocrinology,* edited by D. T. Krieger and J. C. Hughes, pp. 44–58. Sunderland, MA: Sinauer Assoc. Inc.

FUXE, K., AGNATI, L. F., GANTEN, D., GOLDSTEIN, M., YUKIMURA, T., JONSSON, G. *et al.* (1981) The role of noradrenaline and adrenaline neuron systems and substance P in the control of central cardiovascular functions. In *Central Nervous System Mechanisms in Hypertension,* edited by J. P. Buckley and C. M. Ferrario, pp. 89–113. New York: Raven Press

FUXE, K., GANTEN, D., HOKFELT, T. and BOLME, P. (1976) Immunohistochemical evidence for the existence of angiotensin II-containing nerve terminals in the brain and spinal cord in the rat. *Neuroscience Letters,* **2,** 229–234

GANTEN, D. and SPECK, G. (1978) The brain renin–angiotensin system: a model for the synthesis of peptides in the brain. *Biochemical Pharmacology,* **27,** 2379–2389

GAVRAS, H., HATZINIKOLAOU, P., NORTH, W. G., BRESNAHAN, M. and GAVRAS, I. (1982) Interaction of the sympathetic nervous system with vasopressin and renin in the maintenance of blood pressure. *Hypertension,* **4,** 400–405

GORDON, F. J., BRODY, M. J., FINK, G. D., BUGGY, J. and JOHNSON, A. K. (1979) Role of central catecholamines in the control of blood pressure and drinking behavior. *Brain Research,* **178,** 161–173

GREGORY, T. J., WALLIS, C. J. and PRINTZ, M. J. (1982) Regional changes in rat brain angiotensinogen following bilateral nephrectomy. *Hypertension,* **4,** 827–838

GUILLEMIN, R. (1980) Hypothalamic hormones: releasing and inhibiting factors. In *Neuroendocrinology, A Hospital Practice Book,* edited by D. T. Krieger and J. C. Hughes, pp. 23–32. Sunderland, MA: Sinauer Assoc. Inc.

HADDY, F. J. (1982) Natriuretic hormone–the missing link in low renin hypertension? *Biochemical Pharmacology,* **31,** 3159–3161

HAEUSLER, G., FINCH, I. and THOENEN, H. (1972) Central adrenergic neurones and the initiation and development of experimental hypertension. *Experientia,* **28,** 1200–1203

HARTLE, D. K., LIND, R. W., JOHNSON, A. K. and BRODY, M. J. (1982) Localization of the anterior hypothalamic angiotensin II pressor system. *Hypertension,* **4** (Suppl. II), II-159–II-165

HAYWARD, J. N. and VINCENT, J. D. (1970) Osmosensitive single neurons in the hypothalamus of unanesthetized monkeys. *Journal of Physiology (London),* **210,** 947–972

HENRY, J. P., GAUER, O. H. and REEVES, J. L. (1956) Evidence of the atrial location of receptors influencing urine flow. *Circulation Research,* **4,** 85–90

HENRY, J. P. and PEARCE, J. W. (1956) The possible role of cardiac atrial stretch receptors in the induction of changes in urine flow. *Journal of Physiology (London),* **131,** 572–585

HEYNDRICKX, G. R., BOETTCHER, D. H. and VATNER, S. F. (1976) Effects of angiotensin, vasopressin, and methoxamine on cardiac function and blood flow distribution in conscious dogs. *American Journal of Physiology,* **231,** 1579–1587

HILTON, S. M. (1975) Ways of viewing the central nervous control of the circulation–old and new. *Brain Research,* **87,** 213–219

HIROSE, S., YOKOSAWA, H. and INAGAMI, T. (1978) Immunochemical identification of renin in rat brain and distinction from acid proteases. *Nature (London),* **274,** 392–393

HOWE, P. R. C., COSTA, M., FURNESS, J. B. and CHALMERS, J. P. (1980) Simultaneous demonstration of phenylethanolamine *N*-methyltransferase immunofluorescent and catecholamine fluorescent nerve cell bodies in the rat medulla oblongata. *Neuroscience Letters,* **5,** 2229–2238

HUSAIN, A., BUMPUS, F. M., SMEBY, R. R., BROSNIHAN, K. B., KHOSLA, M. C., SPETH, R. C. and FERRARIO, C. M. (1983) Evidence for the existence of a family of biologically active angiotensin I-like peptides in the dog central nervous system. *Circulation Research,* **52,** 460–464

HUTCHINSON, J. S., CSICSMANN, J., KORNER, P. I. and JOHNSTON, C. I. (1978) Characterization of immunoreactive angiotensin in canine cerebrospinal fluid as des-Asp[1] Ang II. *Clinical Science and Molecular Medicine,* **54,** 147–151

ITO, T., EGGENA, P., BARRETT, J. D., KATZ, D., METTER, J. and SAMBHI, M. P. (1980) Studies on angiotensin of plasma and cerebrospinal fluid in normal and hypertensive human subjects. *Hypertension,* **2,** 432–436

JEWELL, P. A. and VERNEY, E. B. (1957) An experimental attempt to determine the site of the neurohypophysial osmoreceptors in the dog. *Philosophical Transactions of the Royal Society of London,* **B240,** 197–324

JOHNSTON, C. I., NEWMAN, M. and WOOD, R. (1981) Role of vasopressin in cardiovascular homeostasis and hypertension. *Clinical Science,* **61,** 129S–139S

KATCHALSKY, A. and REHOVOTH, A. O. (1971) Mechanochemical conversion. In *Handbook of Sensory Physiology, Vol. 1,* edited by W. R. Loewenstein, pp. 1–17. Berlin: Springer-Verlag

KATHOLI, R. E., WHITLOW, P. L., WINTERNITZ, S. R. and OPARIL, S. (1982) Importance of the renal nerves in established two-kidney, one-clip hypertension. *Hypertension,* **4** (Suppl. II), II-166–II-174

KLEEMAN, C. R. and BERL, T. (1979) The neurohypophysial hormones: vasopressin. In *Endocrinology, Vol. 1,* edited by L. J. DeGroot *et al.,* pp. 253–275. New York: Grune and Stratton

KNIGGE, K. M., HOFFMAN, G. E., JOSEPH, S. A., SCOTT, D. E., SLADEK, C. D. and SLADEK, J. R. JR (1980) Recent advances in structure and function of the endocrine hypothalamus. In *Handbook of the Hypothalamus,* edited by P. J. Morgane and J. Panksepp, pp. 63–164. New York and Basel: Marcel Dekker, Inc.

KOIZUMI, K. and YAMASHITA, H. (1978) Influence of atrial stretch receptors on hypothalamic neurosecretory neurones. *Journal of Physiology (London),* **285,** 341–358

KORNER, P. I. and HEAD, G. A. (1983) Cardiovascular functions of central noradrenergic and serotonergic neurons in conscious rabbits. *Chest,* **83** (Suppl.), 335S–338S

KRAKOFF, L., NICOLIS, G. and AMSEL, B. (1975) Pathogenesis of hypertension in Cushing's syndrome. *American Journal of Medicine,* **58,** 216–220

KRAKOFF, L. R., SELVADURA, R. and SUTTER, E. (1975) Effect of methylprednisolone upon arterial pressure and the renin–angiotensin system in the rat. *American Journal of Physiology,* **228,** 613–617

KRIEGER, E. M., SALGADO, H. C. and MICHELINI, L. C. (1982) Resetting of the baroreceptors. In *International Review of Physiology, Vol. 26, Cardiovascular Physiology IV,* edited by A. C. Guyton and J. E. Hall, pp. 119–146. Baltimore: University Park Press

LeROITH, D., SHILOACH, J., BERELOWITZ, M., FROHMAN, L. A., LIOTTA, A. S., KREIGER, D. T. and ROTH, J. (1983) Are messenger molecules in microbes the ancestors of the vertebrate hormones and tissue factors? *Federation Proceedings,* **42,** 2602–2607

LIARD, J. F., DERIAZ, O., TSCHOPP, M. and SCHOUN, J. (1981) Cardiovascular effects of vasopressin infused into the vertebral circulation of conscious dogs. *Clinical Science,* **61,** 345–347

LIARD, J. F. and SILENZIO, R. (1982) Baroreceptor reflex influence on peripheral circulations in salt-loading hypertension in dogs. *Hypertension,* **4,** 597–603

LOEWY, A. D. and McKELLAR, S. (1980) The neuroanatomical basis of central cardiovascular control. *Federation Proceedings,* **39,** 2495–2503

LOEWY, A. D. and McKELLAR, S. (1981) Serotonergic projections from the ventral medulla to the intermediolateral cell column in the rat. *Brain Research,* **211,** 146–152

LOEWY, A. D., McKELLAR, S. and SAPER, C. B. (1979) Direct projections from the A5 catecholamine cell group to the intermediolateral cell column. *Brain Research,* **174,** 309–314

LOHMEIER, T. E. and CARROLL, R. G. (1982) Chronic potentiation of vasoconstrictor hypertension by adrenocorticotropic hormone. *Hypertension,* **4** (Suppl. II), II-138–II-148

LOHMEIER, T. E. and KASTNER, P. R. (1982) Chronic effects of ACTH and cortisol excess on arterial pressure in normotensive and hypertensive dogs. *Hypertension,* **4,** 652–661

MAJEWSKI, H., RAND, M. J. and TUNG, L. H. (1981) Activation of prejunctional beta-adrenoceptors in rat atria by adrenaline applied exogenously or released as a co-transmitter. *British Journal of Pharmacology,* **73,** 669–679

MANN, J. F. E., PHILLIPS, M. I., DIETZ, R., HAEBARA, H. and GANTEN, D. (1978) Effects of central and peripheral angiotensin blockade in hypertensive rats. *American Journal of Physiology,* **234,** H629–H637

MANNING, R. D. JR, GUYTON, A. C., COLEMAN, T. G. and McCAA, R. E. (1979) Hypertension in dogs during antidiuretic hormone and hypotonic saline infusion. *American Journal of Physiology,* **236,** H314–H322

MARAN, J. W. and YATES, E. (1977) Cortisol secretion during intrapituitary infusion of angiotensin II in conscious dogs. *American Journal of Physiology,* **233,** E273–E285

MARK, A. L., LAWTON, W. J., ABBOUD, F. M., FITZ, A. E., CONNOR, W. E. and HEISTAD, D. D. (1977) Effects of high and low sodium intake on arterial pressure and forearm vascular resistance in borderline hypertension. *Circulation Research,* **36–37,** (Suppl. I), 194–198

MARSON, O., RIBEIRO, A. B., TUFIK, S., FILHO, G. A., SARAGOCA, M. A. S. and RAMOS, O. L. (1981) Role of the anteroventral third ventricle region and the renin angiotensin system in methylprednisolone hypertension. *Hypertension,* **3** (Suppl. II), II-142–II-146

MATSUGUCHI, H., SHARABI, F. M., GORDON, F. J., JOHNSON, A. K. and SCHMID, P. G. (1982) Blood pressure and heart rate responses to microinjection of vasopressin into the nucleus tractus solitarius region of the rat. *Neuropharmacology,* **21,** 687–694

McCUBBIN, J. W. (1974) Peripheral effects of angiotensin on the autonomic nervous system. In *Angiotensin,* edited by I. H. Page and F. M. Bumpus, pp. 418–423. Berlin, New York: Springer-Verlag

McCUBBIN, J. W., GREEN, J. H. and PAGE, I. H. (1956) Baroreceptor function in chronic renal hypertension. *Circulation Research,* **4,** 205–210

McCUBBIN, J. W. and PAGE, I. H. (1963) Neurogenic component of chronic renal hypertension. *Science,* **139,** 210–215

McEWEN, B. S., DAVIS, P. G., PARSONS, B. and PFAFF, D. W. (1979) The brain as a target for steroid hormone action. *Annual Review of Neuroscience,* **2,** 65–112

McKELVY, J. F., GLASEL, J. A. and FOREMAN, M. (1980) Biochemical aspects of hypothalamic function. In *Handbook of the Hypothalamus,* edited by P. J. Morgane and J. Panksepp, pp. 1–62. New York and Basel: Marcel Dekker, Inc.

MICHELINI, L. C., BARNES, K. L. and FERRARIO, C. M. (1983) Arginine vasopressin modulates the central action of angiotensin II in the dog. *Hypertension,* **5,** (Suppl. V), V-94–V-100

MOHRING, J. (1978) Neurohypophyseal vasopressor principle: vasopressor hormone as well as antidiuretic hormone? *Klinische Wochenschrift,* **56** (Suppl. I), 71–79

MOHRING, J., KINTZ, J. and SCHOUN, J. (1979) Studies on the role of vasopressin in blood pressure control of spontaneously hypertensive rats with established hypertension (SHR, stroke-prone strain). *Journal of Cardiovascular Pharmacology,* **1,** 593–608

MOHRING, J., MOHRING, B., PETRI, M. and HAACK, D. (1977) Vasopressor role of ADH in the pathogenesis of malignant DOC hypertension. *American Journal of Physiology,* **232,** F260–F269

MOHRING, J., MOHRING, B., PETRI, M. and HAACK, D. (1978) Plasma vasopressin concentrations and effects of vasopressin antiserum on blood pressure in rats with malignant two-kidney Goldblatt hypertension. *Circulation Research,* **42,** 17–22

MONTANI, J. P., LIARD, J. F., SCHOUN, J. and MOHRING, J. (1980) Hemodynamic effects of exogenous and endogenous vasopressin at low plasma concentrations in conscious dogs. *Circulation Research,* **47,** 346–355

MOORE, R. Y. and BLOOM, F. E. (1978) Central catecholamine neuron systems: anatomy and physiology of the dopamine systems. *Annual Review of Neuroscience,* **1,** 129–169

MOORE, R. Y. and BLOOM, F. E. (1979) Central catecholamine neuron systems: anatomy and physiology of the norepinephrine and epinephrine systems. *Annual Review of Neuroscience,* **2,** 113–168

NASHOLD, B. S., MANNARINO, E. and WUNDERLICH, M. (1961) Pressor–depressor blood pressure response in the cat after intraventricular injection of drugs. *Nature,* **193,** 1297–1298

OLDENDORF, W. H. (1981) Blood brain barrier permeability to peptides: pitfalls in measurements. *Peptides,* **2** (Suppl. II), 109–111

ONOYAMA, K., BRAVO, E. L. and TARAZI, R. C. (1979) Sodium, extracellular fluid volume, and cardiac output changes in the genesis of mineralocorticoid hypertension in the intact dog. *Hypertension,* **1,** 331–336

OSMAN, M. Y., SMEBY, R. R. and SEN, S. (1979) Separation of dog brain renin-like activity from acid protease activity. *Hypertension,* **1,** 53–60

OVERBECK, H. W. and GRISSETTE, D. E. (1982) Sodium pump activity in arteries of rats with Goldblatt hypertension. *Hypertension,* **4,** 132–139

PADFIELD, P. L., BROWN, J. J., LEVER, A. F., MORTON, J. J. and ROBERTSON, J. I. S. (1981) Blood pressure in acute and chronic vasopressin excess. *New England Journal of Medicine,* **304,** 1067–1070

PAGE, I. H. and McCUBBIN, J. W. (1965) The physiology of arterial hypertension. In *Handbook of Physiology: Circulation,* pp. 2163–2208. Washington, DC: American Physiological Society

PAGE, I. H. and McCUBBIN, J. W. (Eds.) (1968) *Renal Hypertension.* Chicago: Year Book Medical Publishers

PALAY, S. L. (1957) The fine structure of the neurohypophysis. In *Ultrastructure and Cellular Chemistry of Neural Tissue,* edited by H. Walsh, pp. 31–44. New York: Paul B. Hoeber, Inc.

PAMNANI, M., HUOT, S., BUGGY, J., CLOUGH, D. and HADDY, F. (1981) Demonstration of a humoral inhibitor of the Na^+–K^+ pump in some models of experimental hypertension. *Hypertension,* **3** *(Suppl. II),* II-96–101

PEACH, M. J., BUMPUS, F. M. and KHAIRALLAH, P. A. (1969) Inhibition of norepinephrine uptake in hearts by angiotensin II and analogs. *Journal of Pharmacology and Experimental Therapeutics*, **167**, 291–299

PETTY, M. A. and REID, J. L. (1979) Catecholamine synthesizing enzymes in brain stem and hypothalamus during the development of renovascular hypertension. *Brain Research*, **163**, 277–288

PHILLIPS, M. I., FELIX, D., HOFFMAN, W. E. and GANTEN, D. (1977) Angiotensin-sensitive sites in the brain ventricular system. In *Neuroscience Symposia*, Vol. 2, edited by W. Cowan and J. A. Ferendelli, pp. 308–339. Bethesda MA: Society for Neuroscience

PRINTZ, M. P. and GREGORY, T. J. (1981) Brain angiotensinogen: evidence for an independent and functional central angiotensin system. In *Central Nervous System Mechanisms in Hypertension*, edited by J. P. Buckley and C. M. Ferrario, pp. 311–326. New York: Raven Press

PRINTZ, M. P., PRINTZ, J. M. and GREGORY, T. J. (1978) Identification of angiotensinogen in animal brain homogenates. *Circulation Research*, **43**, 1-21–27

QUILLEN, E. W. JR and COWLEY, A. W. JR (1983) Influence of volume changes on osmolality–vasopressin relationships in conscious dogs. *American Journal of Physiology*, **244**, H73–H79

QUINLAN, J. T. and PHILLIPS, M. I. (1981) Immunoreactivity for an angiotensin-like peptide in the human brain. *Brain Research*, **205**, 212–218

RABITO, S. F., CARRETERO, O. A. and SCICLI, A. G. (1981) Evidence against a role of vasopressin in the maintenance of high blood pressure in mineralocorticoid and renovascular hypertension. *Hypertension*, **3**, 34–38

REICHLIN, S. (1981) Neuroendocrinology. In *Textbook of Endocrinology*, edited by R. H. Williams, pp. 589–645. Philadelphia: W. B. Saunders Co.

REID, I. A., BROOKS, V. L., RUDOLPH, C. D. and KEIL, L. C. (1982) Analysis of the actions of angiotensin on the central nervous system of conscious dogs. *American Journal of Physiology*, **243**, R82–R91

REID, I. A. and GANONG, W. F. (1977) Control of aldosterone secretion. In *Hypertension*, edited by J. Genest, E. Koiw and O. Kuchel, pp. 265–292. New York: McGraw-Hill Book Co.

REID, J. L., ZIVIN, J. A. and KOPIN, I. J. (1975) Central and peripheral adrenergic mechanisms in the development of deoxycorticosterone-saline hypertension in rats. *Circulation Research*, **37**, 569–579

REIS, D. J. (1981) The brain and arterial hypertension: evidence for a neural-imbalance hypothesis. In *Disturbances in Neurogenic Control of the Circulation*, edited by F. A. Abboud, H. A. Fozzard, J. P. Gilmore and D. J. Reis, pp. 87–104. Bethesda, Maryland: American Physiological Society, Williams and Wilkins

REIS, D. J., JOH, T. H., NATHAN, M. A., RENAUD, B., SNYDER, D. W. and TALMAN, W. (1979) Nucleus tractus solitarii: catecholaminergic innervation in normal and abnormal control of arterial pressure. In *Nervous System and Hypertension*, edited by P. Meyer and H. Schmitt, pp. 147–164. New York: John Wiley Inc.

RODRIGUEZ, E. (1976) The cerebrospinal fluid as a pathway in neuroendocrine integration. *Journal of Endocrinology*, **71**, 407–443

ROSENZWEIG, J. L., LeROITH, D., LESNIAK, M. A., MacINTYRE, I., SAWYER, W. H. and ROTH, J. (1983) Two distinct insulins in the guinea pig: the broad relevance of these findings to evolution of peptide hormones. *Federation Proceedings,* **42,** 2608–2614

ROSS, C. A., ARMSTRONG, D. M., RUGGIERO, D. A., PICKEL, V. M., JOH, T. H. and REIS, D. J. (1981) Adrenaline neurons in the rostral ventrolateral medulla innervate thoracic spinal cord: a combined immunocytochemical and retrograde transport demonstration. *Neuroscience Letters,* **25,** 257–262

ROTSZTEJN, W. H. (1980) Neuromodulation in neuroendocrinology. *Trends in Neuroscience,* **3,** 67–70

RUBIN, B., ANTONACCIO, M. J. and HOROVITZ, Z. P. (1981) The antihypertensive effects of captopril in hypertensive animal models. In *Angiotensin Converting Enzyme Inhibitors,* edited by Z. P. Horovitz, pp. 27–54. Baltimore, Munich: Urban and Schwarzenberg

SAAVEDRA, J. M. (1979) Brain catecholamines during development of DOCA-salt hypertension in rats. *Brain Research,* **179,** 121–127

SAAVEDRA, J. M., CORREA, E. M. and IWAI, J. (1980) Discrete changes in adrenaline-forming enzyme activity in brain stem areas of genetic salt-sensitive hypertensive (Dahl) rats. *Brain Research,* **193,** 299–303

SAAVEDRA, J. M., GROBECKER, H. and AXELROD, J. (1976) Adrenaline-forming enzymes in brain stem: elevation in genetic and experimental hypertension. *Science,* **191,** 483–484

SAAVEDRA, J. M., KVETNANSKY, R. and KOPIN, I. J. (1979) Adrenaline, noradrenaline and dopamine levels in specific brainstem areas of acutely immobilized rats. *Brain Research,* **160,** 271–280

SAITO, T., YAJIMA, Y. and WATANABE, T. (1981) Involvement of AVP in the development and maintenance of hypertension in rats. In *Antidiuretic Hormone,* edited by S. Yoshida, L. Share and K. Yagi, pp. 215–225. Baltimore: University Park Press

SAWCHENKO, P. E. and SWANSON, L. W. (1982) Immunohistochemical identification of neurons in the paraventricular nucleus of the hypothalamus that project to the medulla or the spinal cord in the rat. *Journal of Comparative Neurology,* **205,** 260–272

SCHARRER, E. and SCHARRER, B. (1954) Hormones produced by neurosecretory cells. *Recent Progress in Hormone Research,* **10,** 183–240

SCHOLKENS, B. A., JUNG, W., LANG, R. E., RASCHER, W., UNGER, TH. and GANTEN, D. (1982) The role of neuropeptides in central mechanisms of blood pressure regulation. In *Endocrinology of Hypertension,* edited by F. Mantero, E. G. Biglieri and C. R. W. Edwards, pp. 339–362. London and New York: Academic Press

SCOGGINS, B. A., COGHLAN, J. P., CONGIU, M., DENTON, D. A., GRAHAM, W. F., McKINLEY, M. J. *et al.* (1982a) Alterations in osmotic but not pressor responses to ACTH by optic recess lesions in sheep. *Hypertension,* **4** (Suppl. II), II-154–II-158

SCOGGINS, B. A., COGHLAN, J. P., DENTON, D. A., MASON, R. T. and WHITWORTH, J. S. (1982b) A review of mechanisms involved in the production of steroid induced hypertension with particular reference to ACTH dependent hypertension. In *Endocrinology of Hypertension,* edited by F. Mantero, E. G. Biglieri and C. R. W. Edwards, pp. 41–68. London, New York: Academic Press

SEMPLE, P. F., McCRAE, W. A. and MORTON, J. J. (1980) Angiotensin II in human cerebrospinal fluid may be an immunoassay artifact. *Clinical Science,* **59** (Suppl. 6), 61S–64S

SHARE, L. (1976) Role of cardiovascular receptors in the control of ADH release. *Cardiology,* **61** (Suppl. I), 51–64

SHARE, L. and LEVY, M. N. (1962) Cardiovascular receptors and blood titer of antidiuretic hormone. *American Journal of Physiology,* **203,** 425–428

SLADEK, C. D. and JOHNSON, A. K. (1983) Effect of anteroventral third ventricle lesions on vasopressin release by organ-cultured hypothalamo-neurohypophyseal explants. *Neuroendocrinology,* **37,** 78–84

SLADEK, C. D. and KNIGGE, K. M. (1977) Osmotic control of vasopressin release by rat hypothalamo-neurohypophyseal explants in organ culture. *Endocrinology,* **101,** 1834–1838

SLATER, E. E. (1981) Brain renin: progress in research. In *Central Nervous System Mechanisms in Hypertension,* edited by J. P. Buckley and C. M. Ferrario, pp. 293–300. New York: Raven Press

SMITH, M. J. JR, COWLEY, A. W. JR, GUYTON, A. C. and MANNING, R. D., JR. (1979) Acute and chronic effects of vasopressin on blood pressure, electrolytes, and fluid volumes. *American Journal of Physiology,* **237,** F232–F240

SOFRONIEW, M. V. (1980) Projections from vasopressin, oxytocin and neurophysin neurons to neural targets in the rat and human. *Journal of Histochemistry and Cytochemistry,* **28,** 475–478

SOFRONIEW, M. V. and SCHRELL, U. (1981) Evidence for a direct projection from oxytocin and vasopressin neurons in the hypothalamic paraventricular nucleus to the medulla oblongata: immunohistochemical visualization of both the horseradish peroxidase transported and the peptide produced by the same neurons. *Neuroscience Letters,* **22,** 211–217

SONGU-MIZE, E., BEALER, S. L. and CALDWELL, R. W. (1982) Effect of AV3V lesions on development of DOCA-salt hypertension and vascular Na^+-pump activity. *Hypertension,* **4,** 575–580

SOWERS, J. R., NYBY, M. and JASBERG, K. (1982) Dopaminergic control of prolactin and blood pressure: altered control in essential hypertension. *Hypertension,* **4,** 431–438

SPETH, R. C., VALLOTTON, M. B., CHERNICKY, C., KHOSLA, M. C. and FERRARIO, C. M. (1983) Angiotensin II receptors in dog brain. *Federation Proceedings,* **42,** 494

STEINBUSCH, H. W. M. (1981) Distribution of serotonin-immunoreactivity in the central nervous system of the rat cell bodies and terminals. *Neuroscience,* **6,** 557–618

SUZUKI, H., FERRARIO, C. M., SPETH, R. C., BROSNIHAN, K. B. and SMEBY, R. R. (1983) Alterations in plasma and cerebrospinal fluid norepinephrine and angiotensin II during the development of renal hypertension in conscious dogs. *Hypertension,* **5** (Suppl. I), I-139–I-148

SWANSON, L. W. and SAWCHENKO, P. E. (1980) Paraventricular nucleus: a site for the integration of neuroendocrine and autonomic mechanisms. *Neuroendocrinology*, **31**, 410–417

SWARTZ, S. L., WILLIAMS, G. H., HOLLENBERG, N. K., LEVINE, L., DLUHY, R. G. and MOORE, T. J. (1980) Captopril-induced changes in prostaglandin production. *Journal of Clinical Investigation*, **65**, 1257–1264

SZILAGYI, J. E. and FERRARIO, C. M. (1981) Central opiate system modulation of the area postrema pressor pathway. *Hypertension*, **3**, 313–317

SZILAGYI, J. E., MASAKI, Z., BROSNIHAN, K. B. and FERRARIO, C. M. (1981) Neurogenic suppression of carotid sinus reflexes by vagal afferents in sodium depleted dogs. *American Journal of Physiology*, **241**, H255–262

TAKESHITA, A., TANAKA, S., KUROIWA, A. and NAKAMURA, M. (1975) Reduced baroreceptor sensitivity in borderline hypertension. *Circulation*, **51**, 738–742

TAKISHITA, S. and FERRARIO, C. M. (1982) Altered neural control of cardiovascular function in sodium-depleted dogs. *Hypertension*, **4** (Suppl. II), II-175–II-182

TANAKA, T., SEKI, A. and FUJII, J. (1982) Effect of high and low sodium intake on norepinephrine turnover in the cardiovascular tissues and brain stem of the rabbit. *Hypertension*, **4**, 294–298

TANAKA, T., SEKI, A., FUJII, J., KURIHARA, H. and IKEDA, M. (1982) Norepinephrine turnover in the cardiovascular tissues and brainstem of the rabbit during development of one-kidney and two-kidney Goldblatt hypertension. *Hypertension*, **4**, 272–278

TARAZI, R. C., FOUAD, F. M. and FERRARIO, C. M. (1983) Can the heart initiate some forms of hypertension? *Federation Proceedings*, **42**, 2681–2697

TOBIAN, L. (1977) Salt and hypertension. In *Hypertension*, edited by J. Genest, E. Koiw and O. Kuchel, pp. 423–433. New York: McGraw-Hill

UNGER, T., ROCKHOLD, R. W., KAUFMANN-BUHLER, I., HUBNER, D., SCHULL, B., SPECK, G. and GANTEN, D. (1981) Effects of angiotensin-converting enzyme inhibitors on the brain. In *Angiotensin-Converting Enzyme Inhibitors*, edited by Z. P. Horovitz, pp. 55–80. Baltimore, Munich: Urban and Schwarzenberg

VAN AMERINGEN, M. R., deCHAMPLAIN, J. and IMBEAULT, S. (1977) Participation of central noradrenergic neurons in experimental hypertension. *Canadian Journal of Physiology and Pharmacology*, **55**, 1246–1251

VARMA, S., BHUWANESHWAR, P. J. and BHARGAVA, K. P. (1969) Mechanism of vasopressin-induced bradycardia in dogs. *Circulation Research*, **24**, 787–792

VECSEI, P., HACKENTHAL, E. and GANTEN, D. (1978) The renin–angiotensin–aldosterone system. *Klinische Wochenschrift*, **56** (Suppl. I), 5–21

VERNEY, E. B. (1947) The antidiuretic hormone and the factors which determine its release. *Proceedings of the Royal Society of London*, **B135**, 25–106

VETTER, W., VETTER, H., BECKERHOFF, R., REDLICH, B., COTTIER, P. and SIEGENTHALER, W. (1976) The effect of saralasin (1-sar-8-ala-angiotensin II) on blood pressure in patients with Cushing's syndrome. *Klinische Wochenschrift*, **54**, 661–663

WAEBER, B., GAVRAS, H., GAVRAS, I. *et al.* (1982) Evidence for a sodium-induced activation of central neurogenic mechanisms in one-kidney, one-clip renal hypertensive rats. *Journal of Pharmacology and Experimental Therapeutics*, **223**, 510–515

WALLIS, C. J. and PRINTZ, M. P. (1980) Adrenal regulation of regional brain and angiotensinogen content. *Endocrinology,* **106,** 337–342

WESTFALL, T. C. (1980) Neuroeffector mechanisms. *Annual Review of Physiology,* **42,** 383–397

WINTERNITZ, S. R., KATHOLI, R. E. and OPARIL, S. (1982) Decrease in hypothalamic norepinephrine content following renal denervation in the one-kidney, one-clip Goldblatt hypertensive rat. *Hypertension,* **4,** 369–373

WOODS, R. L. and JOHNSTON, C. I. (1982) Role of vasopressin in hypertension: studies using the Brattleboro rat. *American Journal of Physiology,* **242,** F727–F732

YAMADA, S., YAMAMURA, H. I. and ROESKE, W. R. (1980) Alterations in central and peripheral adrenergic receptors in deoxycorticosterone/salt hypertensive rats. *Life Sciences,* **27,** 2405–2416

YAMASHITA, H. and KOIZUMI, K. (1979) Influence of carotid and aortic baroreceptors on neurosecretory neurons in supraoptic nuclei. *Brain Research,* **170,** 259–277

ZANCHETTI, A. (1979) Overview of cardiovascular reflexes in hypertension. *American Journal of Cardiology,* **44,** 912–918

ZIMMERMAN, E. A., STILLMAN, M. A., RECHT, L. D., ANTUNES, J. L., CARMEL, P. W. and GOLDSMITH, P. C. (1977) Vasopressin and corticotropin releasing factor: an axonal pathway to portal capillaries in the zona externa of the median eminence containing vasopressin and its interaction with adrenal corticoids. *Annals of the New York Academy of Sciences,* **297,** 405–419

2
Is epinephrine the cause of essential hypertension?

Morris J. Brown

PHYSIOLOGICAL BACKGROUND

Among its contemporaries, epinephrine (EPI) has long seemed the Cinderella of hormones. Indeed, there is a paradoxical gulf between the role of epinephrine (adrenaline) in common parlance ('the adrenaline ran in his veins') and the cold shoulder shown to it by endocrinologists. No disease state of epinephrine deficiency is known, and epinephrine replacement is not required after adrenalectomy. Conversely, the greater interest of phaeochromocytoma to clinical pharmacologists than endocrinologists symbolizes the prevalent view that the known actions of epinephrine are of pharmacological rather than physiological importance.

The reasons for this disinterest are probably two-fold. First, since the discovery that the neurotransmitter of the sympathetic nervous system was not epinephrine but norepinephrine (NE), the latter has rightly been assumed to play the more important role physiologically; although the adrenal medulla is undoubtedly an endocrine organ, most of its functions in mammals have been subsumed by the sympathetic nervous system, and the adrenal medulla therefore belongs functionally to this as a minor if not vestigial part.

The second more mundane reason for physiological disinterest in epinephrine is that physiological levels of epinephrine in the circulation are very low – generally less than 1 nmol – and much lower than those of noradrenaline. The analytical details of how epinephrine may be measured accurately will be of little interest to the general reader. It is worth explaining, however, that neither norepinephrine nor epinephrine may currently be measured by a radioimmunoassay technique such as is used for other hormones. This is because their small molecular size makes it difficult to raise antibodies specific for each catecholamine and not cross-reacting with their metabolites. Fortunately nature has compensated for this by providing, in a number of tissues including the mammalian liver, abundant concentrations of an enzyme, catechol-o-methyltransferase (COMT), which is employed to measure its catechol substrates. The technique of radioenzymatic assay is used in which the catecholamine of unknown concentration is converted to a radiolabelled methylated derivative in the presence of COMT and a radiolabelled methyl donor (s-adenosyl-L-methionine) (Engelman, Portnoy and Lovenberg, 1968). In principle, the amount of radioactivity counted at the end of the assay is proportional to the unknown concentration of catecholamine present at the start. In practice, however, other variables determine the outcome, since the efficiency of methylation varies among biological samples, and the recovery of methylated amines after the incubation (in particular, from the chromatography stage required to separate the various methylated amines) is both low and variable (Da Prada and Zurcher, 1976). We have used a double-isotope technique in which a ^{14}C-tracer corrects for both variable methylation and recovery (Brown and Jenner, 1981), but the assay cannot be regarded as either simple or cheap, and would not be a feasible proposition for routine chemical pathology laboratories – even those with radioimmunoassay facilities. Some laboratories are becoming acquainted with HPLC techniques (using electrochemical or fluorescent detection), but in our experience these are less reliable for epinephrine than norepinephrine analysis, and cannot be used for animal experiments where there is a limit to the total volume of blood samples.

With regard to the question of the involvement of epinephrine in hypertension, there is yet another reason why it has not until recently been taken seriously. This is the well-known pharmacological observation that when epinephrine is infused in man, mean arterial pressure actually falls; systolic pressure rises but this is outweighed by the fall in diastolic pressure (Clutter *et al.*, 1980; Fitzgerald *et al.*, 1980).

The impetus to 'review' the possible pressor role of epinephrine came from the discovery of presynaptic receptors. The release of norepinephrine from sympathetic nerve endings is under the control of various feedback circuits mediated through adrenoceptors (and, perhaps, other receptors) on the neuronal side of the synaptic cleft (Langer, 1981). A negative feedback loop (according to the theory) is mediated through a receptor with some of the characteristics of an alpha (α-)adrenoceptor: it has been designated an α_2-adrenoceptor since it has a greater affinity for agonists such as clonidine than for methoxamine (an α_1-agonist), and greater for antagonists such as yohimbine and phenoxybenzamine than for prazosin and phentolamine. The endogenous agonist is, of course, norepinephrine, which has a similar affinity for both α_1 (mainly postsynaptic) and α_2 (mainly presynaptic) adrenoceptors. When norepinephrine is released from sympathetic nerve endings it not only stimulates the postsynaptic receptors (be they alpha or beta) on the effector tissue but also inhibits its own release by stimulation of the presynaptic α_2-receptors.

In addition to the inhibitory or negative feedback loop mediated through the presynaptic α_2-receptor, there is also evidence of a positive feedback loop mediated through a presynaptic β-receptor (Adler-Graschinsky and Langer, 1975; Stjarne and Brundin, 1975). Although this receptor is less well characterized than the presynaptic α-receptor, it seems to have the attributes of a β_2-receptor in so far as it has a several hundred-fold greater affinity for epinephrine than for norepinephrine (Dahlof, 1981; Majewski, Rand and Tung, 1981). The typical method of demonstrating the positive feedback loop *in vitro* is to measure the release of norepinephrine from a tissue (such as isolated rat atria) during sympathetic nerve stimulation and show that this release is increased in the presence of a β-receptor agonist such as isoproterenol. Alternatively it may be shown that the release of norepinephrine is reduced in the presence of a β-receptor antagonist. However, in this latter case it has been found in most experiments that significant reduction is caused only if the tissue has previously been incubated with epinephrine. It has been known for a long time that epinephrine can enter sympathetic nerve endings via the same neuronal transport process as exists (teleologically speaking) to promote rapid removal of norepinephrine from the synaptic cleft. The epinephrine may be stored in the vesicles and re-released along with norepinephrine by subsequent nervous impulses. What is now proposed is that the 'uptake and re-release' process is not just an epiphenomenon of the neuronal transport process but is used by epinephrine to allow it to be converted from hormone to neurotransmitter: a 'co-transmitter' – released along with noradrenaline – whose principal site of action is the pre-synaptic β-receptor.

THE HYPOTHESIS

Having outlined the physiology, I shall now expound the hypothesis to which it has led and then consider the evidence (Brown and Macquin, 1981).

There are three limbs to the hypothesis:

(1) That epinephrine, released in paroxysms from the adrenal medulla in response to 'stress', is accumulated in sympathetic nerve endings via the neuronal uptake process and re-released by subsequent sympathetic stimulation.
(2) That this neuronally released epinephrine is the physiological agonist at the presynaptic β-receptor, acting to promote a chronic increase in sympathetic neuronal activity.
(3) That this increased sympathetic neuronal activity leads, over many years, to a sustained increase in blood pressure as a result of a chronic elevation in peripheral resistance and/or cardiac output.

Before discussing each of these propositions in detail, I shall consider the general attractions of the hypothesis. For many years the sympathetic nervous system has been considered a possible candidate as a cause of essential hypertension. It is thought to be of importance in the normal control of blood pressure – certainly in the erect position, and probably to some extent in the supine position, since drugs which reduce norepinephrine release reduce supine blood pressure. Excessive release of norepinephrine from a tumour certainly elevates blood pressure; and although patients with essential hypertension have much lower circulating norepinephrine levels than most phaeochromocytoma patients, one must remember that in the former group norepinephrine is not released directly into the circulation and might reach a high synaptic cleft concentration without a similar elevation of its plasma concentration. There have, of course, been numerous studies of plasma norepinephrine concentration in essential hypertension; there is little consensus about the result (Goldstein, 1981). However, it is generally agreed that plasma norepinephrine concentration in normotensive people is age-related (Lake *et al.*, 1977; Sever *et al.*, 1977), while this age-relation may be absent in hypertensives (Goldstein, 1983; Sever *et al.*, 1977). Indirectly this suggests that plasma norepinephrine is elevated in young hypertensives, and this would fit the hemodynamic observations of increased heart rate and cardiac output early in the genesis of hypertension (De Quattro and Chan, 1972; Julius and Conway, 1968).

One of the 'attractions' of the sympathoadrenal system as the prime cause of hypertension is that one need look no further for an explanation of both increased cardiac output and peripheral resistance. If one incriminates other pressor systems not only do they fail to account for the elevated cardiac output early in hypertension but might, on the contrary, be expected to be associated with a compensatory reduction.

But if the sympathetic system were indeed proved to be involved in the development of hypertension, this would in a sense only push back one step the object of enquiry: what is the cause of the elevated sympathetic activity? (This dilemma would, of course, apply to most putative endocrine causes of hypertension, but less acutely perhaps than for a neurotransmitter, whose release is subject to more stringent control than that of a hormone.) If it is in response to external 'stress' this is unlikely to be more than an intermittent stimulus. What the present hypothesis would explain is the link between intermittent exposure to 'stress' and a sustained increase in sympathetic activity: *paroxysms of epinephrine release during periods of stress result in a chronic increase in neuronal epinephrine concentration which results in a sustained increase in epinephrine release by the positive feedback mechanism already described.*

So much for the 'general attractions' of the hypothesis. I shall turn now to the evidence – acquired or desired – for the individual propositions of the hypothesis.

Epinephrine secretion in hypertension

How should this be measured? There are several problems. The most tedious to the general reader, but probably the most important, is the methodological one of measuring epinephrine. The two techniques acceptable today are radioenzymatic assay and HPLC with electrochemical detection. For each method there are almost as many modifications as there are laboratories performing the assays. The first quality control study has only recently been performed, and the results are still awaited. Pending these, my experience from our own comparisons of methods is that HPLC is less specific against interference from unknown compounds, and (at least for plasma) insufficiently sensitive to compare values accurately at the lower end of the physiological range (Causon *et al.*, 1983). On the other hand, I have never understood how most modifications of the radioenzymatic assay method cope with a ten to twelve stage assay without using any internal tracer in the sample to correct for inevitable losses and variation therein; but this can be circumvented using a double-isotope technique and this is my own preference (Brown and Jenner, 1981).

The second question is what samples should be used for the estimation of epinephrine secretion. It is fashionable in the studies of sympathetic activity in hypertension to estimate plasma norepinephrine concentration; and, of course, plasma hormone concentrations seem the obvious method for investigating any putative endocrine cause of hypertension. However, the hypothesis is intended, it will be recalled, precisely to explain how epinephrine may be important even when its circulating level is not elevated, and it is either the neuronal epinephrine concentration or an integrated measure of adrenomedullary secretion that is required. Ideally both measurements would be of value, whereas in practice neither is directly available. However, a compromise worth considering is the use of platelet epinephrine concentration, for platelets accumulate catecholamines in storage vesicles by a process not dissimilar to (though not identical to) that of neuronal transport, so that their concentration will reflect epinephrine output during the lifespan of the platelet (Born and Smith, 1970; Da Prada and Picotti, 1979). This lifespan is a little longer than the likely turnover time of epinephrine in sympathetic nerve endings; but this is an error on the right side and would indicate whether neuronal epinephrine concentration is elevated sufficiently to activate the positive feedback loop.

To my knowledge, no comparison of platelet epinephrine concentration between normotensives and hypertensives has been performed. Indeed, at the present early stage of investigation into the hypothesis, the platelet measurements seem best deferred in favour of a simpler index that can be performed in large numbers of subjects. Such an index is urinary epinephrine measurements, performed on 24-hour samples (or longer). Four consecutive samples are currently being collected and analyzed on coded samples from over 500 untreated hypertensives and matched controls in the MRC Trial for Mild Hypertension. Such is the number estimated by the MRC statisticians as necessary to provide the power necessary to give a negative result the desired degree of significance. Whatever the possible disadvantages of urine versus plasma measurements may be, these seem far outweighed by force of numbers since the logistics of collecting plasma epinephrine samples are complicated by the special precautions required. Despite the large number of studies of catecholamine secretion in hypertension, there has been no previous study of the scale that may be necessary to detect small elevations of epinephrine secretion. And yet some of the small studies have found elevated values of both plasma and urine epinephrine in hypertension. I shall, for the sake of completeness, report these studies, but their conclusion could be correct only fortuitously. It must be remembered that a significant result in a small number of subjects should be easily reproduced – if genuine – in larger groups. If this is not the case, this suggests either methodological problems or differences in the groups studied. Conditions of sampling and matching of control groups have both been found to be of crucial importance when measuring catecholamines – especially in plasma. Even if the groups are matched it may transpire that only studies with a high proportion of young hypertensives will reveal a difference in epinephrine secretion. Such a trend has been observed in studies of plasma norepinephrine in hypertension (Goldstein, 1983). In the case of epinephrine the hypothesis requires elevated epinephrine secretion only in the early stages of hypertension, although there is no obvious reason why this should disappear later. However, the one group of hypertensives where there is already evidence of raised epinephrine secretion is the so-called borderline hypertensives (Cuche *et al.*, 1974; Cousineau, DeChamplain and Lapointe, 1978). These patients are often younger than the average patient with hypertension and the interesting but unresolved question is whether they represent an early stage of essential hypertension.

This highlights the other problem of small studies, that they will not identify subgroups. If, as seems likely, hypertension proves to be a heterogeneous entity, then only a proportion of any group of hypertensives can be expected to provide evidence of a particular abnormality, endocrine or otherwise, and this must be taken into account when designing the size of a study. Paradoxically, the scatter of data may be less in a small study if the abnormal subgroup happens not to be represented; and this artifactually low scatter will then give the false impression of the statistical power of a negative result.

Plasma epinephrine in hypertension

Two studies are often cited as evidence of elevated epinephrine secretion in essential hypertension. The first report was from Franco-Morselli *et al.* (1977). Their comparison of hypertensives and normotensives is reproduced in *Figure 2.1*. The second report was from Bertel *et al.* (1980), who reported a plasma epinephrine of 70 ± 10 pg/ml in 24 hypertensives compared with 42 ± 4 in 20 normotensives; this difference was significant at the 5% level. However, in both

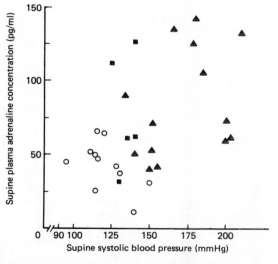

Figure 2.1 Relation between plasma epinephrine concentration and systolic blood pressure in supine position. No significant relation was found for the three groups considered separately; when values were considered together a positive correlation was observed ($r - 0.479$; $P<0.01$). ○ controls; ▲ sustained hypertensives; ■ labile hypertensives. (From Franco-Morselli *et al.*, 1977)

Table 2.1 Plasma epinephrine in resting, supine patients with essential hypertension and in normotensive controls. Each line represents one study in the literature, comparing plasma epinephrine (EPI) concentration in hypertensive (H) and normotensive (N) subjects. (HR = heart rate, MAP = mean arterial pressure) (From Goldstein, 1983)

Reference	H/N (no.)	Age H/N (years)	MAP H/N (mmHg)	HR H/N (bpm)	Assay	EPI H/N (pg/ml)	SD H/N (pg/ml)
Amann et al. (1981)	20/16	48/48	120/80	73/63*	C	30/19*	22/12
Beretta-Piccoli et al. (1980a)	34/25	39/41	109/88	67/66	C	45/31*	28/21
Beretta-Piccoli et al. (1980b)	45/26	42/39	116/89	69/63	C	44/35*	26/17
Bertel et al. (1980)	24/20	—	—	67/62	C	54/35*	39/18
Bolli et al. (1981)	18/15	47/49	118/83	72/60*	C	37/15*	23/14
Buhler et al. (1980)	86/38	—	—	—	C	55/27*	42/17
Corea et al. (1979)	19/7	38/34	128/85	78/67*	F	32/15*	16/3
Cousineau, DeChamplain and Lapointe (1978)	46/28	41/39	114/89	87/75*	P,C	160/89*	128/74
DeChamplain et al. (1981)	67/36	34/29	106/86	75/64*	C	38/31*	—
Eide et al. (1979)	7/7	40/36	109/89	73/74	F	38/46	32/45
Eng, Huber-Smith and McCann (1980)	20/17	47/34	114/90	85/—	C	50/30*	26/18
Esler et al. (1977)	21/11	—	—	—	F	66/69	38/43
Franco-Morselli, Baudouin-Legros and Meyer (1978)	27/12	—	104/87	80/70*	C	87/45*	87/58
Franco-Morselli et al. (1977)	19/11	43/45	116/90	82/71*	C	83/41*	34/18
Fujiki and Tsutsumi (1980)	56/33	53/47	—	—	C	42/37	28/21
Henquet et al. (1981)	25/25	35/35	108/89	73/63*	C	70/90	101/146
Hjemdahl and Eliasson (1978)	7/7	40/40	101/87	72/74	H	123/68	—
Ibsen et al. (1980)	33/31	—	115/91	72/64*	C	30/40	—
Kjedlsen et al. (1981)	20/19	51/52	135/99	—	C	70/35*	25/175
Meier et al. (1981)	24/22	35/37	106/88	65/63	C	43/29*	20/19
Messerli et al. (1981)	72/38	—	94/86	70/68	C	71/80	185/89
Millar et al. (1981)	8/14	—	—	—	C	26/40	21/28
Miura and De Quattro (1975)	34/25	—	142/97	—	C	67/58	52/28
Pedersen and Christiansen (1975)	19/32	41/40	101/86	—	C	34/47	—
Robertson et al. (1979)	9/10	25/27	116/90	69/63*	C	51/36*	24/20
Schiffl et al. (1981)	39/37	42/40	134/110	—	C	45/32*	24/17
Skrabal et al. (1981)	69/19	38/40	119/92	76/74	C	44/37	47/30
Vlachakis (1979)	38/14	48/49	—	—	C	47/40	20/19
Vlachakis and Aledort (1979)	22/13	50/44	—	—	C	45/35	32/10
Vlachakis and Mendelowitz (1980)	60/23	48/46	116/88	—	C	49/40	29/23
Weidmann et al. (1978)	79/90	46/37	123/89	—	C	58/62	69/62

* Statistically significant hypertensive–normotensive difference in heart rate or epinephrine, with $P < 0.05$.
C = COMT radioenzymatic; P = PNMT radioenzymatic; H = HPLC; F = fluorimetric.

studies, no mention was made of the matching of the control subjects, and experience of the early studies of plasma norepinephrine in hypertension showed that controls were often chosen from laboratory personnel unless specifically stated otherwise. Such controls are much less likely to be stressed by blood sampling and participation in an experiment, often being accustomed to the procedures. Several other investigators have not observed any difference in plasma epinephrine between hypertensives and controls. As already discussed, such disagreement is not surprising, and little attention can be paid to either positive or negative results. The present position is summarized in *Table 2.1*, reproduced from Goldstein's latest analysis.

Urine epinephrine in hypertension

There have been fewer studies of this than of plasma epinephrine, at least since the advent of radioenzymatic assay. In some ways this is a little surprising since the concentration of epinephrine in urine is much higher than in plasma; and although urine samples require to be diluted approximately 50-fold before radioenzymatic assay, there are rarely any problems of sensitivity with the assay. (One potential problem, however, with the urine assay is interference from the large amount of dopamine; this is around 2% and may give rise to slight overestimates of urine epinephrine excretion values unless a correction for the interference is applied.) In a small study comparing ten hypertensive and normotensive patients, Christensen observed no difference in epinephrine excretion (Pedersen and Christensen, 1975). In another study he described a group of hypertensive patients with borderline hypertension and some of the clinical features of paroxysmal catecholamine excess reminiscent of phaeochromocytoma, in whom there was marked elevation of epinephrine excretion (Christensen, 1977). Smith and Bing (1982) also have described a group of hypertensives with elevated epinephrine excretion (92 ± 33 versus 66 ± 27 nmol/24 hr); in this study the authors proposed that their 'hyperadrenergic' group may represent an early stage of patients with sustained hypertension.

As I mentioned earlier, it at last appears likely that the controversy will be resolved under the auspices of the current MRC trial for mild blood pressure, the machinery of which is being used to mount a large-scale study of catecholamine excretion in hypertension.

What if this study proves negative – will this disprove the hypothesis? It may be argued theoretically that the population which should be studied is not one with established hypertension but patients likely to develop hypertension – either first degree offspring of hypertensives or adolescents tracking in the highest blood pressure percentiles. In practice, clinical research is the art of the possible, and prospective studies conducted over the decades required for the development of hypertension are a hurdle unlikely to be attempted until a hypothesis has already acquired a high degree of probability. I doubt whether the epinephrine hypothesis (or probably any other hypothesis which implicates sympathetic activity in the pathogenesis of hypertension) could survive a totally negative set of results in the current MRC-based study.

Epinephrine as agonist at presynaptic β-receptors

The evidence for this second limb of the hypothesis is, or will be, of a rather different nature from that for the first limb. The theory of presynaptic receptors (sceptics would say presynaptic receptors themselves) is the creation of pharmacologists; and it is they who have reported experiments such as those described at the beginning of this chapter in support of the theory. In the models of the pharmacologists there is no doubt that epinephrine can facilitate nor-epinephrine release from sympathetic nerve endings during sympathetic nerve firing. For the purposes of the epinephrine hypothesis of hypertension it is not critical what the mechanism of this facilitation is, although, of course, a full explanation of the pathogenesis of hypertension will require to explain each step in the process. However, more contentious than the question of whether presynaptic receptors exist and perform the role ascribed to them is the problem of demonstrating that in whole animals, and in particular man, epinephrine secretion leads to a facilitation of norepinephrine release. Again, it is not critical for the epinephrine hypothesis of hypertension that such facilitation works through presynaptic receptors. However, the assumption that this is the mechanism of epinephrine-induced facilitation of norepinephrine release has, as will become clear, proven an advantage rather than a hindrance in obtaining evidence of this facilitation in man.

   Superficially, it might seem a simple matter to infuse epinephrine and determine whether this causes an increase in plasma norepinephrine concentration, but in practice no such increase occurs; and, if it did, it could not be ascribed with certainty to presynaptic receptor facilitation rather than a baroreceptor response to the fall in mean arterial pressure observed during adrenaline infusion in man. The reader will recall that one of the reasons for the previous lack of interest in epinephrine as a possible cause of hypertension is the fact that infusion of epinephrine has a depressor effect when mean arterial pressure is considered. In studies performed in our department, this problem has been circumvented in two ways. In man, we have concentrated on the haemodynamic and biochemical changes persisting *after* the infusion of epinephrine. Epinephrine has a very short half-life in plasma of around one minute, so most long-lasting effects are unlikely to be due to stimulation of receptors by circulating epinephrine, but may be due to re-release of epinephrine into the synaptic cleft following uptake into sympathetic nerve endings during its infusion. Early in our studies we obtained evidence that this postulated neurotransmitter action of epinephrine might indeed occur in man when we found that a 2-hour infusion of epinephrine at $0.1\,\mu g/kg/min$ caused a tachycardia of approximately 25 beats/min which declined only slowly over the subsequent 2½ hours, although plasma epinephrine concentration returned to normal within a few minutes of the end of the infusion (*Figure 2.2*) (Brown and Macquin, 1982). This persistence of the tachycardia was reduced or abolished if subjects were pretreated with desmethylimipramine 50 mg daily for 1 week to inhibit the uptake of epinephrine into sympathetic nerve endings during its infusion (*Figure 2.3*). Recently we have shown that an infusion of isoprenaline at $0.02\,\mu g/kg/min$ caused a similar tachycardia as the epinephrine during its infusion

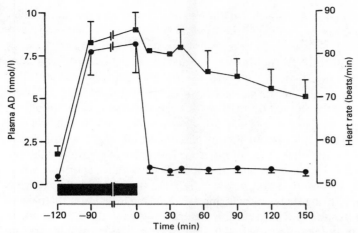

Figure 2.2 Heart rate and plasma epinephrine concentration during and after epinephrine infusion. Epinephrine was infused at 0.1 μg/kg/min for 2 hours (▬◀▮▶▬) in six healthy volunteers. Heart rate (■——■) and plasma epinephrine (●——●) were measured during and for 2½ hours after the infusion

but this tachycardia disappeared within 15–30 min of terminating the infusion (Brown, Brown and Murphy, 1983). Isoprenaline is not a substrate for the neuronal uptake pump so that this difference after the infusions of epinephrine and isoprenaline seemed to confirm that the tachycardia after epinephrine infusion requires its accumulation within sympathetic nerve endings.

This is not the forum to enter a lengthy discussion on the problems of using plasma norepinephrine concentration as an index of its release from sympathetic nerve endings. As already mentioned in this chapter, norepinephrine is a neurotransmitter, not a hormone, and there are no feedback mechanisms controlling its plasma concentration (Silverberg *et al.*, 1978). Only a small,

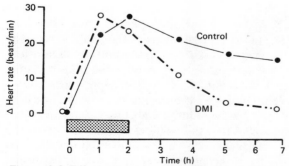

Figure 2.3 Effect of neuronal uptake blockade on post-epinephrine tachycardia. Three normal volunteers were infused with epinephrine 0.025 μg/kg/min or 0.05 μg/kg/min for 2 hours (▦) after receiving desmethylimipramine (DMI) 50 mg daily for 1 week. The change in heart rate during and after infusion (○–· ·–○) is compared with control values (●——●) observed in the same subjects when infused with epinephrine 0.1 μg/kg/min *without* desmethylimipramine pretreatment

undetermined, and probably variable percentage of norepinephrine spills over from synaptic clefts into plasma and the resulting level of circulating norepinephrine is determined not only by this spillover rate but also by the rate of clearance of norepinephrine from the circulation. This rate of clearance approximates to cardiac output and is very sensitive to any factors which modulate cardiac output – for instance, in the present context, epinephrine. It has long seemed to us a possibility that the failure to observe a rise in plasma norepinephrine concentration during epinephrine infusion is due to a simultaneous rise in norepinephrine clearance. Measurement of norepinephrine clearance in man is not usually possible if arterial blood sampling and infusion of tritium labelled norepinephrine are regarded as ethically unjustified. Such an experiment has, however, been recently reported in rabbits by Majewski, who showed that there is an increase in norepinephrine release rate during epinephrine infusion if the plasma norepinephrine concentration is corrected for the epinephrine-induced increase in norepinephrine clearance (Majewski, Hedler and Starke, 1982). While arterial measurements are essential for measuring norepinephrine clearance (otherwise one is measuring mainly clearance of norepinephrine by the limb whose venous drainage is used for sampling (Brown *et al.*, 1981a)), it remains an unresolved issue how reliable venous norepinephrine measurements are even as crude measures of sympathetic activity. As I have already said, the clearance of catecholamines is of the order of cardiac output, with most catecholamines being extracted during one passage through the circulation, so that the risk exists that venous values may reflect mainly local rather than systemic changes in sympathetic nervous activity. In the dog we have found that infusion of epinephrine causes an increase in arterial but not venous norepinephrine concentration. We attempted to circumvent the problem of obtaining arterial samples in our volunteers by using arterialized venous samples but were still unable to detect an increase in norepinephrine concentration during epinephrine infusions.

Almost by chance, however, we discovered the likely explanation for the constancy of norepinephrine values during adrenaline infusion. We were investigating the mechanism of epinephrine-induced hypokalaemia using a selective β_2-antagonist, ICI 118551. We noted that plasma norepinephrine concentration fell during the infusion of epinephrine in subjects who had received this drug, and remained low for some 30 minutes after termination of the infusion. The fall in plasma norepinephrine concentration during adrenaline infusion could have been baroreceptor-induced since the β-antagonist converts epinephrine into a pressor agent, and heart rate also fell. However, after termination of the infusion, there was an immediate reversal of this bradycardia, possibly signifying an end of baroreceptor activation, and we suspected that the persistent reduction in plasma norepinephrine concentration was therefore due to unopposed stimulation by epinephrine of the inhibitory presynaptic α-receptors (Brown, Brown and Murphy, 1983). About this time, Rand published a paper showing that in the isolated heart stimulation of the facilitatory presynaptic β-receptor can be masked by simultaneous and opposing stimulation of the inhibitory presynaptic α-receptor (Majewsky and Rand, 1981). Addition of the α-blocking drug phentolamine then unmasks or enhances the facilitatory β-receptor stimulation. We have, therefore, repeated epinephrine infusions in six subjects who were pretreated with either placebo or a selective α_2-receptor antagonist, RX 781094. This study has only recently been completed. In six subjects the α_2-receptor antagonist unmasked an increase in plasma norepinephrine concentration during epinephrine infusion. Furthermore, this increase declines only slowly after termination of the infusion in parallel with the offset of the tachycardia whereas, as usual, the plasma epinephrine concentration falls within seconds (*Figure 2.4*). So these results, if confirmed, are

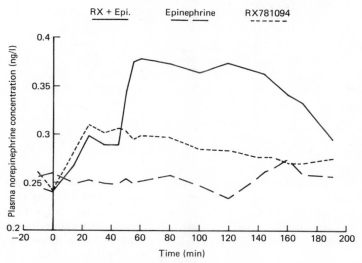

Figure 2.4 Effect of epinephrine on plasma norepinephrine concentration. Six normal volunteers were infused with epinephrine for 95 min 45 min after receiving intravenously either RX 781094 (an α_2-receptor antagonist) 0.2 mg/kg (——) or vehicle (— —). The dose of epinephrine was initially increased at 5 min intervals from 0.025 to 0.075 μg/kg/min, and thereafter infused at 0.05 μg/kg/min. On a third occasion, subjects received a vehicle infusion alone 45 min after intravenous administration of RX 781094 (---). The RX 781094 (or vehicle) was given at time zero

consistent with the hypothesis that the persistent tachycardia after epinephrine infusion is due to accumulation of epinephrine within nerve endings during its infusion and subsequent behaviour as a co-transmitter to facilitate increase of norepinephrine from the nerve endings. This facilitation continues as long as there is an increased amount of epinephrine within the nerve endings even when there is no longer any detectable increase in circulating epinephrine concentration.

The final way in which we have attempted to test this hypothesis *in vivo* was the infusion of epinephrine in subjects who had previously received α-methylparatyrosine. This pharmacological agent inhibits the synthesis of nor-epinephrine, leading to a depletion of norepinephrine stores in both sympathetic nerve endings and in the brain, although the drug therefore has marked central side-effects such as sedation and sometimes depression. Only the peripheral effects of the drug would alter responses to epinephrine infusion since epinephrine itself does not cross the blood–brain barrier. We predicted that if the persistent tachycardia after adrenaline infusion leads to presynaptic stimulation, then the tachycardia would be dependent upon the presence of normal stores of endogenous norepinephrine and would therefore be abolished or inhibited by α-methylparatyrosine. In a pilot experiment in the dog, this inhibition was indeed achieved following a dose of 40 mg/kg/day for 48 hours (*Figure 2.5*). However, in the volunteers, central side-effects limited the dose to less than half that used in the dog – with a similar reduction in the number of volunteers. For one or both reasons we failed to observe any significant effect of the drug in man.

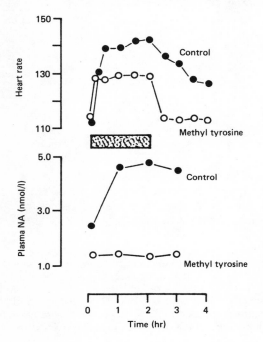

Figure 2.5 Effect of α-methyl-*p*-tyrosine (αMPT) on epinephrine induced tachycardia in the dog. Two dogs received epinephrine 0.1 μg/kg/min for 2 hours ( ) on a control occasion and after oral treatment with αMPT 40 mg/kg b.d. for 48 hours. Heart rate and arterial plasma norepinephrine concentration were measured during and after the infusion

Does a sustained increase in sympathetic activity cause hypertension?

We move on now to consider this last proposition of the hypothesis. On the face of it, this may seem the least contentious of the propositions, or at least the most self-evident. Despite this, the existing evidence is mainly indirect and it would be difficult to reproduce a controlled chronic increase in sympathetic activity. The evidence that a chronic increase in norepinephrine release will elevate blood pressure is of two forms. The first is patients with phaeochromocytoma in whom excessive release of norepinephrine causes prolonged hypertension. The second form of evidence is almost the reverse of this; namely the efficacy of a variety of sympatholytic drugs in the long-term treatment of hypertension. I shall consider each of these forms in turn.

A phaeochromocytoma differs from the possible situation in essential hypertension in that norepinephrine is released directly into the vasculature as a circulating hormone and is secreted by an autonomously functioning gland that has lost most of the mechanisms controlling synthesis and release. The direct release into plasma of the norepinephrine is part of the reason why the ratio of plasma norepinephrine concentration to blood pressure is much higher in phaeochromocytoma than in essential hypertension; in the former the concentration gradient for norepinephrine is downhill from plasma to synaptic cleft, whereas in the latter the reverse is the case, and we just do not know whether the synaptic cleft concentration of norepinephrine in vascular smooth muscle is as high in essential hypertension as the plasma concentration is in phaeochromocytoma. But there are two arguments against this possibility. The first is that patients with phaeochromocytoma are much more susceptible to antihypertensive treatment by α-receptor blockade than patients with essential hypertension. The second argument is that patients with phaeochromocytoma appear to have down-regulated α-receptors as judged by their reduced pressor response to infused norepinephrine, whereas, if anything, the opposite is true of patients with essential hypertension (Kiowski *et al.*, 1981; Philipp, Distler and Cordes, 1978). This suggests that α-receptor stimulation by excessive release of norepinephrine is less important in the genesis of essential hypertension than of phaeochromocytoma. The objection that sympathetic nervous release of norepinephrine is subject to feedback control, whereas phaeochromocytoma release is not, is perhaps less damaging to the epinephrine hypothesis than other explanations of elevated sympathetic activity, for stimulation of the positive feedback loop may result in increased release of norepinephrine precisely because it competes with opposing negative feedback loops.

The evidence from the efficacy of sympatholytic treatment, in particular clonidine-like drugs, which cause a marked reduction in plasma norepinephrine concentration, also has limitations. Firstly, clonidine reduces blood pressure even in normotensive volunteers; the fall in blood pressure is usually greater after acute administration to hypertensives but this is a general property of most such drugs. Secondly, clonidine lowers blood pressure in phaeochromocytoma patients in whom it does not lower plasma norepinephrine concentration (Bravo *et al.*, 1981). Whatever the explanation for this finding may be (and I suspect that the partial agonist clonidine behaves as an α-receptor antagonist in phaeochromocytoma patients), it demonstrates the caution required before drawing conclusions about the mechanism of a form of hypertension from the pharmacology of the drug shown to be effective in treatment.

The foregoing, fairly negative, critique can, however, be balanced in this section by the most positive evidence in favour of the hypothesis. This is the demonstration by Rand's group that the infusion of low doses of epinephrine to achieve an approximate doubling of plasma epinephrine concentration causes a sustained increase in blood pressure in rats, which persists for a number of weeks after termination of the infusion (Majewski, Tung and Rand, 1981). The data is certainly impressive and consistent with the explanation that the epinephrine infused is sufficient to increase the concentration of epinephrine in sympathetic neurones to a level that activates the positive feedback loop. However, infusions of slightly higher doses of epinephrine in rats did not cause a sustained hypertension and this contrasted with their experience of low-dose angiotensin infusion (Brown *et al.*, 1981b; Brown, Clark and Lever, 1983). There were some differences in the technique employed by the two groups which at the moment is the only explanation of the discrepancy between their results. In man it would, of course, be difficult to study the effects of a long-term increase in circulation epinephrine levels, whether of endogenous or exogenous origin. One interesting possibility, however, is patients with small adrenal phaeochromocytomas, which are diagnosed and removed at a stage when they are secreting solely or mainly epinephrine (Brown *et al.*, 1981a). Most phaeochromocytomas are not a good model for testing the hypothesis because they secrete norepinephrine as well as epinephrine, usually in larger amounts. However, there is no doubt that after removal of most phaeochromocytomas there is an almost complete return of blood pressure to normotensive levels, but in 25% of patients there is some residual hypertension requiring treatment. It may be of interest to determine whether either the absolute or relative amount of epinephrine secretion by tumours at the time of their diagnosis can be correlated with the persistence of hypertension after their removal.

Further tests for the hypothesis

The ultimate test for the hypothesis is to demonstrate that the onset of hypertension can be prevented by physically interfering with an early point in the proposed chain of events. What is required in fact is the ability to reduce either secretion of epinephrine from the adrenal medulla, or its subsequent stimulation of the presynaptic β-receptor to activate the positive feedback loop. Other steps in the chain, such as the uptake of epinephrine into sympathetic nerve endings, could not be inhibited without also affecting what happens to norepinephrine. At present no suitable drug exists but the possibilities seem to be either a selective inhibitor of epinephrine synthesis in the adrenal medulla or a β-receptor antagonist, which is selective for the presynaptic β-receptor. An inhibitor of phenylethanolamine methyl transferase (PNMT) has been developed which does not cross the blood–brain barrier and so affects only adrenal PNMT activity (Pendleton *et al.*, 1982). Unfortunately, the reduction in epinephrine secretion, both basal and stimulated, appears to be small, even at high doses of the drug, so that a future development is still awaited. A selective presynaptic β-receptor antagonist is even further in the future and, of course, begs the question of whether the presynaptic β-receptor, assuming it does exist at all, is different from all other β-receptors. One exciting possible approach to both this latter question and to the role of the receptor in hypertension is the development of specific β-receptor antibodies, which are highly specific for β-receptor subtypes; these have been developed by immunologists using the technique either of monoclonal antibodies or that of anti-idiotypic antibodies. In the latter, the receptor molecule is mimicked by raising an antibody to a β-receptor antagonist. This first antibody (the idiotype) is then used to raise a further anti-idiotypic antibody, and affinity chromatography is used to prise apart antibodies with selectivity for the varying receptor subtypes (Fraser and Venter, 1980; Homcy, Rockson and Haber, 1982; *Lancet* Editorial, 1982).

Even if such specific drugs or probes do become available, the question arises whether they could feasibly be given for long periods of time to subjects at risk of developing hypertension and how such subjects may be identified. Again, I do not regard this as an insuperable problem and studies have already been undertaken in children to determine whether treatment of those tracking in the upper decile of blood pressure is effective in delaying the onset of hypertension. As I said earlier in the chapter, however, it would be improper to study such subjects until or unless the epinephrine hypothesis is on a more solid footing than at present. Another short-term approach to the question may be to use specific probes (such as PNMT inhibitors or presynaptic β-receptor antibodies) in patients with established hypertension from whom antihypertensive treatment is withdrawn. There is surprisingly little data on the natural history of treated hypertension. In some patients on some treatments cessation of therapy leads to an immediate rebound of blood pressure to pretreatment values; in others, blood pressure appears to stay low for long periods of time. It is weeks or months before pretreatment values are regained. Only exceptionally does hypertension disappear; even then one must be certain that either the disappearance was not caused by a myocardial infarction or that the original hypertension had a transient secondary cause such as acute nephritis. But it would certainly be possible to identify some patients in whom antihypertensive therapy can be safely withdrawn for some months, during which the effect of the specific probes could be studied.

One issue which I have so far avoided is the cause of elevated epinephrine secretion in hypertension. I think that it is not too sophistic to regard this question as standing apart from the other questions already considered as comprising the package; in other words the hypothesis could be established as showing both that epinephrine can cause hypertension and that epinephrine secretion is increased in hypertensives, even if the explanation of such an increase were not forthcoming. However, there seem to be three separate possibilities worth considering. The simplest is that the increased secretion occurs intermittently in response to 'stress'. One of the things which has become clear since the advent of radioenzymatic assays for plasma catecholamines is that it is epinephrine rather than norepinephrine which is released when patients are anxious or frightened. A good example of this is the increase in plasma epinephrine noted in medical personnel making presentations in public (Dimsdale and Moss, 1980). We have also noted that patients undergoing invasive procedures often have plasma epinephrine concentrations well into the phaeochromocytoma range (*Figure 2.6*).

On the other hand, it is possible that increased release of epinephrine in hypertension has nothing to do with response to stress, and one intriguing, albeit highly speculative, notion is that hypertensives secrete an increased proportion of epinephrine relative to norepinephrine from the adrenal medulla. The synthesis of epinephrine from norepinephrine is catalyzed by the enzyme PNMT as has already been mentioned in this chapter. This enzyme is interesting in that it is induced by high concentrations of glucocorticoids and the reason for the selective origin of epinephrine from the adrenal medulla and not other chromaffin ganglia is the portocapillary circulation in the adrenal gland, which drains from cortex to medulla, so bathing the cells which synthesize epinephrine in high local

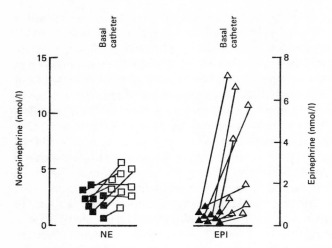

Figure 2.6 Effect of fright on plasma catecholamines. Plasma norepinephrine (NE) and epinephrine (EPI) were measured in nine patients prior to ('basal') and during cardiac catheterization

concentrations of cortisol (Wurtman and Axelrod, 1966). (The major clue to the presence of a tumour in the adrenal gland when adrenal vein sampling is performed in search of a phaeochromocytoma is not the absolute concentration of catecholamines which depends on the adrenal blood flow, but the reversal of the normally predominant ratio of epinephrine to norepinephrine, this reversal being caused by the tumour's disruption of the porto-capillary circulation) (Brown *et al.*, 1981a, 1981c). So in theory the genetic control of PNMT synthesis would offer one explanation of familial trends in hypertension. No evidence exists that an increased proportion of epinephrine is secreted from the adrenal glands of hypertensives, but the proportion of epinephrine in adrenal effluent is certainly variable, between approximately 4:1 and 12:1.

CONCLUSION

Onlookers must sometimes wonder from the large variety of hypotheses to explain hypertension whether any serious progress occurs towards unravelling the problem, and each protagonist, especially of an endocrine cause, seems to favour whichever mediator he is able to measure. I do not believe that it is necessary to be so pessimistic, even without falling back on the excuse that hypertension is likely to be multifactorial. Although there may be as yet some undiscovered pressor agent, it seems unlikely by now that hypertension will prove to be a simple endocrine disease in the way that thyrotoxicosis or Cushing's syndrome can be ascribed solely to high circulating levels of a particular hormone. If the explanation is endocrine, it will be in a more convoluted fashion and it is proper for each endocrine protagonist to explore all the possible roles played by their hormone and use the methodology available to them. Scientific research flourishes when it is designed to investigate a specific hypothesis and so it is both inevitable and healthy that the mutually contradictory hypotheses presented in this book are proposed and investigated. That will not stop me from finishing with a plug for my own hormone, epinephrine. I started this chapter by saying that epinephrine had for long been the Cinderella of hormones; I would finish by suggesting that precisely because of this it may turn out to be a better horse to back than some of its usually more favoured colleagues. Epinephrine is not a hormone essential for life and its plasma concentration may vary several hundred-fold without causing an immediate risk of life. Cinderella left free to look after herself may have given the slip to her more dazzling but chaperoned sisters.

References

ADLER-GRASCHINSKY, E. and LANGER, S. Z. (1975) Possible role of a β-receptor in the regulation of noradrenaline release by nerve stimulation through a feedback mechanism. *British Journal of Pharmacology*, **53**, 43–50

AMANN, F. W., BOLLI, P. B., KIOWSKI, W. and BUHLER, F. R. (1981) Enhanced α-adrenoreceptor-mediated vasoconstriction in essential hypertension. *Hypertension*, **3** (Suppl. 1), 1–19

BERETTA-PICCOLI, C., WEIDMANN, P., KEUSCH, G. et al. (1980a) Renin-hyporesponsiveness in essential hypertension color dissociation between plasma renin and catecholamines or aldosterone following furosemide. *Klinische Wochenschrift*, **58**, 457–466

BERETTA-PICCOLI, C., WEIDMANN, P., MEIR, A., GRIMM, M., KEUSCH, G. and GLUCK, Z. (1980b) Effects of short-term norepinephrine infusion on plasma catecholamines, renin and aldosterone in normal and hypertensive man. *Hypertension*, **2**, 623–630

BERTEL, O., BUHLER, F. R., KIOWSKI, W. and LUTOLD, B. (1980) Decreased β-receptor responsiveness as related to age, blood pressure and plasma catecholamines in patients with essential hypertension. *Hypertension*, **2**, 130–138

BOLLI, P., AMANN, F. W., HULTHEN, L., KIOWSKI, W. and BUHLER, F. R. (1981) Elevated plasma adrenaline reflects sympathetic overactivity and enhanced α-adrenoceptor-mediated vasoconstriction in essential hypertension. *Clinical Science*, **61**, 161S–164S

BORN, G. V. R. and SMITH, J. B. (1970) Uptake, metabolism and release of tritiated adrenaline by human platelets. *British Journal of Pharmacology*, **39**, 765–768

BRAVO, E. L., TARAZI, R. C., FOUAD, F. M., VIDT, D. G. and GIFFORD, R. W. (1981) Clonidine suppression test: a useful aid in the diagnosis of phaeochromocytoma. *New England Journal of Medicine*, **305**, 623–626

BROWN, M. J. and JENNER, D. A. (1981) A novel double-isotope technique for the enzymatic assay of plasma catecholamines, permitting high precision, sensitivity and sample capacity. *Clinical Science*, **61**, 591–598

BROWN, M. J. and MACQUIN, I. (1981) Is adrenaline the cause of essential hypertension? *Lancet*, **2**, 1079–1082

BROWN, M. J. and MACQUIN, I. (1982) Catecholamine neurotransmitters and the heart. *Acta Medica Scandinavica, Suppl.* **660,** 43–39

BROWN, A. J., CLARK, S. A. and LEVER, A. F. (1983) Slow rise and diurnal change of blood pressure with saralasin and angiotensin II in rats. *American Journal of Physiology,* **244,** F84–F88

BROWN, M. J., BROWN, D. C. and MURPHY, M. B. (1983) Adrenaline associated hypokalaemia and tachycardia are selectively antagonised by low dose β$_2$-receptor blockade in man. *Clinical Science,* **64,** 71P

BROWN, M. J., ALLISON, D. J., JENNER, D. A., LEWIS, P. J. and DOLLERY, C. T. (1981a) Increased sensitivity and accuracy of phaeochromocytoma diagnosis achieved by use of plasma adrenaline estimations and a pentolinium suppression test. *Lancet,* **1,** 174–177

BROWN, A. J., CASALS-STENZEL, J., GOFFORD, S., LEVER, A. F. and MORTON, J. J. (1981b) Comparison of fast and slow pressor effects of angiotensin II in the conscious rat. *American Journal of Physiology,* **241,** H381–H388

BROWN, M. J., JENNER, D. A., ALLISON, D. J. and DOLLERY, C. T. (1981c) Variations in individual organ release of noradrenaline measured by an improved radio-enzymatic technique; limitations of peripheral venous measurements in the assessment of sympathetic nervous activity. *Clinical Science,* **61,** 585–590

BUHLER, F. R., KIOWSKI, W., VAN BRUMMELEN, P. *et al.* (1980) Plasma catecholamines and cardiac, renal and peripheral vascular adrenoceptor-mediated responses in different age groups of normal and hypertensive subjects. *Clinical and Experimental Hypertension,* **2,** 409–426

CAUSON, R. C., BROWN, M. J., BOULOUX, P. M. and PERRET, D. (1983) Analytical differences in measurement of plasma catecholamines. *Clinical Chemistry,* **29,** 735–737

CHRISTENSEN, N. J. (1977) Increased excretion of adrenaline in the urine in patients with labile hypertension and episodic tachycardia. *Ugeskrift for Laeger,* **139,** 2938–2940

CLUTTER, W. E., BIER, D. M., SHAH, S. D. and CRYER, P. E. (1980) Epinephrine plasma metabolic clearance rates and physiological thresholds for metabolic and haemodynamic actions in man. *Journal of Clinical Investigation,* **66,** 94–101

COREA, L., MIELE, N., BENTIVOGLIO, M., BOSCHETTI, E., AGABITI-ROSEI, E. and MUIESAN, G. (1979) Acute and chronic effects of nifedipine on plasma renin activity and plasma adrenaline and noradrenaline in controls and hypertensive patients. *Clinical Science,* **57,** 115S–117S

COUSINEAU, C., DECHAMPLAIN, J. and LAPOINTE, L. (1978) Circulating catecholamines and systolic time intervals in labile and sustained hypertension. *Clinical Science,* **55,** 65S–67S

CUCHE, J. L., KUCHEL, O., BARBEAU, A., LANGLOIS, Y., BOUCHER, R. and GENEST, J. (1974) Autonomic nervous system and benign essential hypertension. *Circulation Research,* **35,** 281–289

DA PRADA, M. and PICOTTI, G. B. (1979) Content and subcellular localisation of catecholamines and 5HT in human and animal blood platelets. *British Journal of Pharmacology,* **65,** 653–662

DA PRADA, M. and ZURCHER, G. (1976) Simultaneous radioenzymatic determination of plasma and tissue adrenaline, noradrenaline and dopamine within the femtomole range. *Life Sciences*, **19**, 1161–1174

DAHLOF, C. (1981) Studies on β-adrenoceptor-mediated facilitation of sympathetic neurotransmission. *Acta Physiologica Scandinavica*, **500**, 1–147

DE CHAMPLAIN, J., NADEAU, R. A., LAVALLEE, M. and DENIS, G. (1981) Autonomic dysfunctions in human hypertension. *Hypertension*, **3**, 124

DE QUATTRO, V. and CHAN, S. (1972) Raised catecholamines in some patients with primary hypertension. *Lancet*, **1**, 806–809

DIMSDALE, J. E. and MOSS, J. (1980) Short-term catecholamine response to psychological stress. *Psychosomatic Medicine*, **42**, 493–497

EIDE, I., KOLLOCH, R., DE QUATTRO, V., MIANO, L., DUGGER, R. and VAN DER MUELEN, J. (1979) Raised cerebrospinal fluid norepinephrine in some patients with primary hypertension. *Hypertension*, **1**, 225

ENG, F. W. H. T., HUBER-SMITH, M. and MC CANN, D. S. (1980) The role of sympathetic activity in normal renin essential hypertension. *Hypertension*, **2**, 14–19

ENGELMAN, K., PORTNOY, B. and LOVENBERG, W. (1968) A sensitive and specific double-isotope derivative method for the determination of catecholamine in biological specimens. *American Journal of Medical Science*, **255**, 259–268

ESLER, M., ZWEIFLER, A., RANDALL, O., JULIUS, S. and DE QUATTRO, V. (1977) Agreement among three different indices of sympathetic nervous system activity in essential hypertension. *Mayo Clinic Proceedings*, **52**, 379–382

FITZGERALD, G. A., BARNES, P., HAMILTON, C. A. and DOLLERY, C. T. (1980) The concentration-effect relationships and kinetics of adrenaline in man. *European Journal of Clinical Investigation*, **10**, 401–406

FRANCO-MORSELLI, R., BAUDOUIN-LEGROS, M. and MEYER, P. (1978) Plasma adrenaline and noradrenaline in essential hypertension and after long-term treatment with β-adrenoreceptor-blocking agents. *Clinical Science*, **55**, 97S–100S

FRANCO-MORSELLI, R., ELGHOZI, J. L., JOLY, D., DIGIULIO, S. and MEYER, P. (1977) Increased plasma adrenaline concentrations in benign essential hypertension. *British Medical Journal*, **2**, 1251–1254

FRASER, C. M. and VENTER, J. C. (1980) Monoclonal antibodies to β-receptors. *Proceedings of the National Academy of Sciences of the USA*, **77**, 7034–7038

FUJIKI, H. and TSUTSUMI, E. (1980) Plasma catecholamines and serum dopamine β-hydroxylase activity in essential hypertension. Relation to age and plasma renin activity. *Kumamoto Medical Journal*, **33**, 1

GOLDSTEIN, D. S. (1981) Plasma norepinephrine in essential hypertension. A study of the studies. *Hypertension*, **3**, 48–52

GOLDSTEIN, D. S. (1983) Plasma catecholamines and essential hypertension. An analytical review. *Hypertension*, **5**, 86–99

HENQUET, J. W., KHO, T., SHOLS, M., THIKSSEN, H. and RAHN, K. H. (1981) The sympathetic nervous system and the renin–angiotensin system in borderline hypertension. *Clinical Science*, **60**, 25–31

HJEMDAHL, P. and ELIASSON, K. (1979) Sympatho-adrenal and cardiovascular response to mental stress and orthostatic provocation in latent hypertension. *Clinical Science*, **57**, 189S–191S

HOMCY, C. J., ROCKSON, S. G. and HABER, E. (1982) An anti-idiotypic antibody that recognises the β-adrenergic receptor. *Journal of Clinical Investigation*, **69**, 1147–1154

IBSEN, H., CHRISTENSEN, N. J., HOLLNAGEL, H., LETH, A., KAPPELGAARD, A. M. and GIESE, J. (1980) Plasma noradrenaline concentration in hypertensive and normotensive forty-year-old individuals: relationship to plasma renin concentration. *Scandinavian Journal of Clinical Laboratory Investigation*, **40**, 333–339

JULIUS, S. and CONWAY, J. (1968) Haemodynamic studies in patients,with borderline blood pressure elevation. *Circulation*, **38**, 282

KIOWSKI, W., BUHLER, F. R., VAN BRUMMELEN, P. and AMMAN, F. W. (1981) Plasma noradrenaline concentration and α-adrenoceptor-mediated vasoconstriction in normotensive and hypertensive man. *Clinical Science*, **60**, 483–489

KJELDSEN, S. E., FLAATEN, B., EIDE, I., HELGELAND, A. and LEREN, P. (1981) Increased peripheral release of noradrenaline and uptake of adrenaline in essential hypertension. *Clinical Science*, **61**, 215S–217S

LAKE, C. R., ZIEGLER, M. G., COLEMAN, M. D. and KOPIN, I. J. (1977) Age-adjusted plasma norepinephrine levels are similar in normotensive and hypertensive subjects. *New England Journal of Medicine*, **296**, 208–209

LANCET Editorial (1982) Stress, hypertension and the heart: the adrenal trilogy. *Lancet*, **2**, 1440–1441

LANGER, S. Z. (1981) Presynaptic regulation of the release of catecholamines. *Pharmacological Reviews*, **32**, 37–362

MAJEWSKI, H., HEDLER, L. and STARKE, K. (1982) Noradrenaline release rate in the anaesthetised rabbit. Facilitation by adrenaline. *Naunyn Schmiedeberg's Archives of Pharmacology*, **321**, 20–27

MAJEWSKI, H., RAND, M. J. and TUNG, L.-H. (1981) Activation of prejunctional beta-adrenoceptors in rat atria by adrenaline applied exogenously or released as a co-transmitter. *British Journal of Pharmacology*, **73**, 669–679

MAJEWSKI, H., TUNG, L.-H. and RAND, M. J. (1981) Adrenaline induced hypertension in rats. *Journal of Cardiovascular Pharmacology*, **3**, 179–185

MAJEWSKI, H. and RAND, M. J. (1981) An interaction between prejunctional α-adrenoceptors and prejunctional β-adrenoceptors. *European Journal of Pharmacology*, **69**, 439–498

MEIER, A., WEIDMANN, P., GRIMM, M. *et al.* (1981) Pressor factors and cardiovascular pressor responsiveness in borderline hypertension. *Hypertension*, **3**, 367–372

MESSERLI, F. H., FROHLICH, E. D., SUAREZ, D. H. *et al.* (1981) Borderline hypertension: relationship between age, hemodynamics and circulating catecholamines. *Circulation*, **64**, 760–764

MILLAR, J. A., MCGRATH, B. P., MATTHEWS, P. G. and JOHNSTON, C. I. (1981) Acute effects of captopril on blood pressure and circulating hormone levels in salt-replete and depleted normal subjects and essential hypertensive patients. *Clinical Science*, **61**, 75–83

MIURA, Y. and DE QUATTRO, V. (1975) Biochemical evaluation of sympathetic nerve tone in essential hypertension. *Japanese Circulation Journal*, **39**, 583–589

PEDERSEN, E. B. and CHRISTENSEN, N. J. (1975) Catecholamines in plasma and urine in patients with essential hypertension determined by double isotope derivative techniques. *Acta Medica Scandinavica*, **198**, 373–377

PENDLETON, R. G., GESSNER, G., SAWYER, J., HILLEGASS, L. and MILLER, D. A. (1982) Studies on the long term effects of SK&F 29661 upon adrenal catecholamines. *Naunyn Schmiedeberg's Archives of Pharmacology*, **319**, 22–28

PHILIPP, T., DISTLER, A. and CORDES, U. (1978) Sympathetic nervous system and blood pressure control in essential hypertension. *Lancet*, **2**, 959–963

ROBERTSON, D., SHAND, D. G., HOLLIFIELD, J. W., NIES, A. S., FROLICH, J. C. and OATES, J. A. (1979) Alterations in the responses of the sympathetic nervous system and renin in borderline hypertension. *Hypertension*, **1**, 118

SCHIFFL, H., WEIDMANN, P., MEIER, A. and ZIEGLER, W. H. (1981) Relationship between plasma catecholamines and urinary catecholamine excretion rates in normal subjects and certain diseased states. *Klinische Wochenschrift*, **59**, 837–844

SEVER, P. S., OSIKOWSKA, B., BIRCH, M. and TUNBRIGE, R. D. G. (1977) Plasma noradrenaline in essential hypertension. *Lancet*, **1**, 1078–1081

SILVERBERG, A. B., SHAH, S. D., HAYMOND, M. W. and CRYER, P. E. (1978) Norepinephrine: hormone and neurotransmitter in man. *American Journal of Physiology*, **243**, E252–E256

SKRABAL, F., AUBOCK, J., HORTNAGL, H. and BRUCKE, T. (1981) Plasma epinephrine and norepinephrine concentrations in primary and secondary human hypertension. *Hypertension*, **3**, 373–379

SMITH, A. J. and BING, R. F. (1982) Catecholamines in essential hypertension. *Lancet*, **1**, 112–113

STJARNE, L. and BRUNDIN, J. (1975) Dual adrenoceptor mediated control of noradrenaline secretion from human vasoconstrictor nerves. Facilitation by β-receptors and inhibition by α-receptors. *Acta Physiologica Scandinavica*, **94**, 139–141

VLACHAKIS, N. D. (1979) Blood pressure and catecholamine responses to sympathetic stimulation in normotensive and hypertensive subjects. *Journal of Clinical Pharmacology*, **19**, 458–466

VLACHAKIS, N. D. and ALEDORT, L. (1979) Platelet aggregation in relationship to plasma catecholamines in patients with hypertension. *Atherosclerosis*, **32**, 451–460

VLACHAKIS, N. D. and MENDOLOWITZ, M. (1980) Plasma catecholamines in primary hypertension. *Biochemical Medicine*, **23**, 35–46

WEIDMANN, P., BERETTA-PICCOLI, C., ZIEGLER, W. J., KEUSCH, G., GLUCK, Z. and REUBI, F. C. (1978) Age versus urinary sodium for judging renin aldosterone, and catecholamine levels: studies in normal subjects and patients with essential hypertension. *Kidney International*, **14**, 619–628

WURTMAN, R. J. and AXELROD, J. (1966) Control of enzymatic synthesis of adrenaline in the adrenal medulla by adrenal cortical steroids. *Journal of Biological Chemistry*, **241**, 2301–2305

NOTE: The results from the 2000 catecholamine estimations in the MRC Hypertension Trial are in press in my paper in the *Proceedings of the 9th International Congress of Pharmacology* (Macmillan, 1984).

3
Role of vasopressin in hypertension
Fernando Elijovich and Lawrence R. Krakoff

INTRODUCTION

Arginine vasopressin, a cyclic octapeptide synthesized in the hypothalamus and secreted by the posterior pituitary, is the antidiuretic hormone, the principal circulating factor responsible for conservation of water by the renal collecting ducts. Over the past decade this hormone has been implicated in a number of additional physiological effects occurring at several locations. These include such diverse processes as: regulation of memory and learning (De Wied, 1971), tolerance to opiates (Van Ree and De Wied, 1977), modulation of release of ACTH, growth hormone (Yates, Russell and Moran, 1971) and renin (Johnson, Kinter and Beeuwkes, 1979) and stimulation of formation of intrarenal prostaglandins (Zusman and Kaiser, 1977) and kinins (Fejes-Toth, Zahajszky and Janos, 1980).

The term 'vasopressin' acknowledges an established action of this hormone, that is, the vasoconstrictor and pressor activity of posterior pituitary extracts originally described in 1898 (Howell, 1898). Until recently the pressor action of vasopressin was primarily of pharmacological interest, with doubtful physiological or pathophysiological significance. This view could be justified by the observation that roughly 100 times as much exogenous vasopressin is needed to exert a pressor effect as to exert its antidiuretic action (Guyton et al., 1980). Since the minimum pressor dose of exogenous vasopressin is so far above that producing maximal antidiuresis, it has been considered unlikely that endogenous levels of circulating vasopressin could play a major role in regulation of blood pressure by vasoconstriction in physiological conditions or in disease states.

Moreover, patients with the syndrome of inappropriate secretion of the antidiuretic hormone are usually not hypertensive (Robertson, Aycinena and Zerbe, 1982) and those lacking the hormone, for instance with diabetes insipidus, are rarely hypotensive unless volume-depleted (Streeten, Moses and Miller, 1980). Such clinical observations may account for a lack of past enthusiasm for the view that vasopressin may play a role in the pathogenesis of experimental or clinical hypertension.

Several recent developments call for renewed scrutiny of vasopressin as a participant in the hypertensive process. It has become evident that baroreceptor mechanisms are extraordinarily powerful in diminishing the pressor effect of vasopressin. Baroreceptor denervation in the dog enhances the pressor action of vasopressin by 70-fold (Cowley, Monos and Guyton, 1974). Since defective baroreflex function has often been suspected in hypertension, such an abnormality would enhance the effect of vasopressin. Thus, knowing the plasma concentration of vasopressin might not reveal its pressor activity where baroreflex function is altered.

Interaction of vasopressin and other peptide hormones with local vasoregulatory systems, particularly the prostaglandins, has been extensively studied in recent years (Dunn *et al.*, 1978). It is now evident that the kallikrein kinin system and the prostaglandins participate in regulating the activity of peptide and catecholamine vasoconstrictors in several vascular beds (Carretero and Scicli, 1981). Local modulation altering sensitivity and responsiveness to circulating vasoactive hormones may also play a critical role in long-term elevation of systemic arterial pressure by contributing to raised total peripheral resistance, the hallmark of chronic hypertension.

Precise measurement of circulating vasopressin has been provided by the development of sensitive, specific radioimmunoassays (Robertson, 1977). Such technology has resolved many problems not previously approachable by bioassay. However, determining the vasoconstrictor or pressor activity of the posterior pituitary hormones in relation to measured levels of plasma concentration now depends upon the use of specific blockade through the development of antibodies (Mohring *et al.*, 1977) and peptide analogs of the hormone (Manning and Sawyer, 1982). Specific antagonists of the vasopressor action and of the antidiuretic action of vasopressin have now been developed and are being explored in several laboratories. Thus, tools for analysis of the role of vasopressin in the pathogenesis of experimental and clinical hypertension may now be employed in a manner analogous to the analysis of the renin–angiotensin system through the use of specific radioimmunoassay and pharmacological antagonists. The promising recent developments that are pertinent to understanding the role of vasopressin in clinical hypertension will be the subject of this review.

STORAGE OF VASOPRESSIN

Vasopressin is synthesized in the magnocellular neurons of the supraoptic and paraventricular hypothalamic nuclei together with oxytocin and the specific neurophysins associated with these peptides. The neurophysins may derive from a common precursor and serve as carriers for vasopressin and oxytocin during axonal transport (Gainer, Sarne and Brownstein, 1977). Vasopressin and oxytocin are synthesized in separate neurons. However, immunocytochemical evidence suggests the coexistence of vasopressin and angiotensin II in the same neurons (Kilcoyne,

Hoffman and Zimmerman, 1980). It is not yet known whether the presence of these two peptides in the same neuron is related to any specific physiological relationship. Projections from the supraoptic and paraventricular nuclei extend to the external zone of the median eminence and the neurohypophysis. The latter is the principal storage site for vasopressin from which this hormone is released to the circulation. Multiple other projections of vasopressinergic neurons have been identified in the hypothalamus, thalamus and brain stem (Zimmerman, 1981). Functions of these neurons have not been completely characterized, although their proximity to cardiovascular regulatory centers such as the nucleus tractus solitarii suggest a central modulatory effect for vasopressin on cardiovascular function. It has been observed that direct injection of vasopressin into the nucleus tractus solitarii increases arterial pressure and heart rate (Matsuguchi *et al.*, 1982b).

CONTROL OF VASOPRESSIN SECRETION

Osmolar mechanisms

The role of extracellular fluid osmolality in controlling the release of vasopressin was defined in the classical studies of Verney (1947). A sigmoidal dose–response relationship between intracarotid injection of hypertonic saline and antidiuresis due to pituitary secretion was demonstrated. Quantitative differences in the antidiuretic response to hyperosmolar solutions of different solutes led Verney to conclude that the ability of a solute to generate an osmolar gradient between intracellular and extracellular spaces (membrane permeability) was crucial to determining its potency as a stimulus for vasopressin release: for example, NaCl > glucose > urea. Verney's hypothesis has been supported recently *in vitro* by measuring vasopressin release from hypothalamic explants (Sladek and Knigge, 1977). It has been suggested that the effect of extracellular fluid hyperosmolality in causing increased vasopressin release may be mediated by changes in sodium concentration of ventricular fluid (Andersson and Olsson, 1977).

Quantitative characteristics of the relationship between plasma osmolality and concentration of vasopressin have been studied in several species. The precise nature of the relationship is unsettled. Some studies indicate a strict linear correlation between plasma osmolality and vasopressin (Dunn *et al.*, 1973; Robertson and Athar, 1976). Others suggest an exponential relationship between plasma osmolality and vasopressin concentration averaged over time (Weitzman and Fisher, 1977) to minimize the effect of cyclic secretion (Weitzman *et al.*, 1977a). In normally hydrated human subjects plasma osmolality appears to operate at a 'set point' a few milliosmoles above the threshold osmolality for vasopressin release. A 1% increase in plasma osmolality is sufficient to cause an increase in plasma vasopressin. In comparing the slope of the relationship between plasma vasopressin and osmolality, rodents appear to have a greater sensitivity than primates; that is, the slope is approximately three times greater in rats than in humans (Dunn *et al.*, 1973; Robertson and Athar, 1976).

Volume and pressure stimuli

Non-hypotensive hypovolemia stimulates vasopressin release (Weinstein, Berne and Sachs, 1960). Increases in plasma vasopressin occur at a 10% reduction in blood volume. Furthermore, changes in blood volume modify the sensitivity of the osmolar mechanism for vasopressin release in some species (Robertson, Athar and Shelton, 1977). Hypotensive hemorrhage produces a large increase in plasma vasopressin concentration due to an exponential relationship between vasopressin and volume reduction (Dunn *et al.*, 1973). The level of achieved plasma vasopressin in hypotensive hemorrhage is sufficient to cause direct vasoconstriction and participate in the maintenance of arterial pressure. This has been shown both by decapitation and by use of a specific antagonist of the vascular action of vasopressin (Cowley, Switzer and Guinn, 1980).

The reflex pathways by which changes in arterial pressure and in blood volume control vasopressin release include the arterial high pressure baroreceptors and the low pressure afferent systems located within the chest. While the importance of the high pressure system has been well established (Share, 1976), recent studies emphasize participation of the low pressure system which is sensitive to changes in venous volume and venous return affecting atrial mechanoreceptors. Tonic activity originating from these sites and carried by vagal afferent fibers may be responsible for tonic inhibition of vasopressin release (Thames and Schmid, 1979). In addition, receptors located within the left atria and ventricle may stimulate vasopressin release via afferent pathways travelling in spinal nerves (Thames, Peterson and Schmid, 1980). The significance of these pathways in the response to upright posture is unclear. Some, but not all studies report an increase in plasma vasopressin concentration with upright posture (Baylis and Heath, 1977; Davies, Forsling and Slater, 1977).

Other influences on vasopressin release require integrity of the baroreflexes to exert their effect. Hence, norepinephrine inhibition and isoproterenol stimulation of vasopressin secretion do not occur without intact baroreceptor pathways (Berl *et al.*, 1974a, 1974b). Likewise, stimuli that do not modify arterial pressure, that is, hypoxia and nicotine, are mediated through the afferent baroreflex nerves (Anderson *et al.*, 1978; Cadnapaphornchai *et al.*, 1974).

The central integration of the reflex pathways modulating vasopressin release is not yet well known. Recently, Blessing, Sved and Reis (1982) have shown that norepinephrine containing neurons in the A_1 area of the medulla oblongata exert a major tonic inhibitory influence on vasopressin secretion through hypothalamic projections. Selective destruction of this area is followed by an abrupt increase in arterial pressure and plasma vasopressin. The raised pressure is rapidly lowered by a vasopressin antagonist.

Adrenal steroids

Increased plasma vasopressin concentration has been documented in clinical and experimental adrenal insufficiency (Ahmed *et al.*, 1967; Linas *et al.*, 1980). This is due to both mineralocorticoid and glucocorticoid deficiency. Experimentally, absence of either mineralocorticoids or glucocorticoids results in raised plasma vasopressin concentration which is lowered by replacement of the appropriate steroid (Boykin *et al.*, 1979; Linas *et al.*, 1980). The effect of isolated mineralocorticoid deficiency is best explained by hypovolemia. Glucocorticoid hormones appear to exert a tonic inhibitory influence on vasopressin release. Deficiency of adrenal glucocorticoids results in increased content of vasopressin and its neurophysin, as measured by immunocytochemical techniques, in the zona externa of the median eminence of the rat (Stillman *et al.*, 1977). Administration of glucocorticoids reverses this anatomic alteration (Silverman *et al.*, 1981). Such studies suggest that glucocorticoid action participates in controlling the axonal transport of vasopressin from its site of synthesis to the neurohypophysis where the peptide is released to the circulation.

Endogenous opioids – endorphins, enkephalins

A large number of studies suggest possible roles for endogenous opioids in the control of vasopressin secretion. The evidence is conflicting with studies suggesting that opioids increase or decrease vasopressin release. The possibility that some effects of endogenous opioids are direct has been raised by the detection of high affinity opioid receptors in the rat pituitary (Simantov and Snyder, 1977).

Depending upon the specific experimental protocol, administration of morphine or of beta-endorphin may result in an increase (Weitzman *et al.*, 1977b), no change (Stark *et al.*, 1982) or decrease (van Wimersma-Greidanus *et al.*, 1979) in plasma vasopressin concentration. In some studies, the effect of the opiate is diminished by known opiate antagonists such as naloxone or naltrexone (Grossman *et al.*, 1980). In other studies, the effect of the opiate is not blocked by its 'antagonist' (Van Wimersma-Greidanus *et al.*, 1979). Neuroanatomic studies suggest that leucine enkephalin is closely linked to vasopressin secretion. Rats with hereditary diabetes insipidus have marked reduction in concentration of leucine enkephalin in the pars nervosa of the hypophysis, while the beta-endorphin content of the anterior pituitary is slightly elevated (Rossier *et al.*, 1979). Such results have suggested that enkephalins participate in the control of vasopressin release. However, infusion of a long-acting, enkephalin-like analog to human volunteers has been shown to decrease plasma vasopressin concentration and produce a transient diabetes insipidus-like state (Grossman *et al.*, 1980). There may be several reasons for the confusing results of these studies. Administration of exogenous opiates and opiate-like peptides may not duplicate the effect of endogenous opioid activity at discrete sites in the central nervous system. In addition, the large number and uncertain specificity of opiate receptors and of various antagonists needs to be considered.

Evidence that endogenous opioids participate in mediating the well-known alterations in vasopressin secretion due to osmolar and volume stimuli has become increasingly convincing. It has been shown that both naloxone and oxilorphan blunt the effect of hypertonicity and of hypovolemia upon vasopressin secretion in the rat

(Ishikawa and Schrier, 1982). Recent studies from our laboratory suggest that naloxone may diminish the effect of adrenalectomy upon vasopressin secretion (Elijovich *et al.*, 1983a). These studies emphasize the role of endogenous opioids as local mediators for classical stimuli of vasopressin release.

The renin–angiotensin system

The role of the peripheral or circulating renin–angiotensin system in modulating release of vasopressin is unclear. It has been reported that intravenous infusion of angiotensin II both increases (Bonjour and Malvin, 1970) and does not significantly modify (Cowley, Switzer and Skelton, 1981) the release of vasopressin. Blockade of angiotensin II formation by inhibition of converting enzyme does not modify the increase in plasma vasopressin due to hemorrhage in the dog (Morton *et al.*, 1977). In humans, administration of propranolol inhibits the renin, but not the vasopressin, response to passive tilting (Davies, Forsling and Slater, 1977).

Intracerebroventricular injection of angiotensin II produces a dose-dependent increase in vasopressin secretion (Keil, Summy-Long and Severs, 1975). It has been suggested that this increase in vasopressin is sufficient to account for part of the pressor effect of central angiotensin II (Severs *et al.*, 1970). Prostaglandins may mediate the stimulating effect of angiotensin II upon vasopressin secretion. Intraventricular infusion of PGE_2 also causes vasopressin release (Yamamoto, Share and Shade, 1976). The effect of intraventricular angiotensin II upon vasopressin release is diminished by indomethacin (Yamamoto, Share and Shade, 1978). Isolated explants of the hypothalamus also release vasopressin when stimulated by angiotensin II (Sladek and Joynt, 1979). Injection of subthreshold doses of angiotensin II into the lateral ventricle potentiates the vasopressin releasing effect of intraventricular sodium chloride (Andersson and Westbye, 1970). Such results indicate that the brain renin–angiotensin system may modulate osmotic stimuli for vasopressin release. Linkage of these experiments to a physiological role for the brain renin–angiotensin system is suggested by an experiment in which intracerebroventricular infusion of teprotide, the converting enzyme inhibitor, increases free water clearance in salt-depleted dogs (Brooks and Malvin, 1979). Thus, a sequence of studies suggests that the central renin–angiotensin system participates in regulation of vasopressin secretion.

Other factors modifying vasopressin secretion

A wide variety of stimuli have been shown to increase vasopressin secretion in various studies. Pain, nausea, hyperthermia, stress of various kinds, hypoxia and hypercapnia have all been shown to act as stimuli (Weitzman, 1979). Not all of these factors have been shown to raise vasopressin sufficiently to account for a direct vasopressor action of the peptide. In studies employing a vasopressor antagonist we have found that the pressor effect of pentobarbital anesthesia during surgery for implantation of catheters raises arterial pressure and that a portion of this increase (7 ± 1 mmHg) is attributable to vasopressin. In contrast, conscious, unrestrained normotensive animals have plasma vasopressin levels which are so low that administration of a vasopressin antagonist has no effect on arterial pressure (Elijovich *et al.*, 1983b).

Endogenous opioids, the brain renin–angiotensin system and brain prostaglandins have already been described as possible mediators for control of vasopressin release. In addition, acetylcholine (Hoffman *et al.*, 1977), bradykinin (Hoffman and Schmid, 1978a), histamine (Hoffman and Schmid, 1978b), and catecholamines (Miller *et al.*, 1979) may play some role. Recent experiments suggest that cyclic nucleotides (Schrier, Berl and Anderson, 1979), thyrotropin releasing hormone (Weitzman *et al.*, 1979) and calcium membrane transport (Ishikawa *et al.*, 1981) are additional factors to be considered in the overall control of vasopressin secretion. The degree to which these factors participate in the osmolar, volume and reflex control of vasopressin release remains to be quantified.

METABOLISM OF VASOPRESSIN

Vasopressin secreted from the neurohypophysis rapidly equilibrates into a volume of distribution greater than plasma volume (Wilson, Weitzman and Fisher, 1978). In part, this is due to extravascular binding of the peptide to receptor sites (Weitzman and Fisher, 1978). There is little or no binding of vasopressin to plasma proteins. The normal half-life of vasopressin in the circulation has been reported as ranging from 2 to 40 minutes (Robertson, 1977). Approximately 50% of the total metabolic clearance of vasopressin occurs in the kidneys; much of the remaining metabolism occurs in the liver (Share, Shade and Rabkin, 1978). Renal clearance of vasopressin is dependent upon blood flow and is greater than glomerular filtration rate. Approximately two-thirds of radiolabelled vasopressin passing through the isolated perfused kidney is excreted unchanged in the urine. The remainder is excreted as the desglycinamide metabolite (Walter and Bowman, 1973).

Reductions in renal blood flow to 25% of normal by progressive renal artery constriction have no significant effect upon plasma vasopressin concentration in dogs (Shade and Share, 1977). In contrast, 75% removal of renal mass in the rat causes a progressive and rapid increase in vasopressin production which later falls to levels remaining above normal (Lee-Kwon *et al.*, 1981). Total nephrectomy in the rat increases vasopressin concentration to five-fold above normal in 20 hours (Gavras *et al.*, 1982). This increase is too great to be explained by the reduction in metabolic clearance of the peptide and occurs despite increased blood volume (Elijovich *et al.*, unpublished observations). Increased serum osmolality following nephrectomy is entirely due to retained urea, a permeant solute, which does not stimulate vasopressin release. Other mechanisms accounting for the effect of total nephrectomy upon plasma vasopressin concentration remain to be established.

ACTIONS OF VASOPRESSIN

Water conservation

Fluid conservation due to vasopressin is exerted at the distal portion of the nephron. The collecting duct is impermeable to water in the absence of this hormone. Up to 15% of the glomerular filtrate can be excreted as solute-free water during hydration. When plasma vasopressin is increased by dehydration or hypovolemia, the maximal reabsorption of water that is attained depends upon tubulointerstitial osmolar gradient. This varies with species studied from 1200 mOsmol in man to 4000 mOsmol in rodents. In the presence of vasopressin, permeability of the collecting duct to water permits the existing osmolar gradient to become the major determinant of water reabsorption.

Cellular mechanisms accounting for the action of vasopressin on renal tubular epithelium have become well defined. The peptide binds to receptors on the basolateral surface of collecting duct cells (Grantham and Burg, 1966). Intracellular activation of an adenylcyclase system is initiated, leading to increased cyclic AMP concentration and activation of protein kinases (Dousa, 1977). Ultimately, events mediated by the intracellular second messenger system result in opening of membrane channels, permitting movement of water across the cell to equilibration with interstitial fluid. A direct effect of vasopressin on urea and sodium transport has been demonstrated in some species (Humphreys, Friedler and Earley, 1970; Jaenike, 1961).

Prostaglandins have been shown to inhibit the action of vasopressin upon fluid transport in the kidney (Kirschenbaum *et al.*, 1982). This may be indicative of a physiological local regulation of the action of vasopressin, since this peptide stimulates synthesis and release of PGE_2 by renomedullary cells (Zusman and Kaiser, 1977). Inhibitors of prostaglandin synthetase enhance the antidiuretic action of vasopressin which has clinical utility in the management of partial diabetes insipidus (Robertson, 1977).

Effects on vascular smooth muscle

The effect of vasopressin on vascular smooth muscle is mediated by calcium ion transport rather than the adenylcyclase system by which vasopressin exerts its effect upon renal tubular cells. On a molar basis, vasopressin is one of the most potent vasoconstrictors *in vitro* with detectable action at concentrations of 10^{-12}M (Altura and Altura, 1977). The vasoconstrictor effect of vasopressin has been overlooked in studies which measured only changes in arterial pressure. It has recently become apparent that, in dogs, infusion of vasopressin at doses that increase circulating levels within the physiological range produce significant vasoconstriction without an increase in systemic arterial pressure. This is due to substantial reduction in cardiac output as a result of reflex mechanisms (Montani *et al.*, 1980). Stimulation of endogenous vasopressin secretion by hypertonic saline produces a similar hemodynamic sequence in both dog and rat; an increase in total peripheral resistance, reduction in heart rate and cardiac output, and little change in mean arterial pressure (Charocopos *et al.*, 1982; Montani *et al.*, 1980). These changes are reversed by a specific antagonist of the vascular action of vasopressin, indicating the physiological role of the vascular action of this peptide when stimulated by hypertonicity (Charocopos *et al.*, 1982).

When total peripheral resistance is increased to the same extent by angiotensin, methoxamine or vasopressin the latter peptide is associated with a greater reduction in cardiac output (Heyndrickx, Boettcher and Vatner, 1976). This reduction is due to a slower heart rate in animals with normal reflex control or to diminished myocardial contractility in animals with heart rates kept constant by electrical pacing. Baroreflex denervation causes a 70-fold enhancement of the pressor action of vasopressin, a significantly greater effect than observed with norepinephrine or angiotensin II (Cowley, Monos and Guyton, 1974). It thus appears that vasopressin may have a specific effect upon baroreflex function, perhaps mediated by central actions that are not observed with other physiological and pharmacological arteriolar vasoconstrictors.

The prevailing level of plasma vasopressin determines the pressor effect of changes in hormone concentration. Reduction in circulating vasopressin levels by decapitation further enhances the pressor effect of vasopressin administration in baroreflex denervated dogs (Cowley, Monos and Guyton, 1974). Hypophysectomy also increases the sensitivity to vasopressor infusion into the mesenteric vascular bed of the cat (Pang, Wilcox and McNeill, 1979). Such results may be explained by the receptor occupancy hypothesis that has been employed in the analysis of dose–response relationships for angiotensin II (Thurston and Laragh, 1975).

The vasoconstrictor effect of vasopressin is not uniformly distributed throughout the systemic vascular tree. Major sites of vasoconstriction are the coronary, mesenteric, muscular and cutaneous beds (Hoffman, 1980). Cerebral and renal blood flow are relatively unaffected by vasopressin. When compared to vasopressin, angiotensin II is a much more potent vasoconstrictor of the renal vascular bed (Heyndrickx, Boettcher and Vatner, 1976).

Studies have been addressed to interactions between the three major vasoconstrictors: norepinephrine, the sympathetic neurotransmitter, angiotensin II, and vasopressin. Pharmacological blockade of sympathetic nervous transmission reduces the local vasoconstrictor action of vasopressin, suggesting a synergistic relationship between vasopressin and norepinephrine (Leenen and DeJong, 1969). Tonic constriction of the mesenteric vascular bed may be maintained by either angiotensin II, vasopressin or both acting in concert (McNeill, Wilcox and Pang, 1977). Receptors for both peptides are present in this regional circulation (Alexander *et al.*, 1980; Schiffrin and Genest, 1983). Predominance of the action of one peptide appears to reduce the action of the other in this tissue (McNeill, Wilcox and Pang, 1977). During dehydration and hemorrhagic shock, both angiotensin II and vasopressin exert vasoconstrictor action. Blockade or removal of one peptide system shifts maintenance of arterial pressure to the other with varying completeness (Andrews and Brenner, 1981; Schwartz and Reid, 1981). Several studies suggest that the overall vasoconstrictor effect of vasopressin or angiotensin II may diminish the effect of the other peptide. We have observed that infusion of subpressor doses of vasopressin diminishes the pressor effect of angiotensin II. In contrast, the pressor action of norepinephrine is unchanged (Elijovich *et al.*, in press). Infusion of angiotensin II reduces the pressor action of injected vasopressin (Burnier and Brunner, 1983). Inhibition of the renin–angiotensin system by chronic treatment with captopril appears to enhance the vasopressor effect of vasopressin (Spertini *et al.*, 1981). Such studies suggest that the two endogenous peptide vasoconstrictor substances may have a specific interaction not shared with norepinephrine.

Maintenance of arterial pressure in hypotensive and hypovolemic states

The potent vasoconstrictor action of vasopressin contributes to restoration of arterial pressure during hemorrhagic shock in the dog (Cowley, Switzer and Guinn, 1980). Quantification of the pressor action of vasopressin has been achieved by specific antagonists and by decapitation. In these studies, the confounding influences of the renin–angiotensin system and the efferent sympathetic function have been eliminated by nephrectomy and spinal cord transection at C1. After arterial pressure reduction by hemorrhage to half that of control levels, vasopressin increases arterial pressure to 85% of baseline within 3 min, while plasma concentration rises by four-fold. These experiments elegantly display the pressor action of vasopressin in a hypotensive model, entirely independent of other pressor systems. However, the role of vasopressin when the renin–angiotensin system and sympathetic mechanisms are intact to compensate for reduced arterial pressure or blood volume is not defined in these studies.

Andrews and Brenner (1981) demonstrated that rats deprived of water for 48 hours, then anesthetized, had a significant depressor response averaging 18 mmHg to injection of an antagonist of the vascular action of vasopressin. The response was transient with return of arterial pressure to pre-injection levels by 15 minutes. No depressor effect was observed in normally hydrated control animals. In dehydrated rats, the magnitude of the depressor response to vasopressin antagonism was increased by either saralasin or nephrectomy and the duration of the reduction in pressure was substantially prolonged. This study indicates that both the renin–angiotensin system and vasopressin contribute to maintenance of arterial pressure during water deprivation and that angiotensin action can compensate almost completely for loss of vasopressin. Aisenbrey *et al.* (1981) found that a vasopressin antagonist reduced arterial pressure by 14 mmHg in unanesthetized rats deprived of water for 24 hours, in which a 20-fold increase in plasma vasopressin had occurred. Hemodynamic assessment indicated that a reduction in total peripheral resistance accounted for the fall in pressure as cardiac output did not change. It is puzzling to us that no compensatory increase in cardiac output occurred. Perhaps reduced pre-load due to dehydration accounts for the observations.

As indicated previously, increased plasma vasopressin concentration has been observed in Addison's disease (Ahmed *et al.*, 1967) and in experimental deficiencies of either glucocorticoids (Linas *et al.*, 1980) or mineralocorticoids

(Boykin *et al.*, 1979). In adrenal insufficiency a tendency to reduced arterial pressure is accompanied by both lowered serum sodium and osmolar concentration. The water-retaining or antidiuretic effect of vasopressin in this disorder has been quantified directly through the use of a specific antagonist of the action of vasopressin upon renal tubules (Schrier and Ishikawa, 1982). We have quantified the direct pressor effect of vasopressin in experimental adrenal insufficiency. Injection of a specific antipressor antagonist of vasopressin caused a rapid and sustained 10% reduction of arterial pressure in unanesthetized adrenalectomized rats maintained on a high salt intake. Administration of captopril for blockade of the renin–angiotensin system caused an additional sustained reduction in arterial pressure of 19%. No change in pressure occurred with either antagonist in controls (Elijovich *et al.*, 1983c). Thus, in adrenal insufficiency the two peptide pressor systems play a crucial role in maintenance of arterial pressure. Since combined blockade of these systems causes such a profound and long-lasting reduction in pressure, a defect in function of the sympathetic nervous control of the circulation is suggested.

Elevation of plasma vasopressin concentration has been detected in syncope-prone patients (Baylis and Heath, 1977), in diseases with low cardiac output such as myxedema and congestive heart failure (Skowsky and Kikuchi, 1978; Preibisz *et al.*, 1983) and in states with a decreased 'effective' blood volume such as cirrhosis (Bichet *et al.*, 1982). We cannot find evidence that the nephrotic syndrome has been studied in this regard. A possible contribution of vasopressin to maintenance of arterial pressure in these disorders which have diverse hemodynamic alterations has not yet been explored in a direct manner and remains to be elucidated. Availability of a vasopressin antagonist for clinical investigation would be a valuable tool for study of these conditions.

VASOPRESSIN IN EXPERIMENTAL HYPERTENSION

It is evident from the previous discussion that vasopressin participates in maintenance of systemic arterial pressure through several mechanisms, the best known being its role in conservation of water through enhancement of renal tubular reabsorption. The complexity of vasopressin's other effects, vasoconstriction, central nervous system actions on cardiovascular reflexes, and interaction with other vasoconstrictors, pose unique problems for analysis of the participation by this peptide in experimental and clinical hypertension. At the present time, no form of sustained experimental hypertension is entirely attributable to the action of vasopressin. Nonetheless, recent studies have led to the view that there is need for complete characterization of the renal and vascular actions of this peptide in several experimental models as a prerequisite for an analysis of clinical hypertension. Alterations in baroreflex function, the renin–angiotensin system, vascular responsiveness, and renal function occur in experimental hypertension. These alterations may modify the action of vasopressin to elicit its participation in maintenance of elevated arterial pressure to a degree not evident in normal animals.

Experimental renovascular hypertension

There are several models of experimental renovascular hypertension. These differ from each other with respect to the role played by salt retention and the renin–angiotensin system at various phases in the development and maintenance of elevated pressure.

The two-kidney, one-clip Goldblatt preparation is ordinarily considered a renin-dependent model (Brunner *et al.*, 1971), especially in the early phase of its development. In this model plasma vasopressin is increased but the magnitude of the increase is far greater if animals enter the malignant phase of hypertension in which there is reduced blood volume (Mohring *et al.*, 1978). Vasopressin is not indispensable for hypertension as rats with hereditary diabetes insipidus (Brattleboro rats) develop two-kidney, one-clip hypertension similar in magnitude and time-course to controls (Johnston, Newman and Woods, 1981; *see Table 3.5*).

Table 3.1 Vasopressin in experimental renovascular hypertension

Model	Plasma vasopressin	Anti-vasopressin antibodies	Vasopressin antagonists	References
Benign hypertension				
two-kidney, one-clip*	↑	↓	—	Mohring *et al.* (1978); Johnston, Newman and Woods (1981)
one-kidney, one-clip*	↑	—	—	Johnston, Newman and Woods (1981); Pullan *et al.* (1980); Share and Crofton (1982)
Malignant hypertension				
two-kidney, one-clip	↑ ↑	↓	←→†	Mohring *et al.* (1978); Rabito, Carretero and Scicli (1981)
aortic ligature	↑ ↑	—	—	Woods *et al.* (1983)

* Designate the two models of Goldblatt hypertension respectively
† The horizontal arrow indicates no change

The direct vasoconstrictor role of vasopressin in two-kidney, one-clip hypertension remains unclear. Mohring *et al.* (1978) found that injection of antivasopressin antibodies significantly reduced arterial pressure in 50% of rats in the malignant phase (*Table 3.1*). In contrast, Rabito, Carretero and Scicli (1981) have reported that specific antagonists of the vascular action of vasopressin had no effect on arterial pressure in the same model. The difference between the two studies is not readily explained. However, antibody preparations may contain or elicit non-specific effects. Slight differences in the protocols may have led to variations in stress-induced release of vasopressin. Increased vascular reactivity to vasopressin has been suggested as an additional factor (Mohring *et al.*, 1978) in this model, but there is no confirming evidence that this occurs as a specific effect.

Rats with an occluding ligature of the aorta between the renal arteries develop malignant hypertension which is similar to the two-kidney, one-clip model. Although plasma vasopressin concentration is increased in Long Evans rats with aortic ligation, hypertension develops to an equal extent in the Brattleboro strain (Woods *et al.*, 1983) indicating that vasopressin is not required for hypertension in this model.

The one-kidney, one-clip Goldblatt model of experimental hypertension depends largely upon salt and water retention when available, but activation of the renin–angiotensin system maintains elevated pressure in salt-deprived (Gavras *et al.*, 1973), diuretic-treated (Gavras *et al.*, 1975) or adrenalectomized animals (Ribeiro and Krakoff, 1978).

Rats and dogs with one-kidney, one-clip hypertension have elevation in plasma vasopressin which reaches twice normal values (Johnston, Newman and Woods *et al.*, 1981; Pullan *et al.*, 1980). Brattleboro rats lacking vasopressin develop one-kidney, one-clip hypertension but the degree of increase in arterial pressure is less than that of their controls (Share *et al.*, 1982; *see Table 3.5*). Administration of DDAVP, which has the antidiuretic but not the vasoconstrictor action of vasopressin, to one-kidney, one-clip Brattleboro rats causes arterial pressure to increase to the same extent as in controls with endogenous vasopressin (Johnston, Newman and Woods, 1981). Antivasopressin antibodies and antipressor peptide antagonists have not been evaluated in the one-kidney, one-clip model. An alteration in vascular responsiveness to vasopressin has not been documented.

In summary, the antidiuretic effect of vasopressin may play a small additive role in the pathogenesis of benign one-kidney, one-clip hypertension. Reduced renal mass and blood flow with resultant impairment of metabolic clearance of vasopressin could account for the action of this hormone in this model. There is no evidence that osmotic or volume stimuli are present to cause excessive secretion of the hormone by the neurohypophysis.

Experimental renal failure

Vasopressin may play a role in the transient elevation of arterial pressure that occurs in glycerol-induced acute renal failure in the rat. During the first two hours after glycerol administration plasma vasopressin concentration increases 40-fold. This is attributable, in part, to increased serum osmolality as a result of glycerol itself and also to impaired renal conservation of water due to the acquired tubular damage. The elevation of arterial pressure is reversed by antivasopressin antibodies but not by saralasin (Hofbauer *et al.*, 1977). Brattleboro rats have no increase in arterial pressure despite development of more severe renal failure reflected in lesser urine output and higher serum urea concentration (Konrads *et al.*, 1979; *see Table 3.5*). An elevation of arterial pressure due to vasopressin in this setting appears surprising, but may result from the combined effects of the prominent stimuli for vasopressin release and reduced metabolic clearance of the hormone due to the degree of renal damage.

It has previously been mentioned that total nephrectomy in the rat is associated with increased plasma vasopressin concentration and a small increase in mean arterial pressure which can be reduced by administration of specific vasopressin antagonists (Gavras *et al.*, 1982; Elijovich, Leskiw and Krakoff, 1981). These animals have increased blood volume, reduced serum sodium concentration and

Table 3.2 Vasopressin in experimental models of acute or chronic renal failure

Model	Plasma vasopressin	Urine vasopressin	Antivasopressin antibodies	Peptide antagonists	References
Glycerol ATN*	↑↑↑	—	↓ ↓	—	Hofbauer et al. (1977); Konrads et al. (1979)
Partial NX*	↑	—	—	↔†	Di Pette et al. (1982)
Partial NX-salt	↑↑	↑	—	↓ or ↔†	Di Pette et al. (1982); Lee-Kwon et al. (1981)
Total NX	↑	—	—	→	Elijovich, Leskiw and Krakoff (1981); Gavras et al. (1982)
Total NX-salt	↑	—	—	→	Hatzinikolaou et al. (1980; 1981)

* Glycerol ATN: acute renal failure induced by glycerol injection. NX: nephrectomy
† The horizontal arrow indicates no change

increased serum osmolality due to retained urea, a permeant solute. The increased plasma vasopressin concentration observed is then not due to osmotic stimuli or hypovolemia.

In a model of chronic renal failure achieved by subtotal (85%) nephrectomy, plasma vasopressin concentrations twice normal have been measured when rats were given water to drink (*Table 3.2*). When given 1% saline arterial pressure rose significantly and plasma vasopressin was increased to eight times normal. Administration of a vasopressin antagonist reduced arterial pressure substantially (Di Pette *et al.*, 1982). However, Lee-Kwon *et al.* (1981) found that plasma vasopressin concentration was only 2.5 times normal in rats with 75% nephrectomy given saline; a vasopressin antagonist had only a modest effect on arterial pressure (9 ± 2 mmHg). Slight differences in the degree of chronic renal insufficiency might explain the discrepancy between these two studies. In advanced chronic renal failure there may be abnormal stimuli for vasopressin release as well as substantial reduction in renal metabolic clearance of the peptide. Both factors may then account for elevated plasma concentrations which have a pressor effect.

Genetic hypertension

The role of vasopressin in the spontaneous hypertensive rat (SHR) has been extensively investigated. Comparison of the SHR to the WKY controls indicated that the former have increased plasma vasopressin concentration, urine vasopressin excretion and increased neurohypophyseal content of the hormone (Crofton *et al.*, 1978; Mohring, Kintz and Schoun, 1979; *see Table 3.3*). Increases in plasma vasopressin vary from two- to four-fold in the SHR compared to the WKY, with the larger increases observed in stroke-prone SHR with malignant hypertension. Metabolic clearance of vasopressin is not different between the two strains (Mohring, Kintz and Schoun, 1979), suggesting that the differences in plasma concentration result from differences in synthesis and secretion. The stimulus for enhanced secretion of vasopressin in the SHR remains unclear. It has been observed that intracerebroventricular injection of captopril (Crofton *et al.*, 1981b) or PGE_2 (Takahashi and Buñag, 1981) stimulate vasopressin release to a greater extent in the SHR compared to the WKY. This suggests hyper-reactivity to central stimuli which control vasopressin release in this model.

Participation by vasopressin in elevation of arterial pressure in the SHR is suggested by a strong correlation between plasma vasopressin concentration and level of arterial pressure (Mohring, Kintz and Schoun, 1979). More direct evidence for the role of vasopressin in the SHR is found in the demonstration that blood pressure reduction is caused by vasopressin antagonists and vasopressin antibodies in several studies (Crofton *et al.*, 1978; Mohring, Kintz and Schoun, 1979).

Spontaneous hypertensive rats are more sensitive to the pressor effect of exogenous vasopressin compared to the WKY as indicated by a leftward shift of the dose–response curve by a factor of four. This results in a threshold for the pressor effect of vasopressin in the SHR of approximately 4 pg/ml which is well within the range of plasma levels observed in these animals and is about one-fifth the threshold observed in the WKY (Mohring *et al.*, 1981).

Table 3.3 Vasopressin in experimental genetic hypertension

Model	Plasma vasopressin	Urine vasopressin	Antivasopressin antibodies	Peptide antagonists	Vascular responsiveness	References
Benign hypertension						
SHR*	↑	↑	→	→	↑	Crofton et al. (1978); Mohring, Kintz and Schoun (1979); Mohring et al. (1981)
NZGH*	↔†	↔†	—	—	↑	Crofton et al. (1981a)
Na-FED DAHL-S*	↑	↑	—	↔†	↑	Matsuguchi et al. (1981); Share and Crofton (1982)
Malignant hypertension						
SHR	↑↑	—	↓↓	—	↑	Mohring, Kintz and Schoun (1979)

* SHR: Japanese strain of spontaneously hypertensive rats. NZGH: New Zealand strain of genetically hypertensive rats. Na-FED DAHL-S: genetically salt-sensitive rat of the Dahl strain

† The horizontal arrow indicates no change

The increased pressor responsiveness to vasopressin observed in the SHR may not be specific as enhanced responses to other pressor agents have been observed in this model (Rockhold, Crofton and Share, 1980). It has been suggested that increased responsiveness to infused pressor substances in the SHR may be due to impaired buffering by baroreflexes. The bradycardic response to vasopressin, norepinephrine and phenylnephrine is diminished in the SHR compared to the WKY (Mohring *et al.*, 1981). A possible role for central vasopressin has been suggested by the observation that brain stem vasopressin is reduced in SHR (Mohring *et al.*, 1980). This has led to speculation that brain stem vasopressin plays a facilitatory role for central mediation of baroreflex pathways. There is evidence for this view in the observation that injection of vasopressin into the fourth ventricle reduces heart rate and/or arterial pressure (Verma, Jaju and Bhargava, 1969). Theoretically, then, a diminution in brainstem vasopressin could result in impaired baroreflex function, resulting in inadequate buffering of the pressor response to various vasoconstrictors.

Ganten *et al.* (1983) have bred together the stroke-prone SHR and Brattleboro strains, resulting in rats with both hypertension and diabetes insipidus. These results clearly demonstrate that vasopressin is not necessary for the development of elevated arterial pressure in the SHR, whatever the modifying role of this neuropeptide may be when it is present (*see Table 3.5*).

The New Zealand strain of genetic hypertensive rats is also hyper-responsive to the pressor effect of injected vasopressin (*see Table 3.3*). However, urinary excretion and plasma levels of this hormone are not increased (Crofton *et al.*, 1981a), suggesting that excess secretion of the peptide does not occur in this strain.

Dahl S and R rats have almost equal plasma vasopressin levels. A high salt intake raises arterial pressure only in the S strain, with doubling of plasma vasopressin levels. R rats on high salt have no increase in pressure, although plasma concentration of vasopressin increases by 85%. Injection of a vasopressin antagonist does not reduce arterial pressure in hypertensive S rats (Matsuguchi *et al.*, 1981). Share and Crofton (1982) have also found increased plasma vasopressin levels in salt-fed Dahl S rats coupled with increased excretion of the hormone in urine. In this study, a vasopressin antagonist given alone had no effect on arterial pressure. However, after captopril administration vasopressin antagonism reduced arterial pressure. Since the peripheral renin–angiotensin system is suppressed in salt-fed Dahl S rats, these results are not easily interpreted.

Overall there is little evidence that vasopressin is indispensable for the development of hypertension in the several genetic models that have been studied. Additional cross-breeding of the Brattleboro strain with hypertensive and hypertension-prone strains may yield more definitive information, as indicated by the cited report of Ganten *et al.* (1983).

Experimental hypertension due to mineralocorticoid excess

There is a strong rationale for considering a causative role for vasopressin in hypertension due to mineralocorticoid excess with high salt intake, as exemplified by desoxycorticosterone (DOC)–salt hypertension in the rat (*Table 3.4*). Sodium

Table 3.4 Vasopressin in experimental hypertension due to mineralocorticoid excess

Model	Plasma vasopressin	Urine vasopressin	Antivasopressin antibodies	Peptide antagonists	Vascular responsiveness	References
Benign hypertension						
DOC–salt*	↑ or ↔†	↑	↓	↓ or ↔	↑	Mohring et al. (1977); Crofton et al. (1979); Matsuguchi and Schmid (1982a and b); Berecek et al. (1982a and b); Burnier et al. (1983)
Malignant hypertension						
DOC–salt*	↑↑	—	→	↔	↑	Mohring et al. (1977); Rabito, Carretero and Scicli (1981)
AX-REG*	—	—	—	↔	—	Rabito, Carretero and Scicli (1981)

* DOC–salt: deoxycorticosterone +1% saline hypertension in uninephrectomized rats. AX-REG: adrenal regeneration hypertension
† The horizontal arrow indicates no change

retention due to steroid action upon renal tubules should lead to some degree of hyperosmolality in plasma which then stimulates retention of water (volume) by excess secretion of the antidiuretic hormone. It might be expected that as water is retained, arterial pressure increases and pressure natriuresis occurs, a new steady state is reached so that plasma vasopressin is maintained at nearly normal levels. However, measurements of urinary vasopressin excretion and plasma vasopressin concentration tend to be somewhat elevated (two- to four-fold) during both early and late phases of DOC–salt hypertension (Share and Crofton, 1982).

Causes for persistent increase in plasma vasopressin concentration in DOC–salt hypertension are not entirely certain. Elevation of plasma osmolality due to hypernatremia has been found in some (Mohring *et al.*, 1977) but not all studies (Burnier *et al.*, 1983; Matsuguchi *et al.*, 1982a) of DOC–salt hypertension. This form of experimental hypertension is usually produced in uninephrectomized rats. Combination of reduced renal mass plus the renal vascular lesions of hypertension could reduce the metabolic clearance of vasopressin. However, decreased content of vasopressin in the neurohypophysis of the DOC–salt hypertensive rat suggests that hypersecretion does occur (Crofton *et al.*, 1980). Desoxycorticosterone given without salt increases urinary excretion of vasopressin in uninephrectomized rats, which develop little or no increase in arterial pressure (Crofton *et al.*, 1980). A direct effect for this steroid upon vasopressin secretion or metabolism is suggested by these observations.

Rats with acquired diabetes insipidus due to lesions of the median eminence and those with hereditary diabetes insipidus (Brattleboro strain) fail to develop DOC–salt hypertension (Berecek *et al.*, 1982c; Crofton *et al.*, 1979; Friedman, Friedman and Nakashima, 1960). Administration of exogenous vasopressin or DDAVP to Brattleboro rats permits elevation of arterial pressure by DOC–salt treatment (Berecek *et al.*, 1982c; Saito, Yajima and Watanabe, 1980; *see Table 3.5*). Since DDAVP has no vasoconstrictor action, these studies imply that the antidiuretic, volume-retaining effect of vasopressin is the only mechanism whereby this peptide contributes to DOC–salt hypertension. Nonetheless, a direct vasoconstrictor action is suggested by observations that peptide antagonists of the vascular action of vasopressin (Crofton *et al.*, 1979; Matsuguchi and Schmid, 1982a) produce immediate but small reductions in arterial pressure of DOC–salt hypertensive rats. Other investigators have been unable to reproduce these results (Burnier *et al.*, 1983). The reason for the discrepancy between these studies may be found in the degree of elevation of plasma vasopressin in each protocol. Rascher *et al.* (1983) have reported that administration of vasopressin antagonists to DOC–salt hypertensive rats significantly reduces total peripheral resistance with simultaneous increase in cardiac output resulting in no net change in arterial pressure. Thus, participation of the direct vasoconstrictor action of vasopressin in DOC–salt hypertension is still controversial.

Previous studies have documented a participation of the sympathetic nervous system in DOC–salt hypertension in the rat (DeChamplain, Krakoff and Axelrod, 1967). Burnier *et al.* (1983) reported that antagonists of the vascular action of vasopressin only reduced blood pressure in DOC–salt hypertensive rats pretreated with the alpha-adrenergic blocking agent, phentolamine. Rascher *et al.* (1983)

showed that after sinoaortic deafferentation the reduction in total peripheral resistance produced by an antipressor antagonist of vasopressin in DOC–salt hypertensive rats resulted in arterial pressure reduction due to lack of compensation by an increase in cardiac output. These data, taken together, suggest a reciprocal interaction between the sympathetic nervous system and vasopressin in maintenance of blood pressure in the DOC–salt hypertensivé rat, analogous to that between the renin–angiotensin system and salt in the maintenance of hypertension in the one-kidney, one-clip Goldblatt model of experimental hypertension (Gavras *et al.*, 1973).

Hyper-reactivity to the vascular action of vasopressin, angiotensin II and norepinephrine has been reported in the isolated perfused hind limb (Matsuguchi and Schmid, 1982a) and the isolated perfused kidney (Berecek *et al.*, 1982a) of the DOC–salt hypertensive rat. Vascular hyper-reactivity in the kidney occurs as early as three days after DOC–salt treatment preceding the development of hypertension. Brattleboro rats treated with DOC–salt do not develop renal vascular hyper-reactivity (Berecek *et al.*, 1982a), suggesting that endogenous vasopressin is responsible for this phenomenon.

Pressor responsiveness to exogenous vasopressin is also enhanced in DOC–salt rats. However, the development of pressor hyper-responsiveness is time-dependent, occurring at a later stage compared to vascular hyper-reactivity in isolated vascular beds (Crofton *et al.*, 1980). DOC–salt hypertensive rats develop progressive impairment of baroreflex function paralleling the degree of increase in arterial pressure (Matsuguchi and Schmid, 1982b). As previously described, normal animals specifically counteract the vasoconstrictor action of vasopressin by a powerful reflex buffering such that arterial pressure is kept constant. Impaired baroreflex function in DOC–salt hypertension must then be considered as an additional pathogenetic mechanism which accounts for the temporal sequence in which local vascular hyper-reactivity precedes pressor hyper-responsiveness in this model. The sum of both mechanisms may account for the direct pressor action of vasopressin in DOC–salt hypertension in its later phases despite only modest elevations in plasma concentration.

Lesions of the anteroventral area of the third cerebral ventricle (AV3V) prevent DOC–salt induced elevation of arterial pressure and plasma vasopressin concentration and the appearance of renal vascular hyper-reactivity (Berecek *et al.*, 1982b). Administration of exogenous vasopressin, at doses matched to reach plasma concentrations observed in unlesioned DOC–salt hypertensive rats, partially restores elevation of arterial pressure in AV3V-lesioned animals. In contrast, exogenous vasopressin does not permit the development of DOC–salt hypertension in AV3V-lesioned Brattleboro rats in opposition to its action in unlesioned animals in this strain. The difference between DOC–salt treated, AV3V-lesioned Brattleboro and ordinary laboratory rats in their response to exogenous vasopressin may possibly be due to differences in synthesis or content of vasopressin within the brain in areas other than the neurohypophysis.

The malignant form of DOC–salt hypertension in the rat is characterized by a ten-fold increase in circulating levels of vasopressin compared to the two- to four-fold increase observed in benign hypertension (Mohring *et al.*, 1977). It has been suggested that hypovolemia contributes to the marked increase in the circulating levels of this hormone. Antivasopressin antibodies substantially reduce arterial pressure in malignant DOC–salt hypertension while vascular antagonists do not have a significant effect (Mohring *et al.*, 1977; Rabito, Carretero and Scicli, 1981). Rabito, Carretero and Scicli (1981) have also been unable to demonstrate blood pressure reduction by peptide antagonists of the vascular action of vasopressin in malignant hypertension due to adrenal regeneration, another model of experimental hypertension thought to be secondary to mineralocortcoid excess.

Table 3.5 Hypertensive interventions studied in the rat with hereditary hypothalamic diabetes insipidus (Brattleboro strain)

Intervention	Result	References
Two-kidney, one-clip Goldblatt	Same degree of hypertension as Long-Evans controls	Johnston, Newman and Woods (1981)
Aortic ligature	Same degree of hypertension as Long-Evans controls	Woods *et al.* (1983)
One-kidney, one-clip Goldblatt	Less arterial pressure elevation than Long-Evans controls. Antidiuretic analog (DDAVP) restores full development of hypertension	Johnston, Newman and Woods (1981); Share *et al.* (1982)
Glycerol-ATN	Do not develop hypertension	Konrads *et al.* (1979)
SHR/Brattleboro crossbreeding	Same degree of hypertension as SHR	Ganten *et al.* (1983)
DOC–salt	Do not develop hypertension unless given exogenous vasopressin replacement	Crofton *et al.* (1979); Berecek *et al.* (1982a and b)

The discrepancy between the results with antagonists and antibodies is not readily explained. Non-specific effects of the antibody or differences in the degree of elevation of plasma vasopressin concentration (not reported in the study by Rabito, Carretero and Scicli) may account for the various results reported.

VASOPRESSIN IN CLINICAL HYPERTENSION

The first attempt to measure vasopressin production in essential hypertension was reported by Ellis and Grollman (1949) who found that bioassayable vasopressin in urine extracts was greater than normal in 75% of hypertensive men. These authors emphasized the antidiuretic action of the hormone, speculating that vasopressin might contribute to fluid retention in hypertensives. Vasopressin then received little attention in clinical hypertension until the comprehensive study by Padfield *et al.* (1976) in which a radioimmunoassay was used in patients with benign essential hypertension. No elevated plasma vasopressin concentrations were found. 75% of patients had plasma vasopressin within the range of normal subjects and 25% were below normal. The mean plasma vasopressin for the hypertensive group was significantly less than that of normotensive controls. In a more recent study Cowley *et al.* (1981) found plasma vasopressin in essential hypertensives to be nearly twice that of normotensives. Hypertensives tended to have greater increases in plasma vasopressin with high salt intake and when older than 50 years of age compared to normotensives. The hypertensive subjects had a smaller urine sodium concentration compared to normotensive controls, suggesting that a decrease in the concentrating ability of the kidney could be responsible for compensatory oversecretion of vasopressin, which in turn may play a role in maintenance of elevated blood pressure if the hormone concentration in plasma reaches levels sufficient to exert a vasoconstrictor action.

Differences between these studies are not readily explained. They could be partially accounted for by the recent observations of Preibisz *et al.* (1983) that 90% of circulating vasopressin in humans is bound to or within platelets. In normals, vasopressin concentration of platelet-free plasma obtained by special centrifugation techniques was half that measured in routinely spun samples. With these techniques, authors found a positive correlation between serum osmolality and platelet-rich but not platelet-free plasma vasopressin in normal subjects. Abnormalities in benign essential hypertensives included an elevated plasma vasopressin concentration in male hypertensives and elevated platelet-associated vasopressin concentration in hypertensives of both sexes (*Table 3.6*). Patients did not show correlation between serum osmolality and platelet vasopressin as normals did. Hypertensives had an inverse correlation between serum osmolality and plasma vasopressin, not observed in normotensive men. These observations remain to be confirmed and their physiological significance elucidated. However, it is clear that differences in sample preparation may affect results and account for conflicting reports.

A somewhat different approach to determine the role of circulating vasopressin in human hypertension is the measurement of vasopressin-associated neurophysin, which is known to be released in parallel with vasopressin in response to physiological and pharmacological stimuli. Amico *et al.* (1984) have found no increase in vasopressin-associated neurophysin of human hypertensives. They did find that 25% of the hypertensive patients studied had an increase in the oxytocin-associated neurophysin. Whether plasma levels of oxytocin are elevated in these patients and play any role in sodium metabolism as hypothesized by others (Burstyn, Horrobin and Manku, 1972) is as yet a matter of pure speculation.

Urine excretion of vasopressin was measured by Khokhar and Slater (1976) by radioimmunoassay in an attempt to provide information about integrated secretion of the hormone over a period of time. Similar vasopressin excretion rates were found in young benign hypertensives and normotensive controls when both groups were on unrestricted fluid intake, having a urine osmolality between 0 and 400 mOsmol/kg. During water deprivation urine vasopressin increased more in hypertensives than in controls, this difference becoming progressively larger with higher degrees of dehydration. Despite the difference in urine vasopressin response

Table 3.6 Vasopressin in human hypertension

	Source		Normal range	Hypertensives	Reference
Benign essential hypertension	Urine (bioassay)		92–130 U	90–180 U*	Ellis and Grollman (1949)
	Urine (RIA)†	(a)	55 ± 5 fmol/min	54 ± 9 fmol/min	Khokhar and Slater (1976)
		(b)	102 ± 6 fmol/min	167 ± 12 fmol/min	
	Urine (RIA)		74 ± 10 ng/day	48 ± 8 ng/day*	Shimamoto et al. (1979)
	Plasma (RIA)		6.1 ± 0.3 pg/ml	4.9 ± 0.2 pg/ml*	Padfield et al. (1976)
	Plasma (RIA)		4.5 ± 0.2 pg/ml	4.0 ± 0.1 pg/ml*	Shimamoto et al. (1979)
	Plasma (RIA)		4.7 ± 0.4 pg/ml	8.5 ± 1.0 pg/ml*	Cowley et al. (1981)
	Plasma (RIA)	(c)	1.4 ± 1.0 pg/ml	2.3 ± 0.3 pg/ml*	Preibisz et al. (1983)
		(d)	12.9 ± 5.7 pg/ml	9.3 ± 0.9 pg/ml*	
Malignant hypertension	Plasma (RIA)		5.8 ± 0.2 pg/ml	13.0 ± 2.0 pg/ml*	Padfield et al. (1981)
Primary aldosteronism	Plasma (RIA)		6.1 ± 0.3 pg/ml	4.7 ± 0.6 pg/ml*	Padfield (1977)
	Plasma (RIA)		2.3 ± 0.3 pg/ml	1.3 ± 0.3 pg/ml	Ganguly and Robertson (1981)

(a) normally hydrated, (b) dehydrated, (c) platelet-free plasma, (d) platelet-rich plasma
* indicates statistically significant difference between hypertensives and controls
† RIA = radioimmunoassay

to dehydration between hypertensives and normotensives, renal responses were identical in the two groups as assessed by changes in serum osmolality and tubular reabsorption of water. These observations led these authors to speculate that the kidney of hypertensive patients was partially resistant to the action of the antidiuretic hormone. Therefore, a disproportionate increase in secretion rate of this hormone in response to mild dehydration might exert vascular effects contributing to arterial pressure elevation.

Shimamoto *et al.* (1979) observed changes in urine vasopressin excretion in hypertensives opposite to those mentioned above. Urine vasopressin was diminished by 35% in benign essential hypertensives when compared to that of controls. By simultaneous study of plasma vasopressin in these patients they concluded that vasopressin regulation in response to arterial pressure and blood volume changes (obtained by treatment with bedrest and subsequent sodium restriction) was preserved in human hypertensives. They confirmed the reduction of plasma vasopressin concentration observed previously by Padfield in human hypertensives and attributed it to the elevated arterial pressure. Thus, the difference in urine vasopressin between their patients and those of Khokhar and Slater is not readily explained.

In the malignant phase of essential hypertension Padfield *et al.* (1976) reported a mean plasma vasopressin 70% greater than the normal mean, a significant increase. A weak positive correlation was found between plasma vasopressin and plasma angiotensin II concentrations. In another study this group (Padfield *et al.*, 1981) demonstrated that infusion of vasopressin in normal volunteers, at doses that increase plasma concentration by three- to twelve -fold compared to those in malignant hypertensives, do not raise arterial pressure. Similarly, elevated levels of plasma vasopressin in patients with the syndrome of inappropriate antidiuretic hormone excess (SIADH) were not associated with hypertension. It thus seems certain that vasopressin does not cause malignant hypertension but is most likely increased secondary to increased renin and hypovolemia in these patients. However, an exceptional patient has been reported (Khokhar *et al.*, 1980) in whom a hypertensive response to dehydration was noted in the setting of malignant hypertension and concurrent nephrogenic diabetes insipidus. The degree of elevation of diastolic blood pressure and plasma vasopressin during dehydration in this patient was almost identical to that observed in normal volunteers in whom diastolic blood pressure and plasma vasopressin concentration were raised by infusion of the hormone.

There are no systematic studies of the role of vasopressin in secondary forms of hypertension such as renovascular hypertension, pheochromocytoma or chronic renal disease. In patients with primary hyperaldosteronism, plasma vasopressin concentration is diminished (Padfield, 1977) which has been attributed to volume expansion. This is a surprising finding when compared to the evidence for elevated vasopressin production in DOC–salt hypertension in the rat as this experimental model is considered to be a counterpart to mineralocorticoid hypertension in humans. The regulation of plasma vasopressin concentration by osmolar and non-osmolar stimuli has been recently studied by Ganguly and Robertson (1981) in patients with primary hyperaldosteronism compared to essential hypertensives with different plasma renin activity levels. Patients with primary hyperaldosteronism had a tendency to reduced levels of plasma vasopressin. Both these patients and those with low-renin essential hypertension were characterized by an elevated osmolar threshold (7 mOsmol/kg) for vasopressin release in response to hypertonic saline when compared to normals or to patients with high or normal renin essential hypertension. Vasopressin responses to trimetaphan-induced reduction in arterial pressure were not different between the four groups. Volume expansion in primary hyperaldosteronism and as yet unidentified mechanisms in low-renin essential hypertension (reduced angiotensin II?) may account for the resetting of the osmolar control of vasopressin in these two groups.

In summary, abnormalities of plasma concentration and urine excretion of vasopressin have been detected in several forms and stages of human hypertension. They may reflect abnormalities in renal tubular responsiveness to the hormone, or be secondary to increased arterial pressure, angiotensin II or blood volume changes in the diverse forms of human hypertension. Although infusion studies in normal volunteers and findings in patients with the syndrome of inappropriate antidiuretic hormone excess do not strongly support a pathogenetic role for the vascular action of vasopressin in human hypertension, these studies do not address the possibility that vascular responsiveness to vasopressin or baroreflex buffering of its vasoconstrictor action are altered in hypertensive patients, thus amplifying the vascular effect of modest increases in plasma concentration. If the role of vasopressin is to be fully understood, clinical investigations will combine specific pharmacologic blockade with radioimmunoassay in hypertensive subjects. The availability of several antagonists for experimental use indicates the feasibility of this approach for direct quantification of both the antidiuretic and vasoconstrictor actions of vasopressin in clinical hypertension and other diseases such as congestive heart failure.

References

AHMED, A. B. J., GEORGE, B. C., GONZALEZ-AUVERT, C. and DINGMAN, J. F. (1967) Increased plasma arginine vasopressin in clinical adrenocortical insufficiency and its inhibition by glucosteroids. *Journal of Clinical Investigation*, **46**, 111–123

AISENBREY, G. A., HANDELMAN, W. A., ARNOLD, P., MANNING, M. and SCHRIER, R. W. (1981) Vascular effects of arginine vasopressin during fluid deprivation in the rat. *Journal of Clinical Investigation*, **67**, 961–968

ALEXANDER, R. W., HYMAN, S., ATKINSON, W. and GIMBRONE, M. A. (1980) Regulation of angiotensin II receptors in cultured vascular smooth muscle cells. *Circulation*, **62** (Supply. III), 90 (Abstract)

ALTURA, B. M. and ALTURA, B. T. (1977) Vascular smooth muscle and neurohypophyseal hormones. *Federation Proceedings*, **36**, 1853–1860

AMICO, J. A., CORDER, C. N., MCDONALD, R. H. and ROBINSON, A. G. (1984) Levels of the oxytocin-associated and vasopressin-associated neurophysins in plasma and their responses in essential hypertension. *Clinical Endocrinology,* **20**, 289–297

ANDERSON, R. J., PLUSS, R. G., BERNS, A. S. *et al* (1978) Mechanism of effect of hypoxia on renal water excretion. *Journal of Clinical Investigation*, **62**, 769–777

ANDERSSON, B. and OLSSON, K. (1977) Evidence for periventricular sodium-sensitive receptors of importance in the regulation of ADH secretion. In *Neurohypophysis*, edited by A. M. Moses and L. Share, pp. 118–127. Basel: S. Karger

ANDERSSON, B. and WESTBYE, O. (1970) Synergistic action of sodium and angiotensin on brain mechanisms controlling fluid balance. *Life Sciences*, **9**, 601–608

ANDREWS, C. E. and BRENNER, B. M. (1981) Relative contributions of arginine vasopressin and angiotensin II to maintenance of systemic arterial pressure in the anesthetized water-deprived rat. *Circulation Research*, **48**, 254–258

BAYLIS, P. H. and HEATH, D. A. (1977) Influence of presyncope and postural change upon plasma arginine vasopressin concentrations in hydrated and dehydrated man. *Clinical Endocrinology*, **7**, 79–83

BERECEK, K. H., MURRAY, R. D., GROSS, F. and BRODY, M. J. (1982a) Vasopressin and vascular reactivity in development of DOCA hypertension in rats with hereditary diabetes insipidus (DI). *Hypertension*, **4**, 3–12

BERECEK, K. H., BARRON, K. W., WEBB, R. L. and BRODY, M. J. (1982b) Vasopressin-central nervous system interactions in the development of DOCA hypertension. *Hypertension*, **4** (Suppl. II), 131–137

BERECEK, K. H., BARRON, K. W., WEBB, R. L. and BRODY, M. J. (1982c) Relationship between vasopressin and the anteroventral third ventricle region in deoxycorticosterone/salt hypertension. *Annals of the New York Academy of Sciences*, **394**, 392–397

BERL, T., CADNAPAPHORNCHAI, P., HARBOTTLE, J. A. and SCHRIER, R. W. (1974a) Mechanism of stimulation of vasopressin release during beta-adrenergic stimulation with isoproterenol. *Journal of Clinical Investigation*, **53**, 857–867

BERL, T., HARBOTTLE, J. A., CADNAPAPHORNCHAI, P. and SCHRIER, R. W. (1974b) Mechanism of suppression of vasopressin during alpha adrenergic stimulation with norepinephrine. *Journal of Clinical Investigation*, **53**, 219–227

BICHET, D., SZATALOWICZ, V., CHAIMOVITZ, C. and SCHRIER, R. W. (1982) Role of vasopressin in abnormal water excretion in cirrhotic patients. *Annals of Internal Medicine*, **96**, 413–417

BLESSING, W. W., SVED, A. F. and REIS, D. J. (1982) Destruction of noradrenergic neurons in rabbit brainstem elevates plasma vasopressin, causing hypertension. *Science*, **217**, 661–662

BONJOUR, J. P. and MALVIN, R. L. (1970) Stimulation of ADH release by the renin-angiotensin system. *American Journal of Physiology*, **218**, 1555–1559

BOYKIN, J., DE TORRENTE, A., ROBERTSON, G. L., ERICKSON, A. and SCHRIER, R. W. (1979) Persistent plasma vasopressin levels in the hypo-osmolar state associated with mineralocorticoid deficiency. *Mineral and Electrolyte Metabolism*, **2**, 310–315

BROOKS, V. L. and MALVIN, R. L. (1979) An intracerebral, physiological role for angiotensin: effects of central blockade. *Federation Proceedings*, **38**, 2272–2275

BRUNNER, H. R., KIRSHMAN, J. D., SEALEY, J. E. and LARAGH, J. H. (1971) Hypertension of renal origin: evidence for two different mechanisms. *Science*, **174**, 1344–1346

BURNIER, M., BIOLLAZ, J., BRUNNER, D. B., GAVRAS, H. and BRUNNER, H. R. (1983) Alpha and beta-adrenoceptor blockade in normotensive and deoxycortico-sterone (DOC) hypertensive rats; plasma vasopressin and vasopressin pressor effect. *Journal of Pharmacology and Experimental Therapeutics*, **224**, 222–227

BURNIER, M. and BRUNNER, H. R. (1983) Pressor responses of rats to vasopressin: effect of sodium, angiotensin and catecholamines. *American Journal of Physiology*, **244**, H253–H258

BURSTYN, P. G., HORROBIN, D. F. and MANKU, M. S. (1972) Saluretic action of aldosterone in the presence of increased salt intake and restoration of normal action by prolactin or oxytocin. *Journal of Endocrinology*, **55**, 369–376

CADNAPAPHORNCHAI, P., BOYKIN, J. L., BERL, T., MCDONALD, K. M. and SCHRIER, R. W. (1974) Mechanism of effect of nicotine on renal water retention. *American Journal of Physiology*, **227**, 1216–1220

CARRETERO, O. A. and SCICLI, A. G. (1981) Possible role of kinins in circulatory homeostasis. State of the art review. *Hypertension*, **3** (Suppl. I), 4–12

CHAROCOPOS, F., HATZINIKOLAOU, P., NORTH, W. G. and GAVRAS, H. (1982) Systemic and regional hemodynamic effects of endogenous vasopressin stimulation in rats. *American Journal of Physiology*, **243**, H560–H565

COWLEY, A. W., MONOS, E. and GUYTON, A. C. (1974) Interaction of vasopressin and the baroreceptor reflex system in the regulation of arterial blood pressure in the dog. *Circulation Research*, **34**, 505–514

COWLEY, A. W., SWITZER, S. J. and GUINN, M. M. (1980) Evidence and quantification of the vasopressin arterial pressure control system in the dog. *Circulation Research*, **46**, 58–67

COWLEY, A. W., SWITZER, S. J. and SKELTON, M. M. (1981) Vasopressin, fluid, and electrolyte response to chronic angiotensin II infusion. *American Journal of Physiology*, **240**, R130–R138

COWLEY, A. W., CUSHMAN, W. C., QUILLEN, E. W., SKELTON, M. M. and LANGFORD, H. G. (1981) Vasopressin elevation in essential hypertension and increased responsiveness to sodium intake. *Hypertension* **3**, (Suppl. I), 93–100

CROFTON, J. T., SHARE, L., SHADE, R. E., ALLEN, C. and TARNOWSKI, D. (1978) Vasopressin in the rat with spontaneous hypertension. *American Journal of Physiology*, **235**, H361–H366

CROFTON, J. T., SHARE, L., SHADE, R. E., LEE-KWON, W. J., MANNING, M. and SAWYER, W. H. (1979) The importance of vasopressin in the development and maintenance of DOC–salt hypertension in the rat. *Hypertension*, **1**, 31–38

CROFTON, J. T., SHARE, L., WANG, B. C. and SHADE, R. E. (1980) Pressor responsiveness to vasopressin in the rat with DOC–salt hypertension. *Hypertension*, **2**, 424–431

CROFTON, J. T., SHARE, L., BAER, P. G., ALLEN, C. M. and WANG, B. C. (1981a) Vasopressin secretion in the New Zealand genetically hypertensive rat. *Clinical and Experimental Hypertension*, **3**, 975–989

CROFTON, J. T., ROCHOLD, R. W., SHARE, L., WANG, B. C., HOROVITZ, Z. P., MANNING, M. and SAWYER, W. H. (1981b) Effect of intracerebroventricular captopril on vasopressin and blood pressure in spontaneously hypertensive rats. *Hypertension*, **3** (Suppl. II), 71–74

DAVIES, R., FORSLING, M. L. and SLATER, J. D. H. (1977) The interrelationship between the release of renin and vasopressin as defined by orthostasis and propranolol. *Journal of Clinical Investigation*, **60**, 1438–1441

DE CHAMPLAIN, J., KRAKOFF, L. R. and AXELROD, J. (1967) Catecholamine metabolism in experimental hypertension in the rat. *Circulation Research*, **20**, 136–145

DE WIED, D. (1971) Long-term effect of vasopressin on the maintenance of a conditioned avoidance response in rats. *Nature*, **232**, 58

DI PETTE, D. J., GAVRAS, I., NORTH, W. G., BRUNNER, H. R. and GAVRAS, H. (1982) Vasopressin in salt-induced hypertension of experimental renal insufficiency. *Hypertension*, **4** (Suppl. II), 125–130

DOUSA, T. P. (1977) Cyclic nucleotides in the cellular action of neurohypophyseal hormones. *Federation Proceedings*, **36**, 1867–1871

DUNN, F. L., BRENNAN, T. J., NELSON, A. E. and ROBERTSON, G. L. (1973) The role of blood osmolality and volume in regulating vasopressin secretion in the rat. *Journal of Clinical Investigation*, **52**, 3212–3219

DUNN, M. J., GREELY, H. P., VALTIN, H., KINTER, L. B. and BEEUWKES, R. (1978) Renal excretion of prostaglandins E2 and F2 in diabetes insipidus rats. *American Journal of Physiology*, **235**, E624–E627

ELIJOVICH, F., BARRY, C. R., KRAKOFF, L. F. and KIRCHBERGER, M. Differential effect of vasopressin on angiotensin and norepinephrine pressor action in rats. *American Journal of Physiology* (in press)

ELIJOVICH, F., LESKIW, U. A. and KRAKOFF, L. R. (1981) Vasopressin-dependent arterial pressure in the renoprival rat. *Kidney International*, **19**, 166 (Abstract)

ELIJOVICH, F., KIRCHBERGER, M., BARRY, C. R. and KRAKOFF, L. R. (1983a) Effect of naloxone upon maintenance of arterial pressure by vasopressin and renin in adrenal insufficiency. *Clinical Research*, **31**, 329A (Abstract)

ELIJOVICH, F., KIRCHBERGER, M., BARRY, C. R. and KRAKOFF, L. R. (1983b) Vasopressin maintains blood pressure in adrenalectomy. *Kidney International*, **23**, 168 (Abstract)

ELIJOVICH, F., KIRCHBERGER, M., BARRY, C. R. and KRAKOFF, L. R. (1983c) Maintenance of arterial pressure by vasopressin and angiotensin II in adrenalectomy. *Hypertension*, **5**, (Suppl. V), V53–V56

ELLIS, M. E. and GROLLMAN, A. (1949) The antidiuretic hormone in the urine in experimental and clinical hypertension. *Endocrinology*, **44**, 415–419

FEJES-TOTH, G., ZAHAJSZKY, T. and JANOS, F. (1980) Effect of vasopressin on renal kallikrein excretion. *American Journal of Physiology*, **239**, F388–F392

FRIEDMAN, S. M., FRIEDMAN, C. L. and NAKASHIMA, M. (1960) Accelerated appearance of DCA hypertension in rats treated with pitressin. *Endocrinology*, **67**, 752–759

GAINER, H., SARNE, Y. and BROWNSTEIN, M. J. (1977) Neurophysin biosynthesis: conversion of a putative precursor during axonal transport. *Science*, **195**, 1354–1356

GANGULY, A. and ROBERTSON, G. L. (1981) Osmoregulation and baroregulation of vasopressin secretion in normal, high and low renin hypertension. *Proceedings of the 63rd Annual Meeting of the Endocrine Society*, p. 259 (Abstract)

GANTEN, U., RASCHER, W., LANG, R. E., DIETZ, R., RETTIG, R., UNGER, T., TAUGNER, R. and GANTEN, D. (1983) Development of a new strain of spontaneously hypertensive rats homozygous for hypothalamic diabetes insipidus. *Hypertension*, **5** (Suppl. I), 119–128

GAVRAS, H., BRUNNER, H. R., VAUGHAN, E. D. and LARAGH, J. H. (1973) Angiotensin–sodium interaction in blood pressure maintenance of renal hypertensive and normotensive rats. *Science*, **180**, 1369–1372

GAVRAS, H., BRUNNER, H. R., THURSTON, H. and LARAGH, J. H. (1975) Reciprocation of renin dependency with sodium volume dependency in renal hypertension. *Science*, **188**, 1316–1317

GAVRAS, H., HATZINIKOLAOU, P., NORTH, W. G., BRESNAHAN, M. and GAVRAS, I. (1982) Interaction of the sympathetic nervous system with vasopressin and renin in the maintenance of blood pressure. *Hypertension*, **4**, 400–405

GRANTHAM, J. J. and BURG, M. B. (1966) Effect of vasopressin and cyclic AMP on permeability of isolated collecting tubules. *American Journal of Physiology*, **211**, 255–259

GROSSMAN, A., BESSER, G. M., MILLES, J. J. and BAYLIS, P. H. (1980) Inhibition of vasopressin release in man by an opiate peptide. *Lancet*, **2**, 1108–1110

GUYTON, A. C., COWLEY, A. W., SMITH, M. J., MANNING, R. D. and HOCKEL, G. M. (1980) Hypertensive and hypotensive roles of other hormones: vasopressin, prostaglandin, and kallikrein-kinin systems. In *Circulatory Physiology III: Arterial Pressure and Hypertension*, edited by A. C. Guyton, pp. 225–235. Philadelphia: W. B. Saunders

HATZINIKOLAOU, P., GAVRAS, H., BRUNNER, H. R. and GAVRAS, I. (1980) Sodium-induced elevation of blood pressure in the anephric state. *Science*, **209**, 935–936

HATZINIKOLAOU, P., GAVRAS, H., BRUNNER, H. R. and GAVRAS, I. (1981) Role of vasopressin catecholamines, and plasma volume in hypertonic-saline induced hypertension. *American Journal of Physiology*, **240**, H827–H831

HEYNDRICKX, G. R., BOETTCHER, D. H. and VATNER, S. F. (1976) Effects of angiotensin, vasopressin and methoxamine on cardiac function and blood flow distribution in conscious dogs. *American Journal of Physiology*, **231**, 1579–1587

HOFBAUER, K. G., KONRADS, A., BAUEREISS, K., MOHRING, B., MOHRING, J. and GROSS, F. (1977) Vasopressin and renin in glycerol-induced acute renal failure in the rat. *Circulation Research*, **41**, 424–428

HOFFMAN, W. E. (1980) Regional vascular effects of antidiuretic hormone in normal and sympathetic blocked rats. *Endocrinology*, **107**, 334–341

HOFFMAN, W. E., PHILLIPS, M. I., SCHMID, P. G., FALCON, J. and WEET, J. F. (1977) Antidiuretic hormone release and the pressor response to central angiotensin II and cholinergic stimulation. *Neuropharmacology*, **16**, 463–472

HOFFMAN, W. E. and SCHMID, P. G. (1978a) Separation of pressor and antidiuretic effects of intraventricular bradykinin. *Neuropharmacology*, **17**, 999–1002

HOFFMAN, W. E. and SCHMID, P. G. (1978b) Cardiovascular and antidiuretic effects of central histamine. *Life Sciences*, **22**, 1709–1714

HOWELL, W. H. (1898) The physiological effects of extracts of the hypophysis cerebri and infundibular body. *Journal of Experimental Medicine*, **3**, 245–258

HUMPHREYS, M. H., FRIEDLER, R. M. and EARLEY, L. E. (1970) Natriuresis produced by vasopressin or hemorrhage during water diuresis in the dog. *American Journal of Physiology*, **219**, 658–665

ISHIKAWA, S., HANDELMAN, W., SCHRIER, R. W. and BERL, T. (1981) Evidence for a role of cellular calcium (Ca) uptake in the nonosmotic release of arginine vasopressin (AVP) in the conscious rat. *Kidney International*, **19**, 244 (Abstract)

ISHIKAWA, S. and SCHRIER, R. W. (1982) Evidence for a role of opioid peptides in the release of arginine vasopressin in the conscious rat. *Journal of Clinical Investigation*, **69**, 666–672

JAENIKE, J. R. (1961) Influence of vasopressin on the permeability of the mammalian collecting duct to urea. *Journal of Clinical Investigation*, **30**, 144–151

JOHNSON, M. D., KINTER, L. B. and BEEUWKES, R. (1979) Effects of AVP and DDAVP on plasma renin activity and electrolyte excretion in conscious dogs. *American Journal of Physiology*, **236**, F66–F70

JOHNSTON, C. I., NEWMAN, M. and WOODS, R. (1981) Role of vasopressin in cardiovascular homeostasis and hypertension. *Clinical Science*, **61**, 129S–139S

KEIL, L. C., SUMMY-LONG, J. and SEVERS, W. B. (1975) Release of vasopressin by angiotensin II. *Endocrinology*, **96**, 1063–1065

KHOKHAR, A. M. and SLATER, J. D. H. (1976) Increased renal excretion of arginine–vasopressin during mild hydropenia in young men with mild essential benign hypertension. *Clinical Science and Molecular Medicine*, **51**, 691S–694S

KHOKHAR, A. M., SLATER, J. D. H., MA, J. and RAMAGE, C. M. (1980) The cardiovascular effect of vasopressin in relation to its plasma concentration in man and its relevance to high blood pressure. *Clinical Endocrinology*, **13**, 259–266

KILCOYNE, M. M., HOFFMAN, D. L. and ZIMMERMAN, E. A. (1980) Immunocytochemical localization of angiotensin II and vasopressin in rat hypothalamus: evidence for production in the same neuron. *Clinical Science*, **59**, 57S–60S

KIRSCHENBAUM, M. A., LOWE, A. G., TRIZNA, W. and FINE, L. G. (1982) Regulation of vasopressin action by prostaglandins. Evidence for prostaglandin synthesis in the rabbit cortical collecting tubule. *Journal of Clinical Investigation*, **70**, 1193–1204

KONRADS, A., HOFBAUER, K. G., BAUEREISS, K., MOHRING, J. and GROSS, F. (1979) Glycerol induced acute renal failure in Brattleboro rats with hypothalamic diabetes insipidus. *Clinical Science*, **56**, 133–138

LEE-KWON, W. J., SHARE, L., CROFTON, J. T. and SHADE, R. E. (1981) Vasopressin in the rat with partial nephrectomy–salt hypertension. *Clinical and Experimental Hypertension*, **3**, 281–297

LEENEN, F. H. H. and DE JONG, W. (1969) Augmentation of the pressor response to octapressin by autonomic blocking agents in the pithed rat. *European Journal of Pharmacology*, **6**, 45–49

LINAS, S. L., BERL, T., ROBERTSON, G. L., AISENBREY, G. A., SCHRIER, R. W. and ANDERSON, R. (1980) Role of vasopressin in the impaired water excretion of glucocorticoid deficiency. *Kidney International*, **18**, 58–67

MANNING, M. and SAWYER, W. H. (1982) Antagonists of vasopressor and antidiuretic responses to arginine vasopressin. *Annals of Internal Medicine*, **96**, 520–522

MATSUGUCHI, H. and SCHMID, P. G. (1982a) Acute interaction of vasopressin and neurogenic mechanisms in DOC–salt hypertension. *American Journal of Physiology*, **242**, H37–H43

MATSUGUCHI, H. and SCHMID, P. G. (1982b) Pressor response to vasopressin and impaired baroreflex function in DOC–salt hypertension. *American Journal of Physiology*, **242**, H44–H49

MATSUGUCHI, H., SCHMID, P. G., VAN ORDEN, D. and MARK, A. L. (1981) Does vasopressin contribute to salt-induced hypertension in the Dahl strain? *Hypertension*, **3**, 174–181

MATSUGUCHI, H., SHARABI, F. M., O'CONNOR, G., MARK, A. L. and SCHMID, P. G. (1982a) Central mechanisms in DOC–salt hypertensive rats. *Clinical and Experimental Hypertension. Theory and Practice*, **A4**, 1303–1321

MATSUGUCHI, H., SHARABI, F. M., GORDON, F. J., JOHNSON, A. K. and SCHMID, P. G. (1982b) Blood pressure and heart rate responses to microinjection of vasopressin into the nucleus tractus solitarius region of the rat. *Neuropharmacology*, **21**, 687–693

MCNEILL, J. R., WILCOX, W. C. and PANG, C. C. Y. (1977) Vasopressin and angiotensin: reciprocal mechanisms controlling mesenteric conductance. *American Journal of Physiology*, **232**, H260–H266

MILLER, T. R., HANDELMAN, W. A., ARNOLD, P. E., MCDONALD, K. M., MOLINOFF, P. G. and SCHRIER, R. W. (1979) Effect of central catecholamine depletion on the osmotic and nonosmotic stimulation of vasopressin (antidiuretic hormone) in the rat. *Journal of Clinical Invesigation*, **64**, 1599–1607

MOHRING, J., KINTZ, J. and SCHOUN, J. (1979) Studies on the role of vasopressin in blood pressure control of spontaneously hypertensive rats with established hypertension (SHR, stroke-prone strain). *Journal of Cardiovascular Pharmacology*, **1**, 593–608

MOHRING, J., MOHRING, B., PETRI, M. and HAACK, D. (1977) Vasopressor role of ADH in the pathogenesis of malignant DOC hypertension. *American Journal of Physiology*, **232**, F260–F269

MOHRING, J., MOHRING, B., PETRIC, M. and HAACK, D. (1978) Plasma vasopressin concentration and effects of vasopressin antiserum on blood pressure in rats with malignant two-kidney Goldblatt hypertension. *Circulation Research*, **42**, 17–23

MOHRING, J., KINTZ, J., SCHOUN, J. and MCNEILL, R. J. (1981) Pressor responsiveness and cardiovascular reflex activity in spontaneously hypertensive and normotensive rats during vasopressin infusion. *Journal of Cardiovascular Pharmacology*, **3**, 948–957

MOHRING, J., SCHOUN, J., KINTZ, J. and MCNEILL, R. (1980) Decreased vasopressin content in brain stem of rats with spontaneous hypertension. *Naunyn-Schmiedeberg's Archives of Pharmacology*, **315**, 83–84

MONTANI, J. P., LIARD, J. F., SCHOUND, J. and MOHRING, J. (1980) Hemodynamic effects of exogenous and endogenous vasopressin at low plasma concentrations in conscious dogs. *Circulation Research*, **47**, 346–355

MORTON, J. J., SEMPLE, P. F., LEDINGHAM, I. M. *et al.* (1977) Effect of angiotensin-converting enzyme inhibitor (SQ 20881) on the plasma concentration of angiotensin I, angiotensin, II, and arginine vasopressin in the dog during hemorrhagic shock. *Circulation Research*, **41**, 301–308

PADFIELD, P. L. (1977) Vasopressin in hypertension. *American Heart Journal*, **94**, 531–532

PADFIELD, P. L., BROWN, J. J., LEVER, A. F., MORTON, J. J. and ROBERTSON, J. I. S. (1981) Blood pressure in acute and chronic vasopressin excess. Studies on malignant hypertension and the syndrome of inappropriate antidiuretic hormone secretion. *New England Journal of Medicine*, **304**, 1067–1070

PADFIELD, P. L., LEVER, A. F., BROWN, J. J., MORTON, J. J. and ROBERTSON, J. I. S. (1976) Changes of vasopressin in hypertension: cause or effect? *Lancet*, **1**, 1255–1257

PANG, C. C. Y., WILCOX, W. C. and MCNEILL, R. (1979) Hypophysectomy and saralasin on mesenteric vasoconstrictor response to vasopressin. *American Journal of Physiology*, **236**, H200–H205

PREIBISZ, J. J., SEALEY, J. E., LARAGH, J. H., CODY, R. J. and WEKSLER, B. B. (1983) Plasma and platelet vasopressin in essential hypertension and congestive heart failure. *Hypertension*, **5** (Suppl. I), 129–138

PULLAN, P. T., JOHNSTON, C. I., ANDERSON, W. P. and KORNER, P. I. (1980) Plasma vasopressin in blood pressure homeostasis and in experimental renal hypertension. *American Journal of Physiology*, **239**, H81–H87

RABITO, S. F., CARRETERO, O. A. and SCICLI, A. G. (1981) Evidence against a role of vasopressin in the maintenance of high blood pressure in mineralocorticoid and renovascular hypertension. *Hypertension*, **3**, 34–38

RASCHER, W., LANG, R. E., GANTEN, D., MEFFLE, H., TAUBITZ, M., UNGER, T. and GROSS, F. (1983) Vasopressin in deoxycorticosterone acetate hypertension of rats: a hemodynamic analysis. *Journal of Cardiovascular Pharmacology*, **5**, 418–425

RIBEIRO, A. and KRAKOFF, L. R. (1978) Adrenal gland in experimental renal hypertension. *American Journal of Physiology*, **234**, E267–E272

ROBERTSON, G. L. (1977) The regulation of vasopressin function in health and disease. *Recent Progress in Hormone Research*, **33**, 333–375

ROBERTSON, G. L. and ATHAR, S. (1976) The interaction of blood osmolality and blood volume in regulating plasma vasopressin in man. *Journal of Clinical Endocrinology and Metabolism*, **42**, 613–620

ROBERTSON, G. L., ATHAR, S. and SHELTON, R. L. (1977) The osmoregulation of vasopressin. *Kidney International*, **10**, 25–37

ROBERTSON, G. L., AYCINENA, P. and ZERBE, R. L. (1982) Neurogenic disorders of osmoregulation. *American Journal of Medicine*, **72**, 339–353

ROCKHOLD, R. W., CROFTON, J. T. and SHARE, L. (1980) Increased pressor responsiveness to enkephalin in spontaneously hypertensive rats: the role of vasopressin. *Clinical Science*, **59**, 235S–237S

ROSSIER, J., BATTENBERG, E., PITTMAN, Q. *et al.* (1979) Hypothalamic enkephalin neurones may regulate the neurohypophysis. *Nature*, **277**, 653–655

SAITO, T., YAJIMA, Y. and WATANABE, T. (1980) Involvement of AVP in the development and maintenance of hypertension in rats. In *Antidiuretic Hormone*, edited by S. Yoshida, L. Share and K. Yagi, pp. 215–225. Tokyo: Japan Scientific Society Press

SCHIFFRIN, E. L. and GENEST, J. (1983) 3H-Vasopressin binding to the rat mesenteric artery. *Endocrinology*, **113**, 409–411

SCHRIER, R. W., BERL, T. and ANDERSON, R. J. (1979) Osmotic and non-osmotic control of vasopressin release. *American Journal of Physiology*, **236**, F321–F332

SCHRIER, R. and ISHIKAWA, S. (1982) Effect of arginine vasopressin (AVP) antagonist on renal water excretion in glucocorticoid deficient rats. *Kidney International*, **21**, 265 (Abstract)

SCHWARTZ, J. and REID, I. A. (1981) Effect of vasopressin blockade on blood pressure regulation during hemorrhage in conscious dogs. *Endocrinology*, **109**, 1778–1780

SEVERS, W. B., SUMMY-LONG, J., TAYLOR, S. and CONNOR, J. D. (1970) A central effect of angiotensin: release of pituitary pressor material. *Journal of Pharmacology and Experimental Therapeutics*, **174**, 27–34

SHADE, R. E. and SHARE, L. (1977) Renal vasopressin clearance with reduction in renal blood flow in the dog. *American Journal of Physiology*, **232**, F341–F347

SHARE, L. (1976) Role of cardiovascular receptors in the control of ADH release. *Cardiology* (Suppl.), **61**, 51–64

SHARE, L. and CROFTON, J. T. (1982) Contribution of vasopressin to hypertension. *Hypertension*, **4** (Suppl. III), 85–92

SHARE, L., CROFTON, J. T., LEE-KWON, W. J. and SHADE, R. E. (1982) One-clip, one-kidney hypertension in rats with hereditary hypothalamic diabetes insipidus. *Clinical and Experimental Hypertension*, **A4**, 1261–1270

SHARE, L., SHADE, R. E. and RABKIN, R. (1978) Studies on the metabolism of vasopressin with emphasis on the role of the kidney. In *Neurohypophysis*, edited by A. M. Moses and L. Share, pp. 52–64. Basel: S. Karger

SHIMAMOTO, K., ANDO, T., NAKAHASHI, Y. *et al.* (1979) Plasma and urinary ADH levels in patients with essential hypertension. *Japanese Circulation Journal*, **43**, 43–47

SILVERMAN, A. J., HOFFMAN, D., GADDE, C. A., KREY, L. C. and ZIMMERMAN, E. A. (1981) Adrenal steroid inhibition of the vasopressin-neurophysin neurosecretory system to the median eminence of the rat. *Neuroendocrinology*, **32**, 129–133

SIMANTOV, R. and SNYDER, S. H. (1977) Opiate receptor binding in the pituitary gland. *Brain Research*, **124**, 178–184

SKOWSKI, W. and KIKUCHI, T. (1978) The role of vasopressin in the impaired water excretion of myxedema. *American Journal of Medicine*, **64**, 613–621

SLADEK, C. D. and JOYNT, R. J. (1979) Angiotensin stimulation of vasopressin release from the rat hypothalamoneurohypophyseal system in organ culture. *Endocrinology*, **104**, 148–153

SLADEK, C. D. and KNIGGE, K. M. (1977) Osmotic control of vasopressin release by rat hypothalamoneurohypophyseal explants in organ culture. *Endocrinology*, **101**, 1834–1838

SPERTINI, F., BRUNNER, H. R., WAEBER, B. and GAVRAS, H. (1981) The opposing effects of chronic angiotensin-converting enzyme blockade by captopril on the responses to exogenous angiotensin II and vasopressin vs norepinephrine in rats. *Circulation Research*, **48**, 612–618

STARK, R. I., WARDLAW, S. L., DANIEL, S. S. *et al.* (1982) Vasopressin secretion induced by hypoxia in sheep: developmental changes and relationship to β-endorphin release. *American Journal of Obstetrics and Gynecology*, **143**, 204–215

STILLMAN, M. A., RECHT, L. D., ROSARIO, S. L., SEIF, S. M., ROBINSON, G. and ZIMMERMAN, E. A. (1977) The effects of adrenalectomy and glucocorticoid replacement on vasopressin and vasopressin-neurophysin in the zona externa of the median eminence of the rat. *Endocrinology*, **101**, 42–49

STREETEN, D. H. P., MOSES, A. M. and MILLER, M. (1980) Disorders of the neurohypophysis. In *Harrison's Principles of Internal Medicine*, edited by K. J. Isselbacher, R. D. Adams, E. Braunwald, R. G. Petersdorf and J. D. Wilson, pp. 1684–1694. New York: McGraw-Hill

TAKAHASHI, H. and BUÑAG, R. D. (1981) Pressor responses to centrally administered prostaglandin E2 in spontaneously hypertensive rats. *Hypertension*, **3**, 426–432

THAMES, M. D. and SCHMID, P. G. (1979) Cardiopulmonary receptors with vagal afferents tonically inhibit ADH release in the dog. *American Journal of Physiology*, **237**, H299–H304

THAMES, M. D., PETERSON, M. G. and SCHMID, P. G. (1980) Stimulation of cardiac receptors with veratrum alkaloids inhibits ADH secretion. *American Journal of Physiology*, **239**, H784–H788

THURSTON, H. and LARAGH, J. H. (1975) Prior receptor occupancy as a determinant of the pressor activity of infused angiotensin II in the rat. *Circulation Research*, **36**, 113–117

VAN REE, J. M. and DE WIED, D. (1977) Effect of neurohypophyseal hormones on morphine dependence. *Psychoneuroendocrinology*, **2**, 35–41

VAN WIMERSMA-GREIDANUS, T. B., THODY, T. J., VERSPAGET, H. *et al.* (1979) Effects of morphine and β-endorphin on basal and elevated plasma levels of α-MSH and vasopressin. *Life Sciences*, **24**, 579–586

VARMA, S., JAJU, B. P. and BHARGAVA, K. P. (1969) Mechanism of vasopressin-induced bradycardia in dogs. *Circulation Research*, **24**, 787–792

VERNEY, E. B. (1947) The antidiuretic hormone and the factors which determine its release. *Proceedings of the Royal Society of London, Series B*, **135**, 25–105

WALTER, R. and BOWMAN, R. H. (1973) Mechanism of inactivation of vasopressin and oxytocin by the isolated perfused rat kidney. *Endocrinology*, **92**, 189–195

WEINSTEIN, H., BERNE, R. M. and SACHS, H. (1960) Vasopressin in blood: effect of hemorrhage. *Endocrinology*, **66**, 712–718

WEITZMAN, R. E. (1979) Factors regulating the secretion and metabolism of arginine vasopressin (antidiuretic hormone). In *Contemporary Issues in Nephrology. Hormonal Function and the Kidney*, edited by B. M. Brenner and J. H. Stein, pp. 146–168. New York: Churchill Livingstone

WEITZMAN, R. E. and FISHER, D. A. (1977) Log-linear relationship between plasma arginine vasopressin and plasma osmolality. *American Journal of Physiology*, **233**, E37–E40

WEITZMAN, R. E. and FISHER, D. A. (1978) Arginine–vasopressin metabolism in dogs. I. Evidence for a receptor-mediated mechanism. *American Journal of Physiology*, **235**, E591–E597

WEITZMAN, R. E., FIREMARK, H. M., GLATZ, T. H. and FISHER, D. A. (1979) Thyrotropin releasing hormone stimulates release of arginine vasopressin and oxytocin *in vivo*. *Endocrinology*, **104**, 904–907

WEITZMAN, R. E., FISCHER, D. A., DI STEFANO, J. J. and BENNETT, C. M. (1977a) Episodic secretion of arginine vasopressin. *American Journal of Physiology*, **233**, E32–E36

WEITZMAN, R. E., FISHER, D. A., MINICK, S., LING, N. and GUILLEMIN, R. (1977b) Beta-endorphin stimulates secretion of arginine–vasopressin *in vivo*. *Endocrinology*, **101**, 1643–1646

WILSON, K. L., WEITZMAN, R. E. and FISHER, D. A. (1978) Arginine–vasopressin metabolism in dogs. II. Modelling and system analysis. *American Journal of Physiology*, **235**, E598–E605

WOODS, R. L., ABRAHAMS, J. M., KINCAID-SMITH, P. and JOHNSTON, C. I. (1983) Malignant hypertension in Brattleboro (vasopressin deficient) rats. *Journal of Hypertension*, **1**, 37–43

YAMAMOTO, M., SHARE, L. and SHADE, R. E. (1976) Vasopressin release during ventriculocisternal perfusion with prostaglandin F2 in the dog. *Journal of Endocrinology*, **71**, 325–331

YAMAMOTO, M., SHARE, L. and SHADE, R. E. (1978) Effect of ventriculocisternal perfusion with angiotensin II and indomethacin on the plasma vasopressin concentration. *Neuroendocrinology*, **25**, 166–173

YATES, F. E., RUSSELL, D. M. and MARAN, J. W. (1971) Brain adenohypophyseal communication in mammals. *Annual Review of Physiology*, **33**, 393–444

ZIMMERMAN, E. A. (1981) The organization of oxytocin and vasopressin pathways. In *Neurosecretion and Brain Peptides*, edited by J. B. Martin, S. Reichlin and K. L. Bick, pp. 63–75. New York: Raven Press

ZUSMAN, R. M. and KAISER, H. R. (1977) Prostaglandin biosynthesis by rabbit renomedullary interstitial cells in tissue culture. Stimulation by angiotensin II, bradykinin and arginine–vasopressin. *Journal of Clinical Investigation*, **60**, 215–223

4

Salt and essential hypertension

Henry W. Overbeck

INTRODUCTION

Salt and essential hypertension are inextricably linked. Among (Dahl, 1972), and also within (Sasaki, 1964), populations, level of blood pressure has been related to sodium intake. The within-population evidence (for example, the Japanese (Sasaki, 1964)) is more convincing. In otherwise normal populations (both human (Luft et al., 1979) and rat (Meneely, Ball and Youmans, 1957)), extremely high sodium intake elevates blood pressure; in rats this effect of sodium is ameliorated by potassium (Meneely, Ball and Youmans, 1957). Extremely low levels of sodium intake (and high levels of potassium) are accompanied by lack of hypertension in unacculturated societies (Page, Danion and Moellering, 1974) and amelioration of hypertension in patients (Kempner, 1948). A significant proportion of the human population is especially sensitive to the hypertensinogenic effects of dietary salt (Dustan, Bravo and Tarazi, 1973; Kawasaki et al., 1978), a situation analogous to the salt-sensitive rat bred by Louis Dahl (Dahl, Heine and Tassinari, 1962). However, most humans appear resistant to any hypertensive effect of modest increases, or any antihypertensive effect of modest decreases, in salt intake (Simpson, 1979). Elevation of dietary calcium may also attenuate primary hypertension in man and rat (McCarron, Morris and Cole, 1982). These relationships between salt and primary hypertension have been the subject of numerous recent detailed reviews, to which the reader is referred (Freis, 1976; Simpson, 1979; Report of the Hypertension Task Force, 1979c).

The evidence linking sodium and essential hypertension, at least in some humans, is so striking that hypotheses purporting to explain the underlying mechanism abound. The multiplicity of these hypotheses, describing abnormal function of CNS, endocrine, and myogenic systems, among others, is testimony to our deficient understanding and to the fact that, whatever the mechanism, it likely involves multiple systems controlling blood pressure. Indeed, salt may produce hypertension by causing failure in one after another of a number of compensatory mechanisms designed to keep blood pressure at normal levels.

Because abnormal contraction of blood vessels is the common denominator of hypertension, the purpose of this chapter is to examine evidence linking salt to abnormal blood vessel function. Evidence from patients with essential hypertension and also from experimental forms of hypertension, where relevant, is included.

HEMODYNAMICS OF ESSENTIAL HYPERTENSION

To understand how salt might abnormally contract blood vessels producing hypertension, it is necessary first to consider the altered hemodynamic state that characterizes hypertension (Report of the Hypertension Task Force, 1979a; Overbeck *et al.*, 1980). At least in salt-sensitive individuals, salt has been involved in the production of that altered hemodynamic state.

In early stages of many forms of hypertension, including essential, there is evidence for increases in cardiac output (Guyton and Coleman, 1969; Report of the Hypertension Task Force, 1979a; Overbeck *et al.*, 1980), accompanied by increases in central blood volume (Ellis and Julius, 1973; Report of the Hypertension Task Force, 1979a; Overbeck *et al.*, 1980). Total body fluid volumes may not be abnormal (Report of the Hypertension Task Force, 1979a; Overbeck *et al.*, 1980). Such shifts of blood from the peripheral to the central circulation incriminate venous function in hypertension. The increased cardiac output may additionally involve elevations in myocardial contractility (Hawthorne *et al.*, 1974), suggesting an early primary role for abnormal myocardial function. Established essential hypertension, on the other hand, is characterized by a 'normal' cardiac output, and an elevated peripheral vascular resistance (Guyton and Coleman, 1969; Overbeck *et al.*, 1980; Report of the Hypertension Task Force, 1979a). However, the abnormal myocardial function may persist, for as Guyton and Coleman (1969) have pointed out, an elevated systemic resistance should reduce cardiac output under normal operating conditions.

Involvement of the heart and veins, as well as the arteries, may be critical in the process by which salt produces hypertension, by precluding simple compensatory redistribution of abnormal fluid volumes. Thus, elevated arterial resistance, in the absence of enhanced ventricular performance and decreased venous compliance, would simply decrease cardiac output and move blood volume from the arterial to the venous side of the circulation. (This is perhaps why heart failure, which otherwise in many ways resembles hypertension – increased peripheral resistance due to elevated humoral and neurogenic vasoconstriction, abnormal body fluid volumes, decreased venous compliance, as well as vascular wall 'waterlogging' (Zelis and Mason, 1970) is not accompanied by elevated blood pressure. Indeed, if the heart failure is caused by myocardial infarction, previously existing hypertension often disappears.)

The increased peripheral vascular resistance of established hypertension resides in the small terminal arteries and arterioles, and is primarily attributable to reduction in vascular radius, involving both functional and structural components of resistance. With some exceptions the increases in resistance appear to be fairly uniformly distributed among the various vascular beds of the body (Report of the Hypertension Task Force, 1979a; Overbeck *et al.*, 1980), including the renal bed. Without renal involvement, pressure diuresis would reduce intra-arterial pressure to normal and the hypertension would not be sustained (Guyton and Coleman, 1969); this may perhaps be considered to represent another 'failed' compensatory mechanism.

REGULATION OF ARTERIAL RESISTANCE

Neglecting blood viscosity, arterial resistance includes structural and functional components, as shown in *Figure 4.1*. The geometry of the vascular wall, with its smooth muscle completely relaxed, determines the structural component of peripheral resistance (Folkow, 1982); contractile activity of the smooth muscle cells is not involved. Increases in the structural component of resistance, directly or indirectly related to salt, may play a major role in the established phases of hypertension (Folkow, 1982) (*see also Figure 4.1*). But first let us consider functional components of resistance, abnormalities of which have been incriminated as playing the major role early in hypertension.

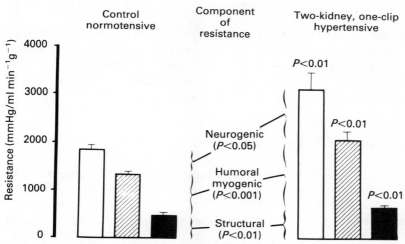

Figure 4.1 Vascular resistances of pump-perfused (blood, 1 ml/min) hindlimbs of 11 control normotensive and six chronic two-kidney, one-clip Goldblatt hypertensive rats. Clear bars represent mean + SEM resistance of intact limbs; cross-hatched bars represent resistance 10 min after acute section of femoral and sciatic nerves supplying the limb; solid bars represent resistance after maximal vasodilatation with sodium nitroprusside. The components of resistance are identified for the two groups: the 'neurogenic' component represents the fall in resistance occurring after acute nerve section; the 'humoral-myogenic' component represents the difference between resistance after nerve section and resistance at maximal vasodilation; and the 'structural' component represents resistance at maximal vasodilation. The *P* values are represented for comparison of resistances in the two groups. (Modified from Bell and Overbeck, 1979)

Functional components of resistance

Functional components of resistance, involving contractile activity of the smooth muscle cells, include (*see Figure 4.1*):

(1) a neurogenic contribution – that portion of resistance attributable to the effects of sympathetic nerve activity;
(2) a humoral contribution – that portion due to the effects of circulating or local vasoactive agents, such as angiotensin, vasopressin, or possibly a putative natriuretic hormone; and
(3) a myogenic contribution – that portion representing the inherent contractile activity of the vascular smooth muscle cell.

It is recognized that, in both health and disease, interactions occur between these functional components of resistance; for example, circulating angiotensin enhances vascular responses to neurogenic stimuli (Zimmerman, 1967) and natriuretic hormone might increase sympathetic discharge as well as enhance myogenic tone. There are also interactions between functional and structural components. In hypertension there is evidence for abnormal increases in each of these functional components of resistance (*see Figure 4.1*). There is also increasing evidence that the relative roles played by these several components vary in different forms and stages of hypertension.

Numerous factors, neural, hormonal and physicochemical (many of which have been incriminated in the mechanisms of salt–hypertension), alter the neurogenic, humoral and myogenic components of vascular resistance. However, one may reduce the effects of these factors to a single common denominator, regulation of the contractile function of the vascular smooth muscle cell.

Contractile function of vascular smooth muscle

Functionally, vascular smooth muscle cells fall into a spectrum ranging between multiunit and single-unit types of smooth muscle, corresponding to the classification of Bozler (Bozler, 1948; Folkow, 1982; Johansson, 1971; Somlyo and Somlyo, 1968a). There is evidence that the major functional type found in a given vessel reflects the mode of control, local or remote, of its contractile state. Multiunit type vascular smooth muscle (Hermsmeyer, 1971; Somlyo and Somlyo, 1971) is characterized by graded depolarization and slow contraction in response to remote neural or humoral stimuli, with little evidence for inherent myogenic activity or propagation. Multiunit smooth muscle is primarily found in large elastic and muscular arteries down to 200 μM outside diameter. In contrast, single-unit type vascular smooth muscle is characterized by rhythmic oscillations of the membrane potential leading to spontaneous action potentials, more primitive than those found in cardiac muscle. These action potentials are propagated from cell to cell and are usually accompanied by relatively rapid phasic contractions ('spontaneous rhythmicity'). Such cells are primarily influenced by the local environment, both chemical and mechanical (Johansson and Mellander, 1975; Johnson, 1978). Single-unit vascular smooth muscle is found primarily in the rhythmically active walls of small resistance and precapillary sphincter vessels, where local regulation of blood flow is of primary importance.

The larger precapillary resistance vessels, controlling peripheral arterial resistance, and, hence, blood pressure, may contain both types of smooth muscle in their walls. Folkow (1982) suggests that there is an outer innervated sheath of multiunit cells responding to extrinsic neural and humoral influences, and an inner portion of single unit cells responding to the local milieu, the positive influence of stretch on these inner cells being balanced by the negative effect of metabolites produced by the tissues. According to Folkow, not only are several functional types of vascular smooth muscle cells represented in a single vessel, but it is also probable that a single smooth muscle cell may be capable of either single-unit or multiunit function, depending on the character of the environment. If remote controlling influences predominate, multiunit function is evoked; if local influences are stronger, the inherent automaticity of these cells may be elicited. Abnormalities in cell salt and water balance induce disequilibria in the delicate balance between these functional types of vascular smooth muscle, involving disturbances in sensitivity, automaticity and propagation of action potentials (Johansson and Somlyo, 1980). Such effects, by altering sarcoplasmic Ca^{2+} levels, change the contractile state of the cells, resistance, and blood pressure.

Regulation of sarcoplasmic calcium ion

As in striated muscle, sarcoplasmic concentration of free calcium ion controls the mechanical interaction of the myofibrils and, thus, force generation in vascular smooth muscle. Threshold activity of actomyosin occurs at sarcoplasmic Ca^{2+} concentrations of approximately 10^{-7} M (Filo, Bohr and Rüegg, 1965). As in striated muscle, Ca^{2+} mediates its effect through regulatory protein, although in vascular smooth muscle calmodulin controlling phosphorylation of myosin light chains (Murphy, 1982), rather than troponin–tropomyosin regulating actin, is involved. Sources and deposits of activator Ca^{2+} in vascular smooth muscle include the extracellular space, the sarcolemma, the sarcoplasmic reticulum, and mitochondria, the latter source apparently of little physiological significance (Somlyo and Somlyo, 1976; Somlyo, 1978). Uptake of calcium by sarcoplasmic reticulum, sarcolemma, and mitochondria are energy-requiring processes about which little is known. Extrusion of Ca^{2+} from the cell by the sarcolemma may involve a Na^+–Ca^{2+} exchange system (Baker *et al.*, 1969; Reuter and Seitz, 1968) as well as ATP-dependent mechanisms (Van Breemen, Aaronson and Loutzenhiser, 1979).

Agonists evoking graded depolarization of vascular smooth muscle increase membrane permeability to monovalent cations (Guignard and Friedman, 1971; Jones, 1973). Graded depolarization (Blaustein, 1977; Droogmans, Raeymaekers and Casteels, 1977), as well as action potentials (Johansson and Somlyo, 1980;

Uvelius, Sigurdsson and Johansson, 1974), probably involve inward trans-sarcolemmal movement of small amounts of Ca^{2+} (Somlyo, Vinall and Somlyo, 1969; Godfraind, 1976) which may, in turn, trigger regenerative discharge of relatively large amounts of Ca^{2+} from the sarcolemma and the sarcoplasmic reticulum (Endo, Tanaka and Ogawa, 1970), evoking the contractile response. Associated with the trans-sarcolemmal movement of Ca^{2+} are influxes of Na^+ and effluxes of K^+ (Guignard and Friedman, 1970; Jamieson and Friedman, 1961). Activity of the sodium pump of the sarcolemma is of critical importance in restoring resting Na^+ and K^+ gradients. The functions of sarcolemmal ion co-transport and counter-transport mechanisms are poorly understood.

The basal myogenic tone constantly present in the single-unit type smooth muscle cells of most resistance vessels distinguishes these smooth muscle cells from cells of cardiac muscle which relax completely between contractions. As pointed out by Blaustein (1977) this resting tension implies that sarcoplasmic concentrations of Ca^{2+} are maintained above $10^{-7}M$ in vascular smooth muscle, the contractile tissue balanced on the rising phase of the $[Ca^{2+}]_i$-tension curve (*Figure 4.2*). Thus, extremely small changes in $[Ca^{2+}]_i$ are capable of evoking immediate response in contractile activity. A matter of considerable interest is how levels of sarcoplasmic Ca^{2+} are precisely controlled in vascular smooth muscle.

Sarcolemmal transport mechanisms for Ca^{2+} in vascular smooth muscle differ fundamentally from those in cardiac muscle. In vascular smooth muscle Ca^{2+} may be released into the sarcoplasm in the total absence of changes in membrane potential; this process has been designated 'non-electrical activation' or 'pharmacomechanical coupling' (Droogmans, Raeymaekers and Casteels, 1977; Evans, Schild and Thesleff, 1958; Somlyo and Somlyo, 1968b). Similar activation mechanisms have not been described in cardiac muscle. A relationship between

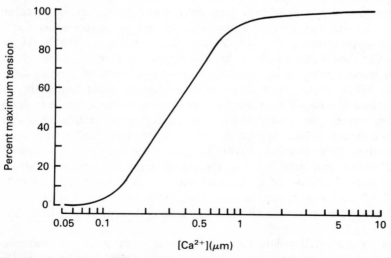

Figure 4.2 Relation of sarcoplasmic ionized Ca^{2+} on the tension developed by glycerinated vascular smooth muscle fibers (hog carotid artery). (From Blaustein, 1977, courtesy of the Publishers, *The American Physiological Society*)

non-electrical activation and membrane permeability may exist (Somlyo, Vinall and Somlyo, 1969), but non-electrical activation is not solely due to calcium influx, because it may occur in the virtual absence of extracellular Ca^{2+} (Devine, Somlyo and Somlyo, 1972). A passive calcium–sodium (Ca^{2+}–Na^+) exchange mechanism may be involved (Blaustein, 1977). The biological role of non-electrical activation in vascular smooth muscle has not been defined, but has been postulated to be of importance (Bohr, 1973).

Non-electrical activation of vascular smooth muscle may operate in parallel with the more familiar mechanism of electromechanical coupling, where transmembrane Ca^{2+} movement is associated with alteration in the electrical state of the sarcolemma induced by chemical or physical stimuli (Johansson, 1971). In contrast to the all-or-none contractions found in cardiac muscle cells, in vascular smooth muscle modulation of contractile state may result from graded depolarization of the membrane. Furthermore, contraction of vascular smooth muscle is often directly initiated by contact of the activating agonist with the plasma membrane. This may also occur in absence of spike potentials. In contrast, in cardiac muscle, agonists do not stimulate contraction directly, but instead alter the contractile process by modulating the response to a propagated action potential that always precedes contraction.

Regulation of membrane potential

The association in vascular smooth muscle of graded contractures with graded membrane depolarization indicates that the precise control of membrane potential is of great importance in the fine regulation of sarcoplasmic Ca^{2+}, and hence of vascular resistance. The major determinant (>60%) of transmembrane potential in vascular smooth muscle (Johansson, 1978), as in cardiac muscle, is the passive diffusion potential resulting from the transmembrane distribution of ions and membrane ion permeability. However, permeability of the sarcolemma to sodium ions is probably higher and permeability to potassium is lower in vascular smooth muscle than in cardiac muscle, accounting for the lower resting membrane potential in the former (in the range -50 to $-75\,mV$ in contrast to $-90\,mV$ in cardiac muscle) (Axelsson *et al.*, 1967; Holman, 1969).

Also, in striking contrast to cardiac muscle, an estimated 10–40% of resting membrane potential in vascular smooth muscle is contributed by the operation of a ouabain-sensitive electrogenic sodium pump in the sarcolemma (Anderson, 1976; Hendrickx and Casteels, 1974). Because each cycle of this pump extrudes more Na^+ than it transports K^+ into the cell, activity of the pump depletes the cell of positive charge, increasing intracellular negativity, thus hyperpolarizing the sarcolemma (Somlyo and Somlyo, 1968a). Pump activity is controlled primarily by extracellular concentrations of potassium ion and by intracellular concentrations of sodium ion, operating via their effects on membrane Na^+, K^+-stimulated ATPase. Cardiac glycosides and temperature also influence pump activity and hence the contractile state of vascular smooth muscle (Anderson, 1976). Because this sodium pump plays a critical role in determining intracellular concentrations of sodium ion, as well as membrane potential, its activity may modify the contractile state of the smooth muscle cell both by voltage effects on membrane slow Ca^{2+} channels and by calcium–sodium exchange mechanisms (Blaustein, 1977; Somlyo and Somlyo, 1968a).

THE VASCULAR SMOOTH MUSCLE CELL IN HYPERTENSION

There is increasing evidence that some of the regulators of contractile function in vascular smooth muscle may be abnormal in hypertension (Report of the Hypertension Task Force, 1979b). Associated with the abnormal vascular contraction in hypertensive animals and patients are increases in spontaneous rhythmicity of the vascular smooth muscle cells (Bandick and Sparks, 1970a; Bohr and Sitrin, 1970), evidence for increases in sensitivity to agonists (Beilin *et al.*, 1970; Berecek and Bohr, 1976, 1977; Bohr and Sitrin, 1970; Collis and Alps, 1975; Doyle and Fraser, 1961; Field, Janis and Triggle, 1972; Finch and Haeusler, 1974; Hansen and Bohr, 1975; Haeusler and Finch, 1972; Hermsmeyer, 1976a; Holloway and Bohr, 1973; Lais and Brody, 1975; McGregor and Smirk, 1970; Mulvany, Aalkjaer and Christensen, 1980), changes in contractility (Bandick and Sparks, 1970a; Bohr and Sitrin, 1970; Clineschmidt *et al.*, 1970; Field, Janis and Triggle, 1972; Hansen, Abrams and Bohr, 1974; Hansen and Bohr, 1975; Horwitz *et al.*, 1974; Shibata, Kurahashi and Kuchii, 1973; Spector *et al.*, 1969) and alterations in relaxation processes (Amer, 1973; Bohr, 1974; Cohen and Berkowitz, 1976; Janis and Triggle, 1973; Levy, 1973, 1974, 1975; Shibata, Kurahashi and Kuchii, 1973; Triner *et al.*, 1975). ('Sensitivity' describes the ease with which a vasoactive agent can cause a response; it is measured as the concentration of agonist that evokes a threshold or a half maximal response. 'Contractility' refers to the maximal contraction obtainable.)

Many of these abnormalities in vasomotion precede or accompany the development of hypertension, suggesting a causal role (Berecek and Bohr, 1977; Collis and Alps, 1975; Shibata, Kurahashi and Kuchii, 1973). These abnormalities incriminate underlying defects in the function of the contractile apparatus of the vascular smooth muscle cell, which might involve any of the components of the contractile system. However, most evidence thus far appears to incriminate membrane function.

Sarcolemmal function

A decrease in the maximum capacity of sarcoplasmic reticulum to sequester Ca^{2+} in spontaneously hypertensive rats (SHR) has been reported by several laboratories (Limas and Cohn, 1977; Webb and Bhalla, 1976). Such an abnormality would tend to increase sarcoplasmic Ca^{2+} concentrations, impeding vascular relaxation. However, the relationship of this abnormality to disease mechanisms in hypertension is questionable, because the hypertensive process involves small changes in the contractile activity of vascular smooth muscle, rather than the failure of maximal relaxing capacity.

Disturbances in sarcolemmal function would be a more likely cause of the changes in the fine regulation of vascular smooth muscle contraction reported to occur in hypertension. Reduced resting membrane potential or enhanced depolarization in response to stimuli such as cold, neural activity or norepinephrine have been reported in hypertensive animals (Friedman and Friedman, 1976; Hermsmeyer, 1976a, 1976b, 1976c; Jones, 1973, 1974a; Jones and Hart, 1975). As noted above, such partial depolarization *in vivo* is accompanied by graded contracture.

Reduction in resting membrane potential could be the result of altered transmembrane ion gradients, ion permeabilities, abnormal operation of the membrane electrogenic sodium pump, or a combination. It is likely that transmembrane ion gradients are altered in hypertension. Elevations of vascular wall water, sodium and potassium content have been repeatedly observed in most forms of hypertension, including essential hypertension (Tobian, 1960). Although most of the water and sodium is bound to extracellular glycosaminoglycans (Hollander *et al.*, 1968), there is evidence that at least some of these increases may be intracellular (Edmondson *et al.*, 1975; Villamil, 1972). However, altered ion concentration gradients across the cell membrane of vascular smooth muscle are probably of small magnitude and are not invariably found in hypertension; thus, changes in gradients probably do not contribute as significantly to abnormalities in membrane function as do changes in membrane kinetics (Jones, 1976).

Regarding kinetics, Jones and his co-workers found increased transmembrane fluxes of K^+, Cl^-, and Na^+ in SHR and DOCA-salt hypertension (Jones, 1974a, 1974b, 1976) and suggested that they reflect underlying increases in membrane permeability to these ions. Changes in membrane permeability may be related to underlying causative mechanisms, because they have been observed to precede the appearance of significant elevations in arterial pressure (Jones and Hart, 1975). This latter observation fails to support the alternative explanation that increased membrane permeability may result from increased intravascular pressure (Friedman and Friedman, 1976), although pressure-induced increases in permeability might later come into play when the hypertension becomes established.

Abnormal erythrocyte membrane co-transport and counter-transport of ions may occur in hypertension (Parker and Berkowitz, 1983). The defects may be genetic variants, but as yet there is insufficient evidence to relate them to the mechanisms of hypertension. There are no reports of defects in co-transport and counter-transport in vascular smooth muscle.

Sodium pump function

An apparent result of the increased membrane permeability of vascular smooth muscle to sodium is an increase in the activity of the membrane sodium pump observed in several forms of hypertension in rats (Friedman, 1979; Folkow, 1982; Göthberg, Jandhyala and Folkow, 1980; Hermsmeyer, 1976a, 1976b). This increased activity may serve to restore cell membrane potential to normal levels (Hermsmeyer, 1976b). Such increased pumping also is observed in arteries excised from normotensive vascular beds in rats with coarctation hypertension (Overbeck *et al.,* 1982). Thus, it is unlikely that pressure-induced increases in sarcolemmal sodium permeability (or pressure-induced tissue hyperplasia/hypertrophy) are involved. It is suggested that increased sodium pumping balances the leaks and serves to maintain cell Na^+ (and hence Ca^{2+}) at near normal levels (Folkow, 1982). Increases in numbers of pump molecules in the sarcolemma, or changes in vascular wall metabolism, for example, of prostaglandins, as well as elevation in cell sodium, may be involved in the increased pumping.

Evidence for a decrease in the activity of the electrogenic sodium pump of the sarcolemma of cardiovascular muscle cells in hypertension also has been reported. Obviously, such changes would impair the ability of the cell to excrete any excess sodium resulting from increased membrane 'leakiness'. In vascular smooth muscle, decreased pumping would additionally alter membrane potential and thereby sarcolemmal Ca^{2+} concentration, promoting vascular contraction.

Three types of evidence indicate decreased sodium pump activity in membranes of cardiovascular cells in hypertension:

(1) The *in vivo* vasodilatory response to small local elevations in plasma K^+ concentration are attenuated in several forms of hypertension, including

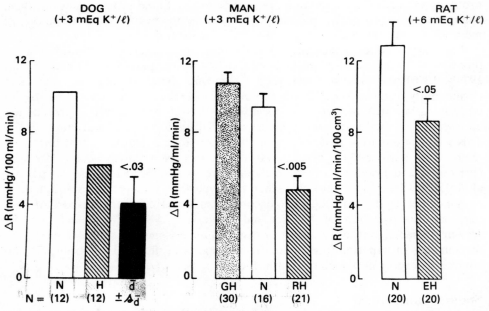

Figure 4.3 Attenuated K^+-induced vasodilation *in vivo* in hypertensive dogs (chronic one-kidney, one-wrapped perinephritic), rats (chronic two-kidney, one-clip Goldblatt), and men (essential). Isotonic KCl solution was infused into brachial (dog, men) or femoral (rat) artery to elevate K^+ in limb arterial plasma by 3–6 mEq/1, while perfusion pressure and flow were monitored. Means (adjusted for covariance effects of initial limb resistance) + SEM and numbers of observations provided. N: normotensive controls; H: perinephritic hypertensive dogs; GH: genetic (New Zealand) hypertensive rats; RH: Goldblatt hypertensive rats; EH: essential hypertensive men. *P* values for comparison of means calculated by analysis of covariance. (From Overbeck 1983, courtesy of the Publishers)

one-kidney, one-wrapped perinephritic hypertension in dogs (Overbeck, 1972), two-kidney, one-clip Goldblatt hypertension in rats (Overbeck and Clark, 1975), and established essential hypertension in man (Overbeck *et al.*, 1974) (*Figure 4.3*). Not all patients with essential hypertension exhibited this abnormality. We were unable to relate the abnormality to duration or severity of hypertension, renal function, or plasma renin activity.

Potassium ion activates the membrane ouabain-sensitive sodium pump, so the attenuated responses in hypertensives suggest impaired pump function, perhaps resulting from fewer pump molecules or from a digitalis-like action. These investigations were conducted *in vivo*, where function of arterioles rather than conduit arteries were observed, and where the effects of a circulating digitalis-like pump inhibitor could be detected. The attenuated responses were specific for K^+ (Overbeck, Daugherty and Haddy, 1969; Overbeck, 1972; Overbeck, Pamnani and Derifield, 1975). Thus, the abnormal responses may be attributed to functional, rather than structural, abnormalities in resistance vessels.

(2) The ouabain-sensitive uptake of Rb^+ by vascular smooth muscle *in vitro* is strikingly diminished in dogs with one-kidney perinephritic hypertension (Overbeck *et al.*, 1976) (*Figure 4.4*) and also, in the hands of one group of investigators, in rats with presumably low-renin, presumably volume-expanded, non-genetic forms of hypertension (Haddy, 1980). Rb^+ substitutes

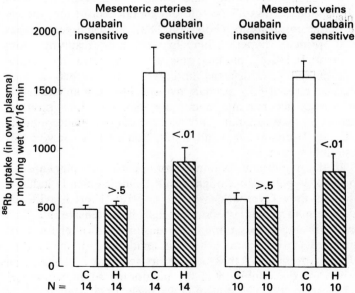

Figure 4.4 Decreased ouabain-sensitive ^{86}Rb uptake *in vitro* by mesenteric arteries and veins from dogs with chronic one-kidney, one-wrapped perinephritic hypertension. Incubation in own plasma. Clear bars represent values in control normotensive dogs, and cross-hatched bars show values in perinephritic hypertensive dogs. Means ± SEM and *N* values provided. *P* values calculated by unpaired Student's *t* test. (From Overbeck, 1983, courtesy of the Publishers)

for K^+, and the ouabain-sensitive portion of its uptake is attributable to activity of the membrane sodium pump (Bernstein and Israel, 1970). This abnormality in membrane function cannot be attributed to the direct effects of elevated intravascular pressure, because it occurred in veins as well as arteries (Overbeck *et al.*, 1976).

(3) Activity of Na,K–ATPase, the enzymatic expression of the membrane sodium pump, is reported to be reduced in sarcolemmal fractions derived from ventricular myocardium of rats with several forms of hypertension (Clough *et al.*, 1977; Haddy, 1980; Lee *et al.*, 1982).

Mechanisms of abnormal membrane function

Because these various abnormalities in sarcolemmal permeability and sodium pump function may be related to underlying causative mechanisms, there has been considerable interest in their pathogenesis. It is proposed that, in forms of hypertension characterized by elevated levels of steroids (Bohr and Sitrin, 1970; Hansen and Bohr, 1975; Jones and Hart, 1975), the steroids, or the interaction of steroids with salt, increase the ion permeability of the sarcolemma of vascular smooth muscle. There might be an underlying abnormality in Ca^{2+} absorption on membrane sites (Jones, 1976), perhaps reflecting changes in surface coat properties of the vascular smooth muscle cells (Jones and Swain, 1972; Langer, 1976; Ooshima *et al.*, 1974). In familial forms of hypertension, genetic factors may induce alterations in cell membrane permeability (Folkow, 1982). Alternatively, it has been suggested that, in primary hypertension, hypocalcemia resulting from hypercalcuria reduces membrane Ca^{2+} binding; this would decrease membrane 'stability', increasing permeability. Thus, the antihypertensive effect of high calcium intake, which has been reported in primary hypertension in man and rat, is attributed to correction of hypocalcemia and membrane 'leakiness'. In support of this suggestion, elevations in extracellular Ca^{2+} concentrations hyperpolarize membrane of smooth muscle (Holman, 1958) and, in rats, relax arteries *in vivo* (H. W. Overbeck, unpublished observation).

Decreases in activity of the membrane sodium pump in cardiovascular muscle, especially in genetic forms of hypertension, might result from genetically induced reduction in number of pump sites (Overbeck *et al.*, 1974, 1976). There is evidence that this might be the case in myocardium of spontaneously hypertensive rats (Lee *et al.*, 1982). Alternatively, in one-kidney renal hypertension, and other forms of low-renin, volume-expanded hypertension, there is evidence for circulating humoral agents that elevate pressure. It has been proposed that such humoral agents may be responsible for the inhibition of the membrane sodium pump in cardiovascular muscle (Blaustein, 1977; Haddy and Overbeck, 1976; MacGregor *et al.*, 1981; Overbeck *et al.*, 1974, 1976).

INTER-RELATIONSHIP BETWEEN CELL SODIUM AND PUMP ACTIVITY

As discussed briefly above, it has been suggested by many investigators that primary increases in cell sodium concentration attributable to increased sarcolemmal ion permeability underlie the elevated sodium pump activity observed by several laboratories in tissues from hypertensives. However, cell sodium was not found elevated in arteries from hypertensive rats which clearly had increased sodium pumping (Overbeck and Grissette, 1982; Overbeck *et al.*, 1982). Furthermore, extensive tissue sodium loading did not increase pump activity of arteries from normotensive control rats to the high rates observed in hypertensive arteries at cell sodiums half as great (Overbeck, Ku and Rapp, 1981; Overbeck and Grissette, 1982). To further study the relation between cell sodium and pump activity in hypertension, total cell sodium was varied over a wide range in both hypertensive and normotensive arteries *in vitro* by using incubating solutions with varying sodium content and monensin, a sodium ionophore which increases the passive permeability of the sarcolemma to sodium (Brock, Smith and Overbeck, 1982). Rats with chronic one-kidney, DOCA-salt hypertension and rats with chronic one-kidney, one figure-eight hypertension were studied; the results in the two forms of hypertension did not differ. There was a sigmoid relationship between ouabain-sensitive ^{86}Rb uptake (an index of sodium pump activity) and levels of total cellular sodium content with a clear difference between hypertensive and normotensive tissue (*Figure 4.5*). For any level of total cell sodium, ouabain-

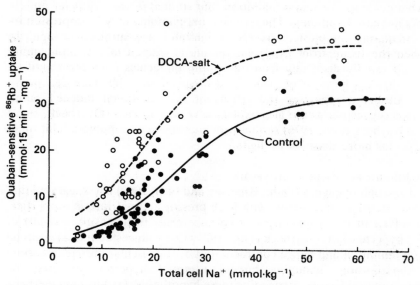

Figure 4.5 Sigmoid relation between total cell Na^+ and *in vitro* ouabain-sensitive ^{86}Rb uptake in thoracic aortas. Values for rats with chronic one-kidney DOCA-salt hypertension and pooled one-kidney normotensive control rats represented as open and closed circles, respectively. Curves computer-generated for sigmoid relation according to equation: Rb uptake = $K/(1 + \exp[-(A \cdot \text{total cell } Na^+ + B)])$, where K = maximal Rb uptake, A = rate of change of upslope of curve, and B = intercept of curve on vertical axis. R^2 for curve in DOCA-salt rats = 0.94; R^2 for curve in normotensive control rats = 0.95. Derived values for normotensive control rats are: K = 31.9 ± 1.7, A = 0.13 ± 0.02, B = 3.14 ± 0.32. Derived values for DOCA-salt hypertensive rats are: K = 43.2 ± 2.6 ($P < 0.001$), A = 0.13 ± 0.03 ($P > 0.05$), B = −2.47 ± 0.41 ($P > 0.05$). (From Overbeck, 1983, courtesy of the Publishers)

sensitive ^{86}Rb uptake was greater in hypertensive tissue. Furthermore, maximal ^{86}Rb uptake was greater in hypertensive tissue. This sigmoid relation is similar to that reported for normal erythrocytes (Garay and Garrahan, 1973) and for arteries from hypertensive (DOCA–salt) and normotensive control rats by Jones (1981). Jones also found increased pumping at each level of cell sodium, and increased maximal pumping, in hypertensive tissue.

Thus, it is unlikely that the increased sodium pump activity of vascular smooth muscle cells from hypertensive rats is merely a response to increased 'leakiness' of the cell membrane, with sodium efflux due to increased pump activity exactly matching the increased sodium influx, total cell sodium remaining normal. Instead, other vascular wall factors, such as prostaglandins, may be involved in pump stimulation (Lockette, Webb and Bohr, 1980). Alternatively, there may be compensatory induction of more pump molecules per unit sarcolemma, perhaps by chronically increased membrane leakiness to sodium, perhaps by a circulating digitalis-like pump inhibitor (*see below*). With regard to induction, increases in cardiac muscle membrane Na,K–ATPase result from chronic digitalis treatment of animals (Bluschke, Bonn and Greef, 1976). This latter explanation would best account for several observations described above, including the fact that in rats there is *in vivo* evidence for pump inhibition, but studied *in vitro* vascular muscle often displays increased pumping. Thus, *in vivo* net pumping may be depressed by a putative circulating inhibitor, if levels of inhibitor are sufficiently high. In contrast, when the tissue from hypertensive rats is studied *in vitro*, the pump inhibitor would rapidly dissociate from the pump molecules (rats are relatively insensitive to digitalis because of such rapid dissociation), the increased pump activity then observed reflecting the effects of the additional induced pump molecules. This suggestion would also explain why both *in vivo* (Overbeck, 1972) and *in vitro* (Overbeck *et al.*, 1976) studies provide evidence for pump inhibition in dogs, a species far more sensitive to digitalis.

CIRCULATING INHIBITORS OF THE SODIUM PUMP

In 1969 Dahl and his colleagues (Dahl, Knudsen and Iwai, 1969) had suggested that a humoral hypertensinogenic factor, with both pressor and natriuretic properties, might be involved in the mechanisms of certain forms (salt-sensitive; renal) of experimental hypertension. Overbeck *et al.* (1974, 1976) suggested that membrane sodium pump inhibition and hence contraction of cardiovascular muscle in certain forms of hypertension, including human essential hypertension, may be attributable to humoral factors. Expanding these hypotheses, Haddy and Overbeck (1976), and shortly thereafter Blaustein (1977), proposed (*Figure 4.6*) that a putative natriuretic hormone, released in response to volume expansion in experimental and human essential hypertension, might be the circulating inhibitor. An agent that both activates the cardiovascular system and also decreases tubular reabsorption of sodium would be attractive on teleological grounds, because such actions would be the best way to rid the body of extra salt and water (the increase in blood pressure would deliver more salt and water to the tubule where it would be rejected).

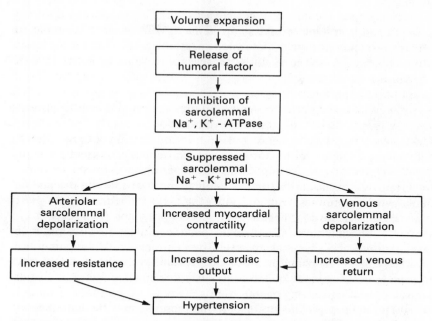

Figure 4.6 Shows the hypothesis relating hypertension to humoral inhibition of the sodium pump in cardiovascular muscle (Overbeck *et al.*, 1976; Haddy and Overbeck, 1976). See text for further description

To explain the observation that salt (volume) loading is not invariably associated with hypertension, for example, in salt-resistant persons or rats, Haddy and Overbeck (1976) suggested that there may be biological variation in one or a combination of the following critical characteristics:

(1) Renal function – those with better renal function would be expected to have lesser increases in body fluid volumes, and hence lesser rises in pressure.
(2) The amount of humoral agent released in response to a given increase in body fluid volumes – those with a lesser release would be expected to have a lesser rise in pressure.
(3) The responsiveness of the cardiovascular muscle cells to the humoral agent – those with a lesser responsiveness would be expected to have a lesser rise in pressure.
(4) The responsiveness of the kidney tubules to the natriuretic effect of the humoral agent – those with a greater responsiveness would be expected to have a lesser rise in pressure.
(5) The chemical form of the released humoral agent – those releasing an agent with a lesser cardiovascular action would be expected to have a lesser rise in pressure.

To these possibilities it might be added that humans (or rats) may also vary in the distribution of body fluid volumes – greater movement of excess fluid volumes from the intravascular to the extravascular space (Overbeck, Ku and Rapp, 1981), or lesser shifts of excess fluid volumes to a critical area, such as the cardiopulmonary circulation, might result in a lesser release of the factor and hence a lesser rise in pressure. It is also possible that, in some persons prone to develop salt hypertension, natriuretic hormone might be autonomously released in the absence of volume expansion.

As discussed in detail in the next chapter, de Wardener and MacGregor (1980) have stressed the possibility that there may be a primary renal defect in humans prone to develop essential, or salt-sensitive, hypertension.

Considerable evidence has accumulated supporting the hypothesis that a circulating digitalis-like factor, with natriuretic properties, depresses sodium pump activity in cell membranes in certain forms of hypertension. In some human essential hypertensives a plasma factor has been found that inhibits the sodium pump in leukocyte membranes (Edmondson *et al.*, 1975; Poston *et al.*, 1981; Thomas *et al.*, 1975). However, there is more recent evidence (Heagerty *et al.*, 1982) that such abnormalities in leukocyte sodium transport also occur in normotensive relatives of essential hypertensive patients and thus may not participate directly in the mechanisms of blood pressure elevation. On the other hand, there is an interesting study of leukocyte ouabain-sensitive sodium transport in pre-eclampsia indicating striking decreases in activity which disappear promptly (within one day) upon termination of pregnancy and resolution of the hypertension (Forrester and Alleyne, 1980).

As discussed in the next chapter, MacGregor *et al.* (1981) found in patients with essential hypertension a plasma factor that stimulates the activity of glucose-6-phosphate-dehydrogenase (G6PD), an enzyme they feel reflects in a reciprocal manner the activity of cell membrane Na,K–ATPase. More recently, Blaustein's group (Hamlyn *et al.*, 1982) found elevated levels of an inhibitor of renal Na,K–ATPase in the plasma of patients with essential hypertension. The levels of this inhibitor correlated well with the blood pressure but not with plasma renin activity or 'endotoxin' levels (*see below*). It is difficult to reconcile this observation of Hamlyn *et al.* (1982) with the currently held concept that 'essential hypertension' is not a homogeneous disease entity, but instead represents a grouping of various, but unidentified, mechanisms.

In animals and patients with low-renin forms of hypertension, Haddy's group (Burris *et al.*, 1982; Haddy, 1980) has found evidence for a heat-stable plasma factor that inhibits sodium pump activity in rat tail artery and leukocytes *in vitro*. They also report (Pamnani *et al.*, 1981b) that this factor reduces membrane potential in vascular smooth muscle of normal tail artery (to the same extent as it is reduced by maximal inhibitory levels of ouabain).

The digitalis-like factor is apparently not present in rats with anteroventral third ventricular (AV3V) lesions, even with acute volume expansion (Pamnani *et al.*, 1981a). It is noteworthy that the AV3V lesion itself is reported to be accompanied by a degree of volume-expansion without hypertension (Brody and Johnson, 1980). The lesion also prevents the development of various forms of volume-expanded experimental hypertensions (Brody and Johnson, 1980), as well as evidence for pump inhibition (Songu-Mize, Bealer and Caldwell, 1982). These observations suggest that the hypothalamus may be involved in the release of a natriuretic hormone and that interplay of neural and humoral influences may be necessary for the development of salt-sensitive, volume-dependent hypertension.

Additionally, Gruber, Whitaker and Buckalew (1980) have found a plasma fraction with natriuretic and Na,K–ATPase inhibitory effects that cross-reacts with digoxin antibodies. Levels are elevated both in acutely volume-expanded animals and also in primates with long-standing spontaneous or Goldblatt hypertension (Gruber, Rudel and Bullock, 1982). They have named this factor 'endoxin'. The same group (Plunkett *et al.*, 1982) found that endoxin increased rat cremaster arteriolar sensitivity to norepinephrine, angiotensin II and vasopressin.

In contrast to leukocytes, studies of erythrocytes have provided more evidence for increased (Garay and Dagher, 1980; Garay, Dagher and Meyer, 1980; Garay *et al.*, 1980; Wambach *et al.*, 1978, 1979, 1980; Woods, Beevers and West, 1981) than decreased (Fadeke Aderounmu and Salako, 1979; Rahman *et al.*, 1982; Rygielski, Kropp and Duran, 1981; Walter and Distler, 1980, 1982) membrane pump activity in hypertension. It is noteworthy that in these studies the erythrocytes were not incubated in plasma; thus it is possible that the circulating inhibitor had been washed off the membrane before sodium pump activity was measured. It is also possible that decreases in erythrocyte pump activity may be associated only with certain specific subtypes of essential hypertension, for example, low-renin varieties (Rahman *et al.*, 1982). In late complicated essential hypertension there is evidence for suppression of the sodium pump of the erythrocyte membrane (Garay *et al.*, 1980), presumably by the circulating pump inhibitors that accompany renal dysfunction.

In this regard, in hypertensives humoral factors other than a putative natriuretic hormone may depress the activity of the membrane sodium pump (Overbeck *et al.*, 1974, 1976). An outstanding example is methylguanidine, body levels of which are elevated in uremia (Stein *et al.*, 1971). Such substances may well play a role in pump inhibition observed in hypertension complicated by renal insufficiency. Other slow-acting humoral vasoconstrictors have been reported in hypertension (see Haddy and Overbeck, 1976; Haddy, 1980), but their relation to sarcolemmal sodium pump function has not yet been investigated.

It must be emphasized that *in vitro* observations of rat vascular smooth muscle from a number of laboratories do not appear to support the hypothesis that the membrane sodium pump is universally inhibited in volume-expanded forms of hypertension. In vascular smooth muscle from animals with benign DOCA-salt hypertension, for example, there have been a number of reports suggesting increased, rather than decreased, sarcolemmal sodium pump activity (*see above*), even if freshly excised arterial tissue is rapidly processed (Brock, Smith and Overbeck, 1982) and incubated in the rat's own plasma (Songu-Mize, Bealer and Caldwell, 1982). In rats with benign, one-kidney, one-clip Goldblatt hypertension and drinking saline, two laboratories have reported elevated ouabain-sensitive Rb^+ uptake by freshly excised conduit arteries (Overbeck and Grissette, 1982; Songu-Mize, personal communication). In contrast, Haddy's laboratory (Haddy, 1980), using essentially identical techniques, reports decreased arterial sodium pump activity in these forms of volume-expanded, low-renin hypertension. A possible explanation for this discrepancy may be that rats in the latter study were in late, complicated stages of hypertension with elevated levels of more tightly bound pump inhibitors such as those characterizing uremia.

Furthermore, in arteries from salt-fed Dahl salt-sensitive rats with documented volume-expansion and chronic hypertension, Overbeck, Ku and Rapp (1981) and Pamnani *et al.* (1980) found increased, rather than decreased, pump activity. This form of experimental hypertension first led Dahl, Knudsen and Iwai (1969) to propose a circulating factor with pressor and natriuretic properties. In this form of hypertension, humoral vasoconstrictor substances have been reported (Tobian *et al.*, 1979) and this form of volume-expanded hypertension is blocked by the AV3V lesion (Brody and Johnson, 1980). Thus, if a natriuretic hormone is generally involved in volume-expanded hypertension, one would certainly have expected to find evidence in the Dahl salt-sensitive rats. More attention to the early developmental stages of these forms of hypertension may provide such evidence.

SODIUM PUMP FUNCTION AND CELL CALCIUM ION IN HYPERTENSION

Two mechanisms have been proposed to explain how sodium pump inhibition would increase sarcoplasmic Ca^{2+} and thereby muscle contractile state in hypertension (Blaustein, 1977; Overbeck *et al.*, 1976). Because the pump is electrogenic, pump inhibition would partially depolarize the sarcolemma. This, in turn, would open voltage-dependent Ca^{2+} channels, thereby increasing sarcoplasmic Ca^{2+} concentrations (Overbeck *et al.*, 1976). Alternatively, Blaustein (1977) has proposed that abnormal Na^+-Ca^{2+} transmembrane exchange may underlie the contraction of vascular smooth muscle in hypertension, even in the absence of changes in cell membrane potential. Small (about 5%) increases in intracellular sodium, resulting from increased permeability and/or decreased pumping, could, by this latter exchange mechanism, elevate sarcoplasmic concentrations of Ca^{2+}.

Relation of membrane function abnormalities and stage of hypertension

Folkow (1982) suggests that inciting stimuli, including changes in vascular smooth muscle permeability to sodium and in membrane sodium pump activity, may be of greatest pathophysiological importance early in the development of hypertension, to be superseded within a very short time by mechanisms involving structural vascular changes. Supporting this suggestion, there is a report of increased sensitivity of the microcirculation to norepinephrine only in the first two weeks of the one-kidney, one-clip Goldblatt hypertension in rats (Joshua *et al.*, 1984).

Also, Gruber and Buckalew's laboratory (personal communication) reports high endotoxin levels in the very early stages of one-kidney, DOCA-salt hypertension in rats; these levels decrease as the hypertension becomes chronic. Overbeck (1984) has recently investigated the possibility that significant levels of pump inhibition occur only in the very early developmental stages of one-kidney, one-clip Goldblatt hypertension in rats.

In rats with chronic (>4 weeks) one-kidney, one-clip hypertension there was no evidence for increased vascular sensitivity to norepinephrine (only evidence for vascular structural changes was present), nor for change in the ouabain-induced shift of the norepinephrine dose–response curve. Such abnormalities would have been expected if there were physiologically (inotropic) significant levels of a circulating ouabain-like pump inhibitor (and/or if the vessels were able to respond in a normal manner to such a circulating inhibitor – that is, had normal numbers of membrane sodium pump molecules). In contrast, in rats with very early one-kidney, one-clip hypertension (<1 week duration), before structural changes develop in the arteries, there may be an increase in norepinephrine sensitivity (H. W. Overbeck, unpublished observation). Thus, early in hypertension there may be mechanisms increasing the contractile state of vascular smooth muscle and elevating blood pressure. Rapidly, however, the arterial smooth muscle may develop compensatory changes, reducing the effect of such mechanisms. Additionally, wall thickening appears in arteries, allowing the body to maintain the needed elevated blood pressure in a more mechanically and thus metabolically efficient manner.

STRUCTURAL COMPONENT OF RESISTANCE IN HYPERTENSION

This considerable evidence suggesting abnormalities in the function of vascular smooth muscle cells in hypertension is matched by equally strong evidence suggesting that the structural component of resistance is also abnormal (*see Figure 4.1*). The structural component of resistance is contributed by the vascular wall, an organ composed of a heterogeneity of elements that clearly vary in the different forms and stages of hypertension. Such structural changes also involve abnormalities in salt metabolism.

Evidence for structural changes in hypertension that may infringe upon the vascular lumen comes from anatomical, biochemical, and hemodynamic studies of the vascular wall. Clearly, the muscular elements of the arterial wall undergo hypertrophy and hyperplasia in hypertension (Aikawa and Koletsky, 1970; Bevan, Van Marthens and Bevan, 1976; Friedman, Nakashima and Mar, 1971; Furuyama, 1962; Hatt, 1972). Additionally there are increased connective tissue components (Bandick and Sparks, 1970b, Ooshima *et al.*, 1974), including salt-binding glycosaminoglycans (Hollander *et al.*, 1968). Elevations of vascular wall water and sodium contents have been repeatedly observed in most forms of hypertension (Tobian, 1960).

Although these compositional changes have been regarded as being the direct result of elevated intravascular pressure, vascular wall 'waterlogging' and growth may also occur in normotensive vascular beds of hypertensive animals, such as the arterial tree downstream to an aortic coarctation, or venous walls (Overbeck, 1979; Pamnani and Overbeck, 1976). Such changes also occur in vascular walls of hypertensive animals with the sympathoadrenergic system ablated (Overbeck, 1979). Thus, humoral or local vascular wall (for example, endothelial cell) influences, as well as pressure or neurogenic influences, may play a pathogenic role.

In addition to this indirect evidence, there is direct evidence that humoral substances may be involved in the vascular wall 'waterlogging' and growth occurring in hypertension. For example, chronic digoxin administration to dogs (Overbeck, Pamnani and Ku, 1980) and rats (Overbeck, 1981) is accompanied by vascular wall 'waterlogging' and, in rats, mild hypertension. Thus, one may speculate that a circulating digitalis-like substance in hypertensives may have the same effect (*see Figure 4.6*). Simon (1979, and personal communication) has reported evidence for a humoral factor in hypertensive dogs that induces increases in glycosaminoglycan, ion and water content of cultured vascular tissue. Of great interest in this regard is the report by Schreiber *et al.* (1981) that rats with coarctation hypertension have circulating digitalis-like factors that may promote growth of myocardial cells. If growth of vascular cells also occurs, this would represent a possible link in hypertension between release of a humoral sodium-pump inhibitor, alteration in smooth muscle function and vascular wall hypertrophy/hyperplasia. The endogenous inhibitor may have stronger growth-producing and weaker inotropic properties. Thus, the former effect of the humoral substance may be far more important than the latter effect in the disease mechanisms of hypertension, and new research should address this possibility.

It is noteworthy that in spontaneous hypertension rats (SHR) cardiovascular wall thickening may occur before there is a rise in blood pressure, or even when the rise in blood pressure is prevented (Cutilletta *et al.*, 1977). Furthermore, for equal elevation in arterial pressure, the magnitude of vascular structural changes in SHR is greater than that occurring in Goldblatt hypertensive rats (Folkow, 1982). On the basis of these observations Folkow (1982) and his co-workers have suggested that there may be a 'genetic propensity' for structural vascular changes in primary forms of hypertension, such as SHR or essential hypertension in man. The biochemical mechanism of such genetic propensity has not been investigated.

The time-course of the development of structural vascular changes in hypertension is quite rapid. Folkow's group reports hemodynamic evidence for such changes within two weeks of the onset of Goldblatt hypertension in rats and we find similar evidence. The nature of these very early changes in vascular thickness has not been investigated. It is possible that increased thickness due to vascular wall edema precedes, and is gradually replaced by, the development of smooth muscle hypertrophy/hyperplasia which subsequently progresses to wall fibrosis.

Such wall thickening, whatever its cause, decreases vascular compliance (Feigl, Peterson and Jones, 1963). Wall thickening would, therefore, explain the findings of numerous hemodynamic investigations that maximal vasodilatation is impaired in most vascular beds, including both arteries and veins, in animals with hypertension (Conway, 1963; Folkow *et al.*, 1973; Overbeck *et al.*, 1971; Overbeck and Clark, 1975; Sivertsson, 1970). In these studies, supramaximal doses of potent vasodilators, such as papaverine or sodium nitroprusside, were administered intra-arterially, sometimes in conjunction with non-oxygenated artificial perfusate. Or, in man, vascular responses to profound active and reactive hyperemia were observed (Conway, 1963; Sivertsson, 1970). It is likely that these maneuvers eliminate all active tone of the vascular smooth muscle and that residual arterial resistance (the 'structural component' of resistance) or residual venous compliance, represents passive vasodilatation responding to transmural pressure.

Folkow and his associates (Folkow, 1982; Folkow *et al.*, 1973) have found that regional flow resistance under such conditions of maximal vasodilatation in established uncomplicated essential and experimental hypertension is increased to approximately the same extent as is the overall systemic resistance. Thus, these investigators postulate that, in established phases of hypertension, structural vascular changes may entirely account for the elevated resting resistance without the need to assume any increased vascular smooth muscle contraction.

These important functional implications of increases in vascular wall-to-lumen ratio due to wall thickening may best be understood in terms of the Law of Laplace. An increase in wall-to-lumen ratio decreases wall tension, conferring a mechanical advantage upon the vessel. Furthermore, contraction of smooth muscle cells situated peripherally in a thickened arterial wall would push an increased mass of tissue into the lumen, even if the degree of muscle shortening were normal. Thus,

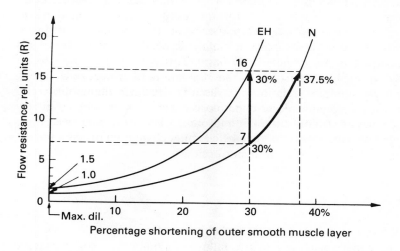

Figure 4.7 Diagram illustrating the changed relationship between degree of vascular smooth muscle shortening and increase in flow resistance, once an adaptive structural change in wall/lumen ratio has occurred in essential hypertension (EH) as compared to normotension (N). Note the increased resistance already present at maximal dilation and the exaggerated resistance increases in essential hypertension for a given smooth muscle shortening. (Modified from Folkow and Neil, 1971, courtesy of the Publishers)

any activation of the smooth muscle would evoke accentuated increases in resistance (*Figure 4.7*). This mechanical advantage of a thickened vascular wall would explain, at least in part, the observed enhanced responsiveness of hypertensives to vasoconstrictor agents (Folkow *et al.*, 1973; Lais and Brody, 1975).

These data offer compelling evidence for the importance of vascular wall thickening in the pathophysiology of established hypertension. This would represent the most metabolically efficient mechanism by which the organism could sustain an elevated vascular resistance and blood pressure over a prolonged period.

In addition to evidence for increases in wall-to-lumen ratio of arteries in hypertension, the geometry of the entire arterial bed may be abnormal. Numbers of small arterioles have been observed to be reduced by 50% in the vascular bed of the cremaster muscle in SHR (Hutchins and Darnell, 1974). The role of arterial rarification in the increased vascular resistance and enhanced responsiveness in hypertension requires further investigation. Also, the mechanism for such rarification, which may be genetic, requires further exploration.

Restructuring of vascular beds is also the basis of 'long-term total body autoregulation' proposed by Guyton, Coleman and their associates (Guyton and Coleman, 1969). Most vascular beds regulate flow by local mechanisms, such as autoregulation and active hyperemia. In the long term, alterations in blood flow through a tissue result in changes in vessel geometry, including vessel wall thickness and vessel density, for example, the development or regression of collateral vessels. Guyton and Coleman and their co-workers propose that vascular restructuring occurs in response to chronic tissue hyperfusion resulting from an increase in cardiac output in early hypertension. (Hyperperfusion is defined as a disproportionately high tissue blood flow for tissue metabolic needs.) This hypothesis is difficult to test adequately on a whole-body basis. This is in part because tissue substrate–metabolite levels, important in the regulation of blood flow, are a function of extremely complex relationships between cellular metabolism and microcirculatory flow, involving blood composition, capillary density, capillary perfusion, transit times, diffusion distances and other variables (Overbeck *et al.*, 1980). Most of these variables have not been well studied even in normal animals, and any one of them may be altered in hypertension.

CONCLUSIONS

It is clear from the preceding discussion that salt-induced hypertension is a multifaceted disorder that appears to involve failure of a number of compensatory mechanisms designed to maintain normal levels of blood pressure. It is also clear that the mechanisms by which salt induces hypertension importantly involve changes in the function of the vascular smooth muscle cell and changes in the structure of the vascular wall, as well as interactions. This mix of mechanisms appears to vary in the various forms and stages of hypertension, and considerable additional work is necessary to precisely define roles. Nevertheless, a current view (*Figure 4.8*) that is intellectually attractive and supported by increasing evidence is that functional cardiovascular (and perhaps neurological) abnormalities play the major role in the initial elevations of resistance and pressure in hypertension. It appears most likely at the present time that abnormalities in cell membrane ion kinetics are involved. In vascular smooth muscle the final common denominator of these abnormalities is an increase in sarcoplasmic Ca^{2+} and, hence, in the contractile state of the muscle.

Such cellular mechanisms are intimately associated with salt metabolism; there are very early increases in sarcolemmal permeabilities to Na^+ and K^+, perhaps genetically induced, perhaps resulting from abnormal levels of steroids, or even

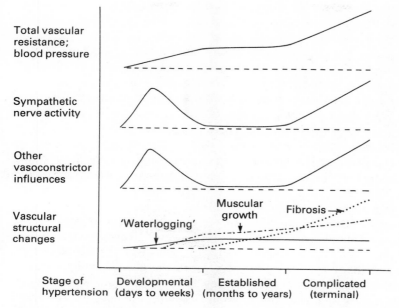

Figure 4.8 Diagram illustrating hypothetical changes in relative contributions of components of vascular resistance in stages of hypertension. 'Other vasoconstrictor influences' would include changes in sarcolemmal ion permeability and in sodium pump activity inducing increases in vascular smooth muscle myogenic tone and in sensitivity to vasoconstrictor influences. Such changes in membrane function may also contribute to increased sympathetic nerve activity. Changing role of vascular wall 'waterlogging', muscular growth, and fibrosis in the 'structural component' indicated. Hatched lines indicate baseline (normotensive) values for each variable

perhaps occurring as a result of transient, neurogenically induced, rises in intravascular pressure. Decreases in membrane sodium extrusion, for example, by defective co-transport mechanisms, may combine with the increased membrane permeability to result in net increases in cell Na^+. In turn the tendency to elevated cell sodium stimulates activity of the ouabain-sensitive sodium–potassium pump of the sarcolemma which serves to extrude the excess Na^+. As pointed out by Folkow (1982), any decrease in sodium pump function at this point would impair this compensatory process. This would tend to increase cell sodium and decrease cell membrane potential, both elevating sarcoplasmic Ca^{2+} levels. On the arterial side resistance would increase and, on the venous side, compliance decrease, the latter promoting venous return and elevating cardiac output (*see Figure 4.6*).

Function of the cell membrane sodium pump in certain patients with essential hypertension might be depressed due to genetically induced membrane abnormalities, such as fewer pump molecules. The decreases in membrane pump activity that have been observed in hypertension have also been associated with circulating digitalis-like substances that inhibit the pump. In turn, there is increasing evidence that, in early phases of hypertension, the circulating inhibitor may be a putative natriuretic hormone. Release of a natriuretic hormone, of course, is postulated to occur in response to salt load-induced volume expansion. Certainly biological variation in factors linking salt loading to volume expansion (at least to expansion in a critical portion of the circulatory tree), and/or linking volume expansion to the release of a vasoconstrictor/natriuretic factor, could account for observed differences in response to salt loading in man.

Increases in cell Na^+ concentration induced by cell membrane 'leakiness', complicated by abnormal sodium pump function, may well have other consequences of major importance for the hypertensive process. For example, such changes in cells of the nervous system may well result in increased firing of vasomotor neurons, decreased re-uptake of neurotransmitter, or both, elevating the neurogenic component of resistance. The circulating pump inhibitor (and/or the elevated cell Na^+, or increased levels of steroids), may well also induce the 'compensatory' formation of new sarcolemmal pump molecules. Induced pump molecules would tend to decrease the functional effects of the permeability increase and pump inhibition. Meanwhile, increased cell Na^+ would likely be accompanied by vascular wall 'waterlogging' (as it is in leukocytes or in vascular walls of animals given digoxin), causing very early increases in the structural component of resistance. Vascular structural changes resulting from vessel wall 'waterlogging' very early in the course of hypertension would be an extremely metabolically efficient means for maintenance of the hypertension. This would in turn perhaps result in a tendency for removal of the stimuli that induced the very early functional changes.

It is also certainly possible that elevated sodium and calcium in cardiovascular cells, interacting with the elevated pressure (and perhaps with a 'genetic propensity' or circulating growth factors), would stimulate cell growth. This would result in the vascular wall hypertrophy/hyperplasia, that characterizes the chronic established uncomplicated phases of hypertension. Although remnants of functional abnormalities may persist at reduced levels in these established phases, it is unlikely that they would contribute significantly to the elevated vascular resistance and pressure.

The late, complicated stages of hypertension are a different matter entirely. Salt-losing nephropathy reduces body fluid volumes, elevating vasoconstrictors such as ADH and angiotensin II, as well as plasma renin activity and aldosterone. Renal insufficiency is accompanied by high body levels of substances such as methylguanidine that are powerful inhibitors of membrane Na,K–ATPase. These may override any induced increases in membrane Na,K–ATPase, depolarizing sarcolemma, and elevating cell sodium, calcium and contractile state. Such pressor influences are considerably more potent, of course, in the presence of thickened vascular walls, resulting in the intense vasoconstriction characteristic of the terminal stages of hypertensive disease.

Acknowledgement

David F. Bohr, MD, kindly reviewed this chapter and provided helpful suggestions.

References

AIKAWA, M. and KOLETSKY, S. (1970) Arteriosclerosis of the mesenteric arteries of rats with renal hypertension. *American Journal of Pathology*, **61**, 293–322

AMER, M. S. (1973) Cyclic adenosine monophosphate and hypertension in rats. *Science*, **179**, 807–809

ANDERSON, D. K. (1976) Cell potential and the sodium–potassium pump in vascular smooth muscle. *Federation Proceedings*, **35**, 1294–1297

AXELSSON, J., WAHLSTRÖM, B., JOHANSSON, B. and JONSSON, O. (1967) Influence of the ionic environment on spontaneous electrical and mechanical activity of the rat portal vein. *Circulation Research*, **21**, 609–618

BAKER, P. F., BLAUSTEIN, M. P., HODGKIN, A. L. and STEINHARDT, R. A. (1969) The influence of calcium on sodium efflux in squid axons. *Journal of Physiology (London)*, **200**, 431–458

BANDICK, N. R. and SPARKS, H. V. (1970a) Contractile response of vascular smooth muscle of renal hypertensive rats. *American Journal of Physiology*, **219**, 340–344

BANDICK, N. R. and SPARKS, H. V. (1970b) Viscoelastic properties of the aorta of hypertensive rats. *Proceedings of the Society for Experimental Biology and Medicine*, **134**, 56–60

BEILIN, L. J., WADE, D. N., HONOUR, A. J. and COLE, T. J. (1970) Vascular hyper-reactivity with sodium loading and with desoxycorticosterone induced hypertension in the rat. *Clinical Science*, **39**, 793–810

BELL, D. R. and OVERBECK, H. W. (1979) Increased resistance and impaired maximal vasodilation in normotensive vascular beds of rats with coarctation hypertension. *Hypertension*, **1**, 78–85

BERECEK, K. H. and BOHR, D. F. (1976) Basis for increased vascular reactivity in experimental hypertension. In *Vascular Neuroeffector Mechanisms, Second International Symposium, Odense, 1975*, edited by J. A. Bevan *et al.*, pp. 199–204. Basel: S. Karger

BERECEK, K. H. and BOHR, D. F. (1977) Structural and functional changes in vascular resistance and reactivity in the deoxycorticosterone acetate hypertensive pig. *Circulation Research*, **40** (Suppl. I), I-146–I-152

BERNSTEIN, J. and ISRAEL, Y. (1970) Active transport of ^{86}Rb in human red cells and rat brain slices. *Journal of Pharmacology and Experimental Therapeutics*, **174**, 323–329

BEVAN, R. D., VAN MARTHENS, E. and BEVAN, J. A. (1976) Hyperplasia of vascular smooth muscle in experimental hypertension in the rabbit. *Circulation Research*, **38** (Suppl. II), II-58–II-62

BLAUSTEIN, M. P. (1977) Sodium ions, calcium ions, blood pressure regulation and hypertension: a reassessment and a hypothesis. *American Journal of Physiology*, **232**, C165–C173

BLUSCHKE, V., BONN, R. and GREEF, K. (1976) Increase in the $(Na^{+}-K^{+})$–ATPase activity in heart muscle after chronic treatment with digoxin or potassium deficient diet. *European Journal of Pharmacology*, **37**, 189–191

BOHR, D. F. (1973) Vascular smooth muscle updated. *Circulation Research*, **32**, 655–672

BOHR, D. F. (1974) Reactivity of vascular smooth muscle from normal and hypertensive rats: effects of several cations. *Federation Proceedings,* **33,** 127–132

BOHR, D. F. and SITRIN, M. (1970) Regulation of vascular smooth muscle contraction. *Circulation Research,* **26/27** (Suppl. II), II-83–II-90

BOZLER, E. (1948) Conduction, automaticity, and tonus of visceral muscles. *Experientia,* **4,** 213–218

BROCK, T. A., SMITH, J. B. and OVERBECK, H. W. (1982) Relationship of vascular $Na^+–K^+$ pump activity to intracellular sodium in hypertensive rats. *Hypertension,* **4** (Suppl. II), II-43–II-48

BRODY, M. J., JOHNSON, A. K. (1980) Role of the anteroventral third ventricle region in fluid and electrolyte balance, arterial pressure regulation, and hypertension. In *Frontiers in Neuroendocrinology,* edited by L. Martini and W, F. Ganong, pp. 249–292. New York: Raven Press

BURRIS, J. F., PAMNANI, M. B., HUOT, S. J., JEMIONEK, J. F., FREIS, E. D. and HADDY, F. J. (1982) Sodium–potassium pump activity in low renin essential hypertension. *Clinical Research,* **30,** 733A (Abstract)

CLINESCHMIDT, B. V., GELLER, R. G., GOVIER, W. C. and SJOERDSMA, A. (1970) Reactivity to norepinephrine and nature of the alpha-adrenergic receptor in vascular smooth muscle of a genetically hypertensive rat. *European Journal of Pharmacology,* **10,** 45–50

CLOUGH, D. L., PAMNANI, M. B., OVERBECK, H. W. and HADDY, F. J. (1977) Decreased Na,K–ATPase in right ventricular myocardium of rats with one-kidney Goldblatt hypertension. *Physiologist,* **20,** 18 (Abstract)

COHEN, M. L. and BERKOWITZ, B. A. (1976) Decreased vascular relaxation in hypertension. *Journal of Pharmacology and Experimental Therapeutics,* **196,** 396–406

COLLIS, M. G. and ALPS, B. J. (1975) Vascular reactivity to noradrenaline, potassium chloride, and angiotensin II in the rat perfused mesenteric vasculature preparation during the development of renal hypertension. *Cardiovascular Research,* **9,** 118–126

CONWAY, J. (1963) A vascular abnormality in hypertension. Study of blood flow in the forearm. *Circulation,* **27,** 520–529

CUTILLETTA, A. F., ERINOFF, L., HELLER, A., LOW, J. and OPARIL, S. (1977) Development of left ventricular hypertrophy in young spontaneously hypertensive rats after peripheral sympathectomy. *Circulation Research,* **40,** 428–434

DAHL, L. K., HEINE, M. and TASSINARI, L. (1962) Effects of chronic excess salt ingestion. Evidence that genetic factors play an important role in susceptibility to experimental hypertension. *Journal of Experimental Medicine,* **115,** 1173–1190

DAHL, L. K., KNUDSEN, K. D. and IWAI, J. (1969) Humoral transmission of hypertension. Evidence from parabiosis. *Circulation Research,* **24/25** (Suppl. I), I-21–I-33

DAHL, L. K. (1972) Salt and hypertension. *American Journal of Clinical Nutrition,* **25,** 231–244

DEVINE, C. E., SOMLYO, A. V. and SOMLYO, A. P. (1972) Sarcoplasmic reticulum and excitation–contraction coupling in mammalian smooth muscles. *Journal of Cell Biology,* **52,** 690–718 de WARDENER, H. E. and MACGREGOR, G. A. (1980) Dahl's hypothesis that a saluretic substance may be responsible for the sustained rise in arterial pressure: its possible role in essential hypertension. *Kidney International,* **18,** 1–9

DOYLE, A. E. and FRASER, J. R. E. (1961) Essential hypertension and inheritance of vascular reactivity. *Lancet,* **2,** 509–511

DROOGMANS, G., RAEMAEKERS, L. and CASTEELS, R. (1977) Electro- and pharmaco-mechanical coupling in the smooth muscle cells of the rabbit ear artery. *Journal of General Physiology,* **70,** 129–148

DUSTAN, H. P., BRAVO, E. L. and TARAZI, R. C. (1973) Volume-dependent essential and steroid hypertension. *American Journal of Cardiology,* **31,** 606–615

EDMONDSON, R. P. S., THOMAS, R. D., HILTON, P. J., PATRICK, J. and JONES, N. F. (1975) Abnormal leukocyte composition and sodium transport in essential hypertension. *Lancet,* **1,** 1003–1005

ELLIS, C. N. and JULIUS, S. (1973) Role of central blood volume in hyperkinetic borderline hypertension. *British Heart Journal,* **35,** 450–455

ENDO, M., TANAKA, M. and OGAWA, Y. (1970) Calcium induced release of calcium from the sarcoplasmic reticulum of skeletal muscle fibres. *Nature (London),* **228,** 34–36

EVANS, D. H. L., SCHILD, H. O. and THESLEFF, S. (1958) Effects of drugs on depolarized plain muscle. *Journal of Physiology (London),* **143,** 474–485

FADEKE ADEROUNMU, A. and SALAKO, L. A. (1979) Abnormal cation composition and transport in erythrocytes from hypertensive patients. *European Journal of Clinical Investigation,* **9,** 369–375

FEIGL, E. O., PETERSON, L. H. and JONES, A. W. (1963) Mechanical and chemical properties of arteries in experimental hypertension. *Journal of Clinical Investigation,* **42,** 1640–1647

FIELD, F. P., JANIS, R. A. and TRIGGLE, D. J. (1972) Aortic reactivity of rats with genetic and experimental renal hypertension. *Canadian Journal of Physiology and Pharmacology,* **50,** 1072–1079

FILO, R. S., BOHR, D. F. and RÜEGG, J. C. (1965) Glycerinated skeletal and smooth muscle: calcium and magnesium dependence. *Science,* **147,** 1581–1583

FINCH, L. and HAEUSLER, G. (1974) Vascular resistance and reactivity in hypertensive rats. *Blood Vessels,* **11,** 145–158

FOLKOW, B. (1982) Physiological aspects of primary hypertension. *Physiological Reviews,* **62,** 347–504

FOLKOW, B. and NEIL, E. (1971) *Circulation.* New York: Oxford University Press

FOLKOW, B., HALLBÄCK, M., LUNDGREN, Y., SIVERTSSON, R. and WEISS, L. (1973) Importance of adaptive changes in vascular design for establishment of primary hypertension, studied in man and in spontaneously hypertensive rats. *Circulation Research,* **22/23** (Suppl. I), I-2–I-16

FORRESTER, T. E. and ALLEYNE, G. A. O. (1980) Leukocyte electrolytes and sodium efflux rate constants in the hypertension of pre-eclampsia. *Clinical Science,* **59,** 199S–201S

FREIS, E. D. (1976) Salt, volume and the prevention of hypertension. *Circulation,* **53,** 589–595

FRIEDMAN, S. M. (1979) Evidence for an enhanced sodium transport in the tail artery of the spontaneously hypertensive rat. *Hypertension*, **1**, 572–582

FRIEDMAN, S. M. and FRIEDMAN, C. L. (1976) Cell permeability, sodium transport, and the hypertensive process in the rat. *Circulation Research*, **39**, 433–441

FRIEDMAN, S. M., NAKASHIMA, M. and MAR, M. A. (1971) Morphological assessment of vasoconstriction and vascular hypertrophy in sustained hypertension in the rat. *Microvascular Research*, **3**, 416–425

FURUYAMA, M. (1962) Histometrical investigations of arteries in reference to arterial hypertension. *Tohoku Journal of Experimental Medicine*, **76**, 388–414

GARAY, R. P. and DAGHER, G. (1980) Erythrocyte Na and K transport systems in essential hypertension. In *Intracellular Electrolytes and Arterial Hypertension*, edited by H. Zumkley and H. Losse, pp. 69–76. Stuttgart, New York: George Thieme Verlag

GARAY, R. P. and GARRAHAN, P. J. (1973) The interaction of sodium and potassium with the sodium pump in red cells. *Journal of Physiology (London)*, **231**, 297–325

GARAY, R. P., DAGHER, G. and MEYER, P. (1980) An inherited sodium ion–potassium ion cotransport defect in essential hypertension. *Clinical Science*, **59**, 191S–193S

GARAY, R. P., DAGHER, G., PERNOLLET, M. G., DEVYNK, M. A. and MEYER, P. (1980) Inherited defect in a Na–K-cotransport system in erythrocytes from essential hypertensive patients. *Nature (London)*, **284**, 281–283

GODFRAIND, T. (1976) Calcium exchange in vascular smooth muscle. Action of noradrenaline and lanthanum. *Journal of Physiology (London)*, **260**, 21–35

GÖTHBERG, G., JANDYALA, B. and FOLKOW, B. (1980) Studies on the role of sodium–potassium activated ATPase as determinant of vascular reactivity in Wistar-Kyoto and spontaneously hypertensive rats. *Clinical Science*, **59**, 187S–189S

GRUBER, K. A., RUDEL, L. L. and BULLOCK, B. C. (1982) Increased circulating levels of an endogenous digoxin-like factor in hypertensive monkeys. *Hypertension*, **4**, 348–354

GRUBER, K. A., WHITAKER, J. M. and BUCKALEW, V. M. JR. (1980) Endogenous digitalis-like substance in plasma of volume-expanded dogs. *Nature*, **287**, 743–745

GUIGNARD, J. P. and FRIEDMAN, S. M. (1970) Intraluminal pressure and ionic distribution in the tail artery of rats. *Circulation Research*, **27**, 505–512

GUIGNARD, J. P. and FRIEDMAN, S. M. (1971) Vascular ionic effects of angiotensin II in the rat. *Proceedings of the Society for Experimental Biology and Medicine*, **137**, 147–150

GUYTON, A. C. and COLEMAN, T. G. (1969) Quantitative analysis of the pathophysiology of hypertension. *Circulation Research*, **24/25** (Suppl. I) I-1–I-19

HADDY, F. J. (1980) Mechanism, prevention and therapy of sodium-dependent hypertension. *American Journal of Medicine*, **69**, 746–758

HADDY, F. J. and OVERBECK, H. W. (1976) The role of humoral agents in volume expanded hypertension. *Life Sciences*, **19**, 935–948

HAEUSLER, G. and FINCH, L. (1972) Vascular reactivity to 5-hydroxytryptamine and hypertension in the rat. *Naunyn-Schmiedeberg's Archives of Pharmacology*, **272**, 101–116

HAMLYN, J. M., RINGEL, R., SCHAEFFER, J. *et al.* (1982) A circulating inhibitor of (Na$^+$ + K$^+$) ATPase associated with essential hypertension. *Nature,* **300,** 650–652

HANSEN, T. R. and BOHR, D. F. (1975) Hypertension, transmural pressure, and vascular smooth muscle response in rats. *Circulation Research,* **36,** 590–598

HANSEN, T. R., ABRAMS, G. D. and BOHR, D. F. (1974) Role of pressure in structural and functional changes in arteries of hypertensive rats. *Circulation Research,* **34,** (Suppl. I) I-101–I-108

HATT, P. Y. (1972) Electron microscopic study of arterial lesions in experimental hypertension. In *Hypertension '72,* edited by J. Genest and E. Koiw, pp. 196–212. Berlin, Heidelberg, New York: Springer-Verlag

HAWTHORNE, E. W., HINDS, J. E., CRAWFORD, W. J. and TEARNEY, R. J. (1974) Left ventricular myocardial contractility during the first week of renal hypertension in conscious instrumented dogs. *Circulation Research,* **34/35** (Suppl. I), I-223–I-234

HEAGERTY, A. M., MILNER, M., BING, R. F., THURSTON, H. and SWALES, J. D. (1982) Leukocyte membrane sodium transport in normotensive populations: dissociation of abnormalities of sodium efflux from raised blood pressure. *Lancet,* **2,** 894–896

HENDRICKX, H. and CASTEELS, R. (1974) Electrogenic sodium pump in arterial smooth muscle cells. *Pflügers Archiv für Gesamte Physiologie,* **346,** 299–306

HERMSMEYER, K. (1971) Contraction and membrane activation in several mammalian vascular muscles. *Life Sciences,* **10,** 223–234

HERMSMEYER, K. (1976a) Electrogenesis of increased norepinephrine sensitivity of arterial vascular muscle in hypertension. *Circulation Research,* **38,** 362–367

HERMSMEYER, K. (1976b) Cellular basis for increased sensitivity of vascular smooth muscle in spontaneously hypertensive rats. *Circulation Research,* **38** (Suppl. II), II-53–II-57

HERMSMEYER, K. (1976c) Ba^{2+} and K$^+$ alteration of K$^+$ conductance in spontaneously active vascular muscle. *American Journal of Physiology,* **230,** 1031–1036

HOLLANDER, W., KRAMSCH, D. M., FARMELANT, M. and MADOFF, I. M. (1968) Arterial wall metabolism in experimental hypertension of coarctation of the aorta of short duration. *Journal of Clinical Investigation,* **47,** 1221–1229

HOLLOWAY, E. T. and BOHR, D. F. (1973) Reactivity of vascular smooth muscle in hypertensive rats. *Circulation Research,* **33,** 678–685

HOLMAN, M. E. (1958) Membrane potentials recorded with high-resistance microelectrodes; and the effects of changes in ionic environment on the electrical and mechanical activity of the smooth muscle of the taenia coli of the guinea pig. *Journal of Physiology (London),* **141,** 464–488

HOLMAN, M. E. (1969) Electrophysiology of vascular smooth muscle. *Ergebnisse der Physiologie,* **61,** 137–177

HORWITZ, D., CLINESCHMIDT, B. V., VAN BUREN, J. M. and OMMAYA, A. K. (1974) Temporal arteries from hypertensive and normotensive man. *Circulation Research,* **34** (Suppl. I), I-109–I-115

HUTCHINS, P. M. and DARNELL, A. E. (1974) Observation of a decreased number of small arterioles in spontaneously hypertensive rats. *Circulation Research,* **34/35** (Suppl. I), I-161–I-165

JAMIESON, J. D. and FRIEDMAN, S. M. (1961) Sodium and potassium shifts associated with peripheral resistance changes in the dog. *Circulation Research,* **9,** 996–1004

JANIS, R. A. and TRIGGLE, D. J. (1973) Effect of diazoxide on aortic reactivity to calcium in spontaneously hypertensive rats. *Canadian Journal of Physiology and Pharmacology,* **51,** 621–626

JOHANSSON, B. (1971) Electromechanical and mechanoelectrical coupling in vascular smooth muscle. *Angiologica,* **8,** 129–143

JOHANSSON, B. (1978) Vascular smooth muscle: biophysics. In *Microcirculation,* edited by B. M. Altura and G. Kaley, pp. 83–117. Baltimore: University Park Press

JOHANSSON, B. and MELLANDER, S. (1975) Static and dynamic components in the vascular myogenic response to passive changes in length as revealed by electrical and mechanical recordings from the rat portal vein. *Circulation Research,* **36,** 76–83

JOHANSSON, B. and SOMLYO, A. P. (1980) Electrophysiology and excitation-contraction coupling. In *Handbook of Physiology, Section on Circulation,* edited by D. F. Bohr, A. P. Somlyo and H. V. Sparks, Volume, 2, Section 2, pp. 301–323. American Physiological Society

JOHNSON, P. C. (1978) Myogenic tone in resistance vessels. In *Mechanisms of Vasodilation,* edited by P. M. Vanhoutte and I. Leusen, pp. 73–78. Basel: S. Karger

JONES, A. W. (1973) Altered ion transport in vascular smooth muscle from spontaneously hypertensive rats. *Circulation Research,* **33,** 563–572

JONES, A. W. (1974a) Altered ion transport in large and small arteries from spontaneously hypertensive rats and the influence of calcium. *Circulation Research,* **34** (Suppl. I), I-117–I-122

JONES, A. W. (1974b) Reactivity of ion fluxes in rat aorta during hypertension and circulatory control. *Federation Proceedings,* **33,** 133–137

JONES, A. W. (1976) Functional changes in vascular smooth muscle associated with experimental hypertension. In *Vascular Neuroeffector Mechanisms,* edited by J. A. Bevan, B. Johansson, R. A. Maxwell and O. A. Nedergaard, pp. 182–189. Basel: S. Karger

JONES, A. W. (1981) Kinetics of active sodium transport in aortas from control and deoxycorticosterone hypertensive rats. *Hypertension,* **3,** 631–640

JONES, A. W. and HART, R. G. (1975) Altered ion transport in aortic smooth muscle during deoxycorticosterone acetate hypertension in the rat. *Circulation Research,* **37,** 333–341

JONES, A. W. and SWAIN, M. L. (1972) Chemical and kinetic analyses of sodium distribution in canine lingual artery. *American Journal of Physiology,* **223,** 1110–1118

JOSHUA, I. G., WIEGMAN, D. L., HARRIS, P. D. and MILLER, F. N. (1984) Progressive microvascular alterations with the development of renovascular hypertension. *Hypertension,* **6,** 61–67

KAWASAKI, T., DELEA, C. S., BARTTER, F. C. and SMITH, H. (1978) The effect of high sodium and low sodium intakes on blood pressure and other related variables in human subjects with idiopathic hypertension. *American Journal of Medicine,* **64,** 193–198

KEMPNER, W. (1948) Treatment of hypertensive vascular disease with rice diet. *American Journal of Medicine,* **4,** 545–577

LAIS, L. T. and BRODY, M. J. (1975) Mechanism of vascular hyper-responsiveness in the spontaneously hypertensive rat. *Circulation Research,* **36** (Suppl. I), I-216–I-222

LANGER, G. (1976) Events at the cardiac sarcolemma: localization and movement of contractile-dependent calcium. *Federation Proceedings,* **35,** 1274–1278

LEE, S.-W., SCHWARTZ, A., ADAMS, R. J., YAMORI, Y. *et al.* (1983) Decrease in Na^+,K^+–ATPase activity and [^3H] ouabain binding sites in sarcolemma prepared from hearts of spontaneously hypertensive rats. *Hypertension,* **5,** 682–688

LEVY, J. V. (1973) Contractile responses of isolated portal veins from normal and spontaneously hypertensive rats. *Clinical Research,* **21,** 237 (Abstract)

LEVY, J. V. (1974) Differences in papaverine inhibition of prostaglandin-induced contraction of aortic strips from normal and spontaneously hypertensive rats (SHR). *European Journal of Pharmacology,* **25,** 117–120

LEVY, J. V. (1975) Verapamil and diazoxide antagonism of agonist-induced contractions of aortic strips from normal and spontaneously hypertensive rats (SHR). *Research Communications Chemistry, Pathology, Pharmacology,* **11,** 387–404

LIMAS, C. J. and COHN, J. N. (1977) Defective calcium transport by cardiac sarcoplasmic reticulum in spontaneously hypertensive rats. *Circulation Research,* **40** (Suppl. I), I-62–I-69

LOCKETTE, W. E., WEBB, R. C. and BOHR, D. F. (1980) Prostaglandins and potassium relaxation in vascular smooth muscle of the rat. The role of the Na–K–ATPase. *Circulation Research,* **46,** 714–720

LUFT, F. C., RANKIN, L. I., HENRY, D. P. *et al.* (1979) Plasma and urinary norepinephrine values at extremes of sodium intake in normal man. *Hypertension,* **1,** 261–266

MACGREGOR, G. A., FENTON, S., ALAGHBAND-ZAADEH, J. *et al.* (1981) Evidence for a raised concentration of a circulating sodium transport inhibitor in essential hypertension. *British Medical Journal,* **283,** 1355–1357

MCCARRON, D. A., MORRIS, C. D. and COLE, C. (1982) Dietary calcium in human hypertension. *Science,* **217,** 267–269

MCGREGOR, D. D. and SMIRK, F. H. (1970) Vascular responses to 5-hydroxytryptamine in genetic and renal hypertensive rats. *American Journal of Physiology,* **219,** 687–690

MENEELY, G. R., BALL, C. O. T. and YOUMANS, J. B. (1957) Chronic sodium chloride toxicity: protective effect of added potassium chloride. *Annals of Internal Medicine,* **47,** 263–273

MULVANY, M. J., AALKJAER, C. and CHRISTENSEN, J. (1980) Changes in noradrenalin sensitivity and morphology of arterial resistance vessels during development of high blood pressure in spontaneously hypertensive rats. *Hypertension,* **2,** 664–671

MURPHY, R. A. (1982) Myosin phosphorylation and cross-bridge regulation in arterial smooth muscle. State-of-the-art review. *Hypertension,* **4** (Suppl. II), II-3–II-7

OOSHIMA, A., FULLER, G. C., CARDINALE, G. J., SPECTOR, S. and UDENFRIEND, S. (1974) Increased collagen synthesis in blood vessels of hypertensive rats and its reversal by antihypertensive agents. *Proceedings of the National Academy of Sciences of the USA,* **71,** 3019–3023

OVERBECK, H. W. (1972) Vascular responses to cations, osmolality, and angiotensin in renal hypertensive dogs. *American Journal of Physiology,* **223,** 1358–1364

OVERBECK, H. W. (1979) Cardiovascular hypertrophy and 'waterlogging' in coarctation hypertension: role of sympathoadrenergic influences and pressure. *Hypertension,* **1,** 486–492

OVERBECK, H. W. (1981) Elevated arterial pressure, vascular wall 'waterlogging', and impaired cardiac growth in rats chronically receiving digoxin. *Proceedings of the Society for Experimental Biology and Medicine,* **167,** 506–513

OVERBECK, H. W. (1983) Function of the sodium pump in vascular smooth muscle in hypertension. In *Pathophysiological Mechanisms of Hypertension,* edited by H. Villareal and M. P. Sambhi. Boston, The Hague, Dordrecht, Lancaster: Martinus Nijhoff

OVERBECK, H. W. (1984) Effect of ouabain on arteriolar responses to norepinephrine in chronic, benign volume-expanded hypertension. *Hypertension,* **6** (Suppl. I), I-82–I-87

OVERBECK, H. W. and CLARK, D. W. J. (1975) Vasodilator responses to K^+ in genetic hypertensive and in renal hypertensive rats. *Journal of Laboratory and Clinical Medicine,* **86,** 973–983

OVERBECK, H. W. and GRISSETTE, D. E. (1982) Sodium pump activity in arteries of rats with Goldblatt hypertension. *Hypertension,* **4,** 132–139

OVERBECK, H. W., DAUGHERTY, R. M. and HADDY, F. J. (1969) Continuous infusion indicator–dilution measurement of limb blood flow and vascular response to magnesium sulfate in normotensive and hypertensive men. *Journal of Clinical Investigation,* **48,** 1944–1956

OVERBECK, H. W., KU, D. D. and RAPP, J. P. (1981) Sodium pump activity in arteries of Dahl salt-sensitive rats. *Hypertension,* **3,** 306–312

OVERBECK, H. W., PAMNANI, M. B. and DERIFIELD, R. S. (1975) Similar vasoconstrictor responses to calcium in normotensive and essential hypertensive men. *Proceedings of the Society for Experimental Biology and Medicine,* **149,** 519–525

OVERBECK, H. W., PAMNANI, M. B. and KU, D. D. (1980) Arterial wall 'waterlogging' accompanying chronic digoxin treatment in dogs. *Proceedings of the Society for Experimental Biology and Medicine,* **164,** 401–404

OVERBECK, H. W., BELL, D. R., GRISSETTE, D. E. and BROCK, T. A. (1982) Function of the sodium pump in arterial smooth muscle in hypertension – role of pressure. *Hypertension,* **4,** 394–399

OVERBECK, H. W., DERIFIELD, R. S., PAMNANI, M. B. and SÖZEN, T. (1974) Attenuated vasodilator responses to K^+ in essential hypertensive men. *Journal of Clinical Investigation,* **53,** 678–686

OVERBECK, H. W., PAMNANI, M. B., AKERA, T., BRODY, T. M. and HADDY, F. J. (1976) Depressed function of an ouabain-sensitive sodium–potassium pump in blood vessels from renal hypertensive dogs. *Circulation Research,* **38** (Suppl. II), II-48–II-52

OVERBECK, H. W., SWINDALL, B. T., COWAN, D. F. and FLECK, M. C. (1971) Experimental renal hypertension in dogs. Forelimb hemodynamics. *Circulation Research*, **29**, 51–62

OVERBECK, H. W., BERNE, R. M., CHIEN, S. *et al.* (1980) Report of the Hypertension Task Force of NHLBI. Current research and recommendations from the subgroup on local hemodynamics. *Hypertension*, **2**, 342–369

PAGE, L. B., DANION, A. and MOELLERING, R. C. JR. (1974) Antecedents of cardiovascular disease in six Solomon Islands societies. *Circulation*, **49**, 1132–1146

PAMNANI, M. B. and OVERBECK, H. W. (1976) Abnormal ion and water composition of veins and normotensive arteries in coarctation hypertension in rats. *Circulation Research*, **38**, 375–378

PAMNANI, M. B., CLOUGH, D. L., HUOT, S. J. and HADDY, F. J. (1980) Vascular Na^+–K^+ pump activity in Dahl S and R rats. *Proceedings of the Society for Experimental Biology and Medicine*, **165**, 440–444

PAMNANI, M., BUGGY, J., HUOT, S., CLOUGH, D. and HADDY, F. (1981a) Vascular Na^+–K^+ pump activity in acutely saline loaded rats with anteroventral (AV3V) lesions. *Federation Proceedings*, **40**, 390 (Abstract)

PAMNANI, M. B., HARDER, D. R., HUOT, S. J., BRYANT, H. J., KUTYNA, F. A. and HADDY, F. J. (1981b) Vascular smooth muscle membrane potentials and the influence of an ouabain-like humoral factor in rats with one-kidney, one-clip hypertension. *Physiologist*, **24**, 6 (Abstract)

PARKER, J. C. and BERKOWITZ, L. R. (1983) Physiologically instructive genetic variants involving the human red cell membrane. *Physiological Reviews*, **63**, 261–313

PLUNKETT, W. C., HUTCHINS, P. M., GRUBER, K. A. and BUCKALEW, V. M. JR. (1982) Evidence for a vascular sensitizing factor in plasma of saline-loaded dogs. *Hypertension*, **4**, 581–589

POSTON, L., SEWELL, R. B., WILKINSON, S. P. *et al.* (1981) Evidence for a circulating sodium transport inhibitor in essential hypertension. *British Medical Journal*, **282**, 847–849

RAHMAN, M., PRIMERA, M. I., QUITANILLA, A. P., HUANG, C. M. and DELGRECO, F. (1982) ATPase activity, Na extrusion and K influx in the red cell in essential hypertension. *Clinical Research*, **30**, 776A (Abstract)

REPORT OF THE HYPERTENSION TASK FORCE (1979a) Volume 3: *Local and Systemic Hemodynamics*. Department of Health, Education and Welfare Publication No. (NIH) 79-1625, pp. 1–236

REPORT OF THE HYPERTENSION TASK FORCE (1979b) Volume 5: *Vascular Smooth Muscle: Contractile Apparatus*. Department of Health, Education and Welfare Publication No. (NIH), 79–1627, pp. 139–245

REPORT OF THE HYPERTENSION TASK FORCE (1979c) Volume 8: *Salt and Water*. Department of Health, Education and Welfare Publication No. (NIH), 79-1630, pp. 115–182

REUTER, H. and SEITZ, H. (1968) The dependence of calcium efflux from cardiac muscle on temperature and external ion composition. *Journal of Physiology (London)*, **195**, 451–470

RYGIELSKI, D. B., KROPP, D. L. and DURAN, W. N. (1981) Hypertension and the Na–K pump. *Federation Proceedings*, **40**, 611 (Abstract)

SASAKI, N. (1964) The relationship of salt intake to hypertension in the Japanese. *Geriatrics,* **19,** 735–744

SCHREIBER, V., KÖLBEL, F., ŠTEPAN, J., GREGOROVÀ, I and PŘIBYL, T. (1981) Digoxin-like immunoreactivity in the serum of rats with cardiac overload. *Journal of Molecular and Cellular Cardiology,* **13,** 107–110

SHIBATA, S., KURAHASHI, K. and KUCHII, M. (1973) A possible etiology of contractility impairment of vascular smooth muscle from spontaneously hypertensive rats. *Journal of Pharmacology and Experimental Therapeutics,* **185,** 406–417

SIMON, G. (1979) Angiopathic serum factor in perinephritic hypertensive dogs. *Hypertension,* **1,** 197–201

SIMPSON, F. O. (1979) Salt and hypertension: a sceptical review of the evidence. *Clinical Science,* **57,** 463S–480S

SIVERTSSON, R. (1970) The hemodynamic importance of structural vascular changes in essential hypertension. *Acta Physiologica Scandinavica,* **79** (Suppl. 343), 5–56

SOMLYO, A. P. (1978) The role of organelles in regulating cytoplasmic calcium in vascular smooth muscle. In *Mechanisms of Vasodilation,* edited by P. M. Vanhoutte and I. Leusen, pp. 21–29. Basel: S. Karger

SOMLYO, A. P. and SOMLYO, A. V. (1968a) Vascular smooth muscle. I. Normal structure, pathology, biochemistry, and biophysics. *Pharmacological Reviews,* **20,** 197–272

SOMLYO, A. V. and SOMLYO, A. P. (1968b) Electromechanical and pharmacomechanical coupling in vascular smooth muscle. *Journal of Pharmacology and Experimental Therapeutics,* **159,** 129–145

SOMLYO, A. V. and SOMLYO, A. P. (1971) Electrophysiological correlates of the inequality of maximal vascular smooth muscle contraction elicited by drugs. In *Vascular Neuroeffector Systems,* edited by J. A. Bevan, R. F. Furchgott, R. A. Maxwell and O. A. Nedergaard, pp. 216–261. Basel: S. Karger

SOMLYO, A. V. and SOMLYO, A. P. (1971) Electrophysiological correlates of the inequality of maximal vascular smooth muscle contraction elicited by drugs. In *Vascular Neuroeffector Systems,* edited by J. A. Bevan, R. F. Furchgott, R. A. Maxwell and O. A. Nedergaard, pp. 216–261. Basel: S. Karger

SOMLYO, A. V., VINALL, O. and SOMLYO, A. P. (1969) Excitation–contraction coupling and electrical events in two types of vascular smooth muscle. *Microvascular Research,* **1,** 354–373

SONGU-MIZE, E., BEALER, S. L. and CALDWELL, R. W. (1982) Effect of AV3V lesions on development of DOCA-salt hypertension and vascular Na^+ pump activity. *Hypertension,* **4,** 575–580

SPECTOR, S., FLEISCH, J. H., MALING, H. M. and BRODIE, B. B. (1969) Vascular smooth muscle reactivity in normotensive and hypertensive rats. *Science,* **166,** 1300–1301

STEIN, I. M., PEREZ, G., JOHNSON, R. and CUMMINGS, N. B. (1971) Serum levels and urinary excretion of methylguanidine in chronic renal failure. *Journal of Laboratory and Clinical Medicine,* **77,** 1020–1024

THOMAS, R. D., EDMONDSON, R. P. S., HILTON, P. J. and JONES, N. F. (1975) Abnormal sodium transport in leukocytes from patients with essential hypertension and the effect of treatment. *Clinical Science Molecular Medicine,* **48,** 169S–170S

TOBIAN, L. (1960) Interrelationship of electrolytes, juxtaglomerular cells and hypertension. *Physiological Reviews,* **40,** 280–312

TOBIAN, L., LANGE, J., IWAI, J., HILLER, K., JOHNSON, M. A. and GOOSENS, P. (1979) Prevention with thiazide of NaCl-induced hypertension in Dahl 'S' rats. Evidence for a Na-retaining humoral agent in 'S' rats. *Hypertension*, **1**, 316–323

TRINER, L., VULLIEMOZ, Y., VEROSKY, M. and MANGER, W. (1975) Cyclic adenosine monophosphate and vascular reactivity in spontaneously hypertensive rats. *Biochemical Pharmacology*, **24**, 743–745

UVELIUS, B., SIGURDSSON, S. B. and JOHANSSON, B. (1974) Strontium and barium as substitutes for calcium on electrical and mechanical activity in rat portal vein. *Blood Vessels*, **11**, 245–259

VAN BREEMEN, C., AARONSON, P. and LOUTZENHISER, R. (1979) Sodium–calcium interactions in mammalian smooth muscle. *Pharmacological Reviews*, **30**, 167–208

VILLAMIL, M. F. (1972) Angiotensin, hypertension and vascular ionic composition. *Medicina*, **32** (Suppl. I), 57

WALTER, U. and DISTLER, A. (1980) Effects of ouabain and furosemide on ATPase activity and sodium transport in erythrocytes of normotensives and of patients with essential hypertension. In *Intracellular Electrolytes and Arterial Hypertension*, edited by H. Zumkley and H. Losse, pp. 170–181. Stuttgart, New York: George Thieme Verlag

WALTER, U. and DISTLER, A. (1982) Abnormal sodium efflux in erythrocytes of patients with essential hypertension. *Hypertension*, **4**, 205–210

WAMBACH, G., HELBER, A., BONNER, G. and HUMMERICH, W. (1978) Natrium–kalium–ATPase aktivitat in Erythrozyten ghost und Electrolytkonzentration in Erythrozyten von Patienten mit essentieller Hypertonie. *Verhandlungen der Deutschen Gesellschaft für Innere Medizin*, **84**, 800–805

WAMBACH, G., HELBER, A., BONNER, G. and HUMMERICH, W. (1979) Natrium–kalium–ATPase aktivitat in Erythrozyten ghosts von Patienten mit essentieller Hypertonie. *Klinische Wochenschrift*, **57**, 169–172

WAMBACH, G., HELBER, A., BONNER, G., HUMMERICH, W., KONRADS, A. and KAUFFMAN, W. (1980) Sodium–potassium ATPase activity in erythrocyte ghosts of patients with primary and secondary hypertension. *Clinical Science*, **59**, 183S–185S

WEBB, R. C. and BHALLA, R. C. (1976) Altered calcium sequestration by subcellular fractions of vascular smooth muscle from spontaneously hypertensive rats. *Journal of Molecular and Cellular Cardiology*, **8**, 651–661

WOODS, K. L., BEEVERS, D. G. and WEST, M. (1981) Familial abnormality of erythrocyte cation transport in essential hypertension. *British Medical Journal*, **282**, 1186–1188

ZELIS, R. and MASON, D. T. (1970) Compensatory mechanisms in congestive heart failure–the role of the peripheral resistance vessels. *New England Journal of Medicine*, **282**, 962–964

ZIMMERMAN, B. G. (1967) Evaluation of peripheral and central components of action of angiotensin on the sympathetic nervous system. *Journal of Pharmacology and Experimental Therapeutics*, **158**, 1–10

5
Natriuretic hormone and essential hypertension

H. E. de Wardener and G. A. MacGregor

NATRIURETIC HORMONE

Whole animal experiments

When the volume of body fluids is expanded the plasma acquires natriuretic properties (de Wardener, 1977) and its capacity to inhibit sodium transport increases (de Wardener and Clarkson, 1982). The principal evidence that the natriuretic activity is due to a circulating substance other than aldosterone which modifies the urinary excretion of sodium comes from experiments in which the fluid volume of an animal that has been given large amounts of salt-retaining steroids is rapidly increased without diminishing the plasma protein concentration or packed cell volume of the animal's blood. In these experiments the presence of the natriuretic substance is simultaneously assayed *in vivo,* either by a denervated or isolated kidney perfused at a controlled pressure, or by a recipient animal cross-circulated with the expanded donor animal. Experiments in which the fluid volume of an animal has been expanded by the administration of saline, Ringer solution or various concentrations of albumin mainly demonstrate that such protocols, which are accompanied by haemodilution, are unsuitable to determine whether the ensuing natriuresis is accompanied by a humoral component.

The ideal way to expand the fluid volume of an animal acutely without causing dilutional change is to expand the animal with blood with which it is in equilibrium. The blood of an animal is continuously exchanged with the contents of a reservoir which is initially primed with a solution of bovine albumin in either Ringer solution or saline. After 1 or 2 hours of such an exchange the blood in the reservoir is in equilibrium with the blood in the animal. The animal's blood volume is then expanded by about 30% in 15–20 min by lowering the fluid level in the reservoir. With a kidney used as the assay system this experiment has been performed by five groups (Bahlmann *et al.*, 1967; Bengele, Houttuin and Pearce, 1972; Blythe *et al.*, 1971; Kaloyanides and Azer, 1971; Knox *et al.*, 1968). The 'assay' kidney is either left *in situ* but is denervated, or it is isolated and perfused in a saline bath (*Figure 5.1*). The perfusion pressure of the 'assay' kidney is controlled. In addition two groups have controlled the renal venous pressure. All workers report that blood volume expansion, performed in this way, induces a 50–100% rise in urinary sodium excretion in the 'assay' kidney. In some experiments there has been a

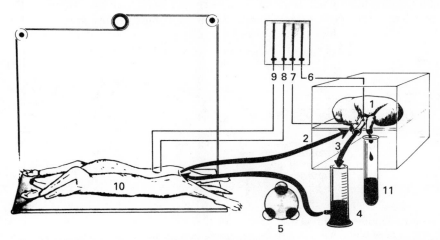

Figure 5.1 Method used to expand an animal's blood volume with blood with which it is in equilibrium. The perfusion pressure to the isolated kidney was controlled by raising and lowering the platform upon which the dog lay. (From Kaloyanides and Azer (1971), courtesy of the Editor and Publishers, *Journal of Clinical Investigation*)

simultaneous fall in glomerular filtration rate and renal blood flow, demonstrating that the rise in urinary sodium excretion is due in part to an overall diminution of tubular sodium reabsorption.

Several other groups have performed almost the same experiment but, instead of using equilibrated blood, the blood volume has been expanded with homologous blood from another animal (Knock, 1980; Lichardus and Nizet, 1972; Lichardus and Ponec, 1970; Sonnenberg, Veress and Pearce, 1972; Tobian, Coffee and McCrea, 1967). Tobian, Coffee and McCrea (1967) perfused an isolated rat kidney, which had been placed between two reservoirs, into one of which flowed arterial blood from a rat, and into the other venous blood from the isolated kidney. When a mixture of two-thirds rat blood and one-third Ringer solution was placed into the venous reservoir, so that it raised the volume of blood in the reservoir without expanding the rat's blood volume, there was no increase in sodium excretion by the isolated 'assay' kidney. But when the same amount of blood/Ringer solution was infused intravenously into the rat there was usually a large rise in urinary sodium excretion. Lichardus and Nizet (1972) transplanted the 'assay' kidney into the dog's neck, where it was perfused at a controlled arterial and venous pressure while the blood volume was expanded about 33% in 15 minutes. Blood volume expansion was associated with a rise in urinary sodium excretion of the transplanted 'assay' kidney.

Others have cross-circulated a donor rat with another recipient 'assay' rat (Knock and de Wardener, 1980; Lichardus and Ponec, 1970; Sonnenberg, Veress and Pearce, 1972) (*Figure 5.2*). The urine of the donor expanded rat was reinfused into its own femoral vein throughout the experiment. When the donor rat was expanded with homologous blood there was a rise in urinary sodium excretion by the recipient 'assay' rat, which was maximal at the end of 1 h and subsided slowly during the next 1–2 hours. This natriuresis was not accompanied by any change in

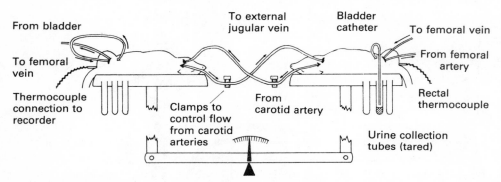

Figure 5.2 Isovolaemic cross-circulation technique. The rat on the left (the donor rat) was given a transfusion of blood without expanding the blood volume of the rat on the right (the recipient rat). (From Sonnenberg, Vereess and Pearce (1972), courtesy of the Editor and Publishers, *Journal of Clinical Investigation*)

glomerular filtration rate or potassium excretion. An exchange transfusion of a similar quantity of blood in and out of the donor rat was not accompanied by a natriuresis in the recipient animal. In such cross-circulation experiments the circulating natriuretic mechanism can only be revealed if the blood volume expansion is sustained, i.e. the loss of sodium and water in the urine is replaced intravenously (Knock and de Wardener, 1980; Lichardus and Ponec, 1970). It is simplest do this by reinfusing the urine. Alternatively, the loss of urinary sodium and water from the expanded donor animal can be prevented by a preceding bilateral nephrectomy (Lichardus and Ponec, 1970).

It must be emphasized that the interpretation of the results of a cross-circulation experiment in which the blood volume of a donor animal is expanded with blood is totally different from that in which the donor animal is expanded with saline. In the first a rise in urinary sodium excretion in the recipient animal is evidence of a change in the circulating concentration of some substance which controls urinary sodium excretion. In the second the administration of saline to the donor animal causes a fall in plasma protein and packed cell volume in the recipient which, although delayed, is of the same order as in the donor animal. If the hypothesis that such dilutional factors are important in the control of urinary sodium excretion is correct, the recipient animal should show a rise in urinary sodium excretion which is comparable with that in the expanded donor animal. Thus the contribution of such an experiment to the study of the natriuretic hormone is not that the recipient animal has a natriuresis but that it is always so much less than that in the donor animal (de Wardener *et al.,* 1961; Johnston and Davies, 1966; Johnston *et al.,* 1967). It was this unexpected anomaly which originally led to the suggestion that the natriuresis of volume expansion might be due in part to circulating factors other than those of dilution (de Wardener *et al.,* 1961). Another cross-circulation experiment of great relevance is expansion of the blood volume of a sodium-deprived rat with equilibrated blood (Pearce *et al.,* 1969). This procedure produces a much smaller natriuresis than when undertaken in a rat that has been given large amounts of deoxycorticosterone (DOC) and sodium chloride. The sodium-depleted rats are then cross-circulated for 1 h with rats that have previously been given deoxycorticosterone and a high intake of sodium. At the end of the hour of cross-circulation blood volume expansion now produces a large rise in sodium excretion in both sodium-depleted rats and the rats given deoxycorticosterone. The altered responsiveness of the salt-depleted rats appears to be due to a change in the concentration of a circulating factor, and cannot be due to a diminution in the concentration of a salt-retaining steroid.

Knock (1980) modified a previous experiment by Pearce, Veress and Sonnenberg (1975) and showed that a very small amount of plasma from a volume-expanded animal when injected into another animal causes a delayed onset but prolonged natriuresis (*Figure 5.3*). It was first shown that blood volume expansion with equilibrated blood in the rat causes a brisk rise in urinary sodium excretion which is maximal at about 1 hour. Blood was removed from the reservoir at the height of the natriuresis, then it was spun and the resultant 1 ml of plasma injected within a few minutes into another rat; 1 ml of plasma obtained from a blood volume expanded rat caused a small but significant natriuresis which began after 1 h and was still increasing 2 h later. This effect was more pronounced if the animal donating the blood had had its urine reinfused. Plasma from a control rat,

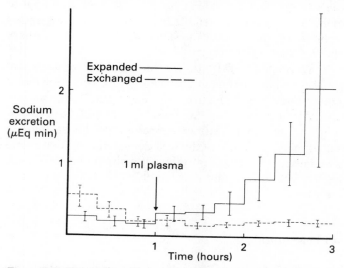

Figure 5.3 Change in urinary sodium excretion of a rat given 1 ml of plasma from another rat whose blood volume had been expanded (————), or had not been expanded (————). (From Knock, 1980, courtesy of the Publishers, *Clinical Science*)

the blood volume of which was not expanded, did not cause a rise in urinary sodium excretion when injected into another rat. Others have also described natriuretic extracts which have a gradual and prolonged effect (Clarkson, Raw and de Wardener, 1976; Pearce, Veress and Sonnenberg, 1975; Sealey, Kirshman and Laragh, 1969). The reason for the delay between injection of the plasma and the onset of the rise in sodium excretion is not known. Pearce, Veress and Sonnenberg (1975) found that the active material in plasma seemed to be contained in the large molecular weight fraction of the plasma. It is possible, as suggested by Clarkson, Raw and de Wardener (1976) that the delay is due to the time for a sufficient quantity of a small active fraction to be metabolized from a large inactive precursor.

Mode of action

The experiments described above demonstrate: (1) that the natriuresis of volume expansion is in part due to a circulating substance; (2) because the natriuresis can occur in spite of a fall in glomerular filtration rate, the substance probably acts directly on the tubule to inhibit sodium reabsorption. This suggestion is supported by experiments which demonstrate that volume expansion is associated with an increase in the capacity of plasma to inhibit net sodium transport directly (Nutbourne *et al.*, 1970). Other experiments show that this change in sodium transport is due to an increased capacity of plasma to inhibit $Na^+-K^+-ATPase$ activity (Clarkson, Talner and de Wardener, 1970). Therefore, the substance in the plasma that causes the natriuresis of volume expansion may inhibit renal tubular $Na^+-K^+-ATPase$.

In the Nutbourne *et al.* (1970) experiment, blood from a dog flowed in and out of a membrane cell that contained a frog skin. When the blood volume was expanded with equilibrated blood, sodium transport across the skin diminished as the urinary excretion of sodium of the dog rose.

Clarkson, Talner and de Wardener (1970) studied fragments of rabbit renal tubules incubated in dog plasma which had been obtained before and after blood volume expansion with equilibrated blood (*Figure 5.4*). The intracellular sodium concentration of the fragments incubated in the plasma obtained after blood volume expansion was higher and the potassium concentration lower than in fragments incubated in control plasma. This was the first demonstration that blood volume expansion causes a change in the concentration of a circulating substance that affects sodium transport in the tubule, and that the effect of this change is an inhibition of net sodium transport.

Circulating $Na^+-K^+-ATPase$ inhibitor

Poston *et al.* (1982) measured the effect on white cell sodium transport of plasma from normal subjects obtained before and after they had been on 9-α-fludrocortisone, and had 'escaped' from its effect. The leukocyte efflux rate

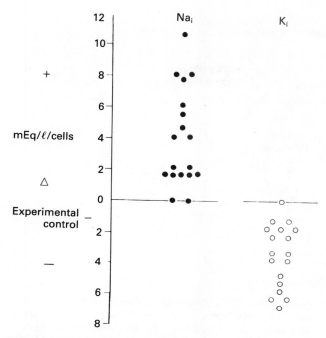

Figure 5.4 Differences (experimental less control) in intracellular sodium (Na_1) and potassium (K_1) concentrations between tubule fragments incubated in plasma taken before (control) and after (experimental) expanding the blood volume. Na_1 ●; K_1 ○. (From Clarkson, Talner and de Wardener, 1970, courtesy of the Publishers, *Clinical Science*)

constant fell substantially due to a significant fall in the ouabain-sensitive efflux rate constant (i.e. due to the activity of Na^+–K^+–ATPase). There was an insignificant fall in the ouabain-insensitive rate constant. Furthermore, the total sodium efflux rate constant of white cells obtained from a normal subject, incubated in the plasma of subjects who had escaped from the effect of 9-α-fludrocortisone, fell significantly. In contrast, the sodium efflux rate constant of white cells from normal control subjects incubated in serum obtained from other normal subjects did not change. These results show that the circulating sodium transport inhibitor demonstrated in the animal experiments is also present in man and affects human white cells by inhibiting Na^+–K^+–ATPase. This conclusion was confirmed by de Wardener *et al.* (1981) who used a cytochemical technique to measure Na^+–K^+–ATPase activity in guinea-pig renal cells *in vitro* (*Figure 5.5*). Purified urinary natriuretic extract inhibited Na^+–K^+–ATPase in intact cells at 6 min in a log-dose linear manner. Human plasma at 1:100 dilution produced maximal inhibition of Na^+–K^+–ATPase. Plasma samples of normal subjects on high and low sodium intakes were tested. The capacity of plasma from subjects on high sodium diet to inhibit the ouabain-sensitive component of Na^+–K^+–ATPase activity was approximately 25 times greater than plasma from sodium-depleted subjects. In addition, inhibition of Na^+–K^+–ATPase is associated with a rise in glucose-6-phosphate dehydrogenase (G6PD) activity (Dikstein, 1971). Fenton *et al.* (1982) have shown that ouabain, plasma and purified natriuretic material from

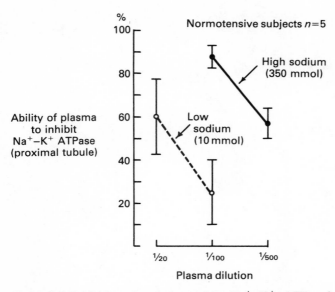

Figure 5.5 Inhibition of ouabain sensitive $Na^+-K^+-ATPase$ by dilutions of plasma from five healthy subjects each on a high (solid circle, solid line) and on a low sodium diet (open circle, solid line) and on a low sodium diet (open circle, broken line). Results are given as per cent inhibition found compared with activity found in segments of the same kidney exposed to the plasma diluent only. (From de Wardener *et al.* (1981), courtesy of the Publishers, *Lancet*)

the urine simultaneously inhibit renal $Na^+-K^+-ATPase$ activity and stimulate G6PD activity of the proximal convoluted tubule *in vitro* in the guinea-pig kidney. The time-course of the changes induced by the natriuretic extract and the plasma are similar, and the rise in G6PD activity induced by a wide range of concentrations of natriuretic extract and plasma are parallel. The identity of these two phenomena suggest that the substance which produces $Na^+-K^+-ATPase$ activity and increases G6PD activity in the natriuretic extract and the plasma are similar. Fenton *et al.* (1982) developed an assay to measure the capacity of biological fluids to stimulate G6PD activity in intact cells *in vitro* as a marker of their ability to inhibit $Na^+-K^+-ATPase$ activity. They found that plasma from salt-loaded subjects stimulated G6PD activity about 20 times more than plasma from the same subjects on a low sodium diet (*Figure 5.6*).

Nature and site of production

Most of the work on the structure of the natriuretic hormone has been carried out on a low-molecular weight (<500) natriuretic substance obtained from the urine, which inhibits $Na^+-K^+-ATPase$ and stimulates G6PD (Clarkson, Raw and de Wardener, 1976; Fenton *et al.*, 1982). The substance is polar and relatively resistant to acid hydrolysis and proteolytic enzymes.

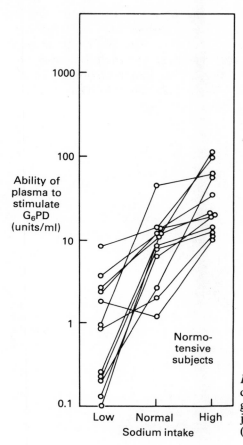

Figure 5.6 Stimulation of glucose-6-phosphate dehydrogenase activity in the proximal tubule of guinea-pig kidney by plasma from normal subjects on low, normal and high sodium intakes. (From de Wardener and MacGregor, 1983)

Natriuretic hormone is probably secreted from the hypothalamus. Kaloyanides, Cohen and DiBona (1977) were unable to obtain a natriuresis from an isolated kidney perfused by blood from a volume-expanded, decapitated dog. The arterial pressure, renal blood flow and glomerular filtration rate of the decapitated dogs were well-maintained. Clarkson *et al.* (1974) found that an extract from bovine hypothalamus contains a natriuretic substance other than vasopressin. Fishman (1979) produced a guinea-pig hypothalamic extract which displaced ouabain from $Na^+–K^+–ATPase$ of brain microsomes and inhibited the uptake of rubidium (^{86}Rb) into human erythrocytes. Haupert and Sancho (1979) prepared a bovine extract of hypothalamus which inhibited active sodium transport across anuran membranes, inhibited ouabain binding to frog urinary bladder and directly inhibited renal $Na^+–K^+–ATPase$ activity. An extract of Lichstein and Samuelov (1980) rat brain inhibited both ouabain binding to rat brain membranes and $Na^+–K^+–ATPase$ activity. Alaghband-Zadeh *et al.* (1983), using the cytochemical assay which measures the ability of biological fluid to stimulate renal glucose-6-phosphate dehydrogenase activity as a marker of $Na^+–K^+–ATPase$

inhibition, found that the hypothalamus was the only site containing G6PD stimulating substance. The G6PD-stimulating activity from hypothalamus was about 10 000 to 100 000 times greater than from plasma. The G6PD stimulating activity of hypothalamic extracts from rats which had been on a high sodium intake for four weeks were approximately 150 times more active than those obtained from rats which had been on low sodium diets (*Figure 5.7*). The G6PD-stimulating activity of the corresponding plasma was six times more active.

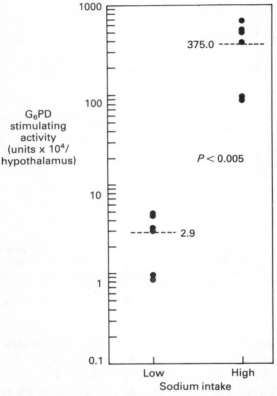

Figure 5.7 Ability of acetone extracts of hypothalami to stimulate renal glucose-6-phosphate dehydrogenase (G6PD) activity (units of G6PD stimulating activity/hypothalamus) in two groups of six male Wistar rats: one group was fed a low sodium (5 mmol/100 g) diet and the other group was fed a high sodium (20 mmol/100 g) diet for four weeks

Afferent system

One of the afferent limbs which monitors blood volume and thus may control the secretion of natriuretic hormone is the intrathoracic blood volume, particularly the left atrial pressure (*Figure 5.8*). The overriding importance of the intrathoracic blood volume, rather than the total blood volume, in causing a rise in urinary sodium excretion has been demonstrated in man by whole-body immersion

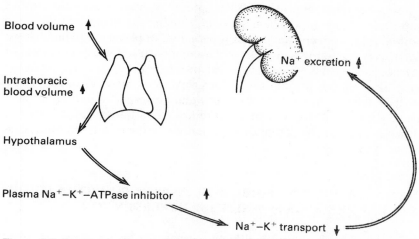

Figure 5.8 Proposed afferent system controlling secretion of circulating sodium transport inhibitor

experiments. This procedure increases the intrathoracic blood volume and causes a sustained rise in urinary sodium excretion that continues despite a gradual fall in total blood volume. Extracts of urine excreted during the natriuresis caused by water immersion are significantly more natriuretic than extracts of control urine (Epstein, Bricker and Bourgoignie, 1978).

RISE IN ARTERIAL PRESSURE IN ACQUIRED HYPERTENSION ASSOCIATED WITH RETENTION OF SODIUM

A circulating natriuretic substance raising the blood pressure was first hypothesized by Dahl, Knudsen and Iwai (1969) to explain the results of parabiotic experiments between salt-sensitive hypertensive and salt-resistant normotensive rats. These investigators stated, 'Many of the apparent anomalies of the angiotensin–aldosterone system in hypertension could be explained if a sodium-excreting hormone were postulated which had the capacity of also inducing hypertension when produced by a hypertension-prone individual'. No notice was taken of this remarkable proposition becaue the concept that a natriuretic substance might cause a rise in blood pressure was not compatible with the contrary observation that a diuretic or a salt-losing state is associated with hypotension. Several years later, Haddy and Overbeck (1976) suggested that a rise in blood pressure could be caused by a circulating sodium transport inhibitor. This proposal was based on Chen *et al.*'s (1972) observations on the vasodilating properties of an intra-arterial infusion of potassium via stimulation of Na^+-K^+-ATPase of arteriolar smooth muscle. Also, the vasodilating effect of potassium was less pronounced in experimental hypertension, in which Na^+-K^+-ATPase activity of arteriolar smooth muscle is possibly impaired. Overbeck *et al.* (1976) then confirmed that, in the one-kidney hypertensive dog, the ouabain sensitive ^{86}Rb uptake of small mesenteric arteries and splanchnic veins is impaired. Pamnani *et al.* (1980) also found that the ^{86}Rb uptake of normal arteries, incubated in the supernatant of plasma obtained from a rat following saline infusion, was depressed. This demonstrated that the plasma of such animals contained an increased concentration of a $Na^+-K^+-ATPase$ inhibitor, supporting the suggestion that the arteriolar abnormalities of $Na^+-K^+-ATPase$ activity might be due to a circulating sodium transport inhibitor. In man the presence of a low molecular weight natriuretic sodium-transport inhibitor has also been demonstrated in the serum of hypertensive patients with chronic renal failure (Bricker *et al.*, 1968).

RELATION OF A CIRCULATING SODIUM-TRANSPORT INHIBITOR TO THE RISE IN ARTERIAL PRESSURE IN ESSENTIAL HYPERTENSION

In rats, there are two forms of essential hypertension: (1) Dahl salt-sensitive and salt-resistant forms, in which the rise in arterial pressure is dependent on a large sodium intake; and (2) the spontaneous form, in which the rise in arterial pressure occurs on a normal sodium diet.

Cross-transplantation experiments

Borst and Borst de Geus (1963) were the first to propose that essential hypertension is due to an impairment in renal control of sodium excretion. Convincing evidence to support this suggestion has come from cross-transplantation experiments in Dahl salt-sensitive hypertensive rats (Dahl and Heine, 1975), in rats of the Milan hypertensive strain (Bianchi *et al.*, 1974), and in Okamoto spontaneously hypertensive rats (Kawabe *et al.*, 1979). In all three 'the hypertension follows the kidney'. For example, if a kidney from a young normotensive strain rat is placed into a young hypertensive strain rat, hypertension does not develop in the hypertensive strain rat. The converse also obtains. This finding implies that all abnormalities of the three forms of inherited hypertension in rats must be secondary to a renal abnormality or unrelated to the mechanism which causes the rise in blood pressure.

Evidence of a renal defect in sodium excretion

When kidneys from 8-week old rats are perfused with blood from normal rats, the kidneys of Dahl sodium-sensitive rats excrete less sodium at each perfusion pressure than the kidneys from normotensive controls (Tobian *et al.*, 1978). In spontaneously hypertensive strains of rat there is a transient period, approximately the 6th–7th week of life, during which the blood pressure rises and the fractional excretion of sodium is lower, the cumulative retention of sodium is greater, and the plasma renin activity is lower than in control normotensive rats (Bianchi *et al.*,

1974; Dietz *et al.*, 1978). In the adult rat, no difference in sodium excretion or plasma renin activity can be discerned. In man, studies of normotensive monozygotic or dizygotic twins show that the renal excretion of sodium is genetically determined (Grim *et al.*, 1979a). In response to an intravenous sodium load, normotensive first-degree relatives of patients with essential hypertension excrete less sodium than control subjects (Grim *et al.*, 1979b).

Salt intake

The relationship between sodium intake and arterial pressure in both human populations and stock colony rats also suggests that the genetic abnormality is expressed as deficient renal sodium excretion. Data from 27 populations show a highly significant correlation between arterial pressure and salt intake in man (Gleiberman, 1973), and those who consume less than 60 mmol of sodium a day have no rise in arterial pressure with age (Gleiberman, 1973).

Accelerated natriuresis

In the spontaneously hypertensive rat (Willis and Bauer, 1978) and in human essential hypertension, the natriuresis following a rapid intravenous infusion of saline begins more rapidly than in normal subjects (Willassen and Offstad, 1980). In rats and man this accelerated natriuresis can be elicited early in life, before the rise in arterial pressure. Such an accelerated natriuresis strongly suggests a state in which there is a need to oppose a persistent tendency to retain sodium. This event also occurs in primary aldosteronism (Rovner *et al.*, 1965) and in normal subjects given aldosterone even when, as in essential hypertension, an increase in extracellular fluid volume cannot be measured.

Evidence for a raised concentration of a circulating sodium transport inhibitor

Leukocytes from normotensive subjects incubated in the serum of hypertensive patients develop impaired sodium transport similar to that found in the leukocytes of hypertensive patients. The ouabain-sensitive component of the sodium efflux rate constant is reduced, whereas the efflux rate constant of normotensive white cells incubated in the serum of another normal subject does not change (Poston *et al.*, 1981a) (*Figure 5.9*). The results suggest that the serum of patients with essential hypertension contains a higher than normal concentration of a substance which inhibits $Na^+-K^+-ATPase$. The intracellular sodium concentration of lymphocytes from normotensive subjects also rises after incubation in the plasma of hypertensive patients (Ambrosioni *et al.*, 1981). The reduction in sodium efflux rate constant is greatest in patients with low renin essential hypertension (Edmondson and MacGregor, 1981). MacGregor *et al.* (1981) measured the ability

White cells from normotensives incubated in:

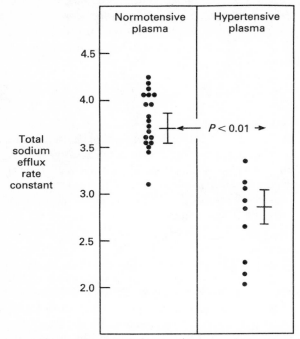

Figure 5.9 Total sodium efflux rate constant of leukocytes from normotensive patients incubated in the plasma of other normotensive subjects or the plasma of hypertensive patients. (From MacGregor and de Wardener (1981), courtesy of the Publishers, *Clinical and Experimental Hypertension*)

of plasma to stimulate G6PD activity of guinea-pig kidney cells as a marker of inhibition of $Na^+-K^+-ATPase$ activity (Fenton *et al.*, 1982). G6PD was stimulated more significantly by the plasma of hypertensive patients than by the plasma of normotensive subjects (*Figure 5.10*). Also, a significant correlation between arterial pressure and the capacity of plasma to stimulate G6PD was observed. In addition, plasma from hypertensive patients with low plasma renin activity stimulated G6PD significantly more than plasma from the other hypertensive patients.

Recently Hamlyn *et al.* (1982) have used a kinetic assay of dog kidney $Na^+-K^+-ATPase$ activity, in which the regulation of enzymatically hydrolyzed ATP is coupled to the oxidation of NADH, so that the action of an inhibitor can be monitored by continuously recording the absorbance of NADH. A significant correlation between mean arterial pressure and $Na^+-K^+-ATPase$ inhibition was found (*Figure 5.11*). Hamlyn *et al.* (1982) were unable to demonstrate a significant elevation of digoxin-like immunoreactivity in plasma samples that inhibited $Na^+-K^+-ATPase$. On the other hand, Gruber, Rudel and Bullock (1982) have claimed that there is an endogenous digoxin-like material in the plasma of hypertensive monkeys.

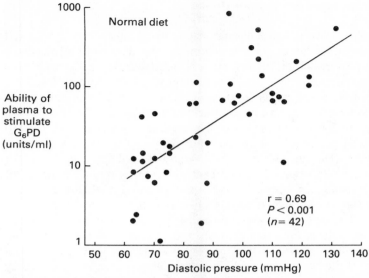

Figure 5.10 Ability of plasma to stimulate guinea-pig renal glucose-6-phosphate dehydro-genase (G6PD) activity *in vitro* plotted against diastolic pressure in 42 individuals taking their normal diet. (From MacGregor *et al.* (1981), courtesy of the Publishers, *British Medical Journal*)

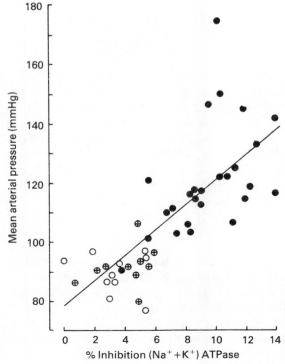

Figure 5.11 The ability of plasma to inhibit $(Na^+ + K^+)$ ATPase activity in 46 individuals plotted against mean arterial pressure. (From Hamlyn *et al.* (1982), courtesy of the Editor and Publishers, *Nature* (*London*))

Evidence for a circulating vasoactive substance

Michelakis *et al.* (1975) injected plasma from hypertensive patients and normotensive subjects into bilaterally nephrectomized rats under the influence of pentolinium. Plasma from hypertensive patients, particularly those with low plasma renin activity, increased the vascular reactivity of the rats to noradrenaline and angiotensin, whereas plasma from normotensive subjects did not have these effects. In the isolated rabbit femoral artery perfused with plasma by means of a constant flow pump the perfusion pressure increased to a greater extent when noradrenaline was added to plasma from hypertensive patients than plasma from normotensive subjects (Bloom, Stein and Rosendorff, 1976). The blood of salt-sensitive hypertensive rats caused a significant rise in the vascular resistance of cross-perfused hindquarters of normotensive salt-resistant rats (Tobian *et al.*, 1979). Greenberg, Gaines and Sweatt (1981) observed that the portal vein of a normotensive strain rat parabiosed to a spontaneously hypertensive rat acquires the properties of the portal vein of the spontaneously hypertensive rat. The portal vein becomes less distensible, medial hypertrophy develops and norepinephrine-induced venous contractility increases. Whether the vasoactive substance causing these vascular changes is the same as the circulating sodium-transport inhibitor is unknown.

Abnormalities of sodium transport

Red cells

Most workers have found that in human essential hypertension (Meyer and Garay, 1981), and in spontaneously hypertensive rats (Losse *et al.*, 1981), red-cell intracellular sodium concentration is raised and that in man it can be reduced to normal by diuretics (Gessler, 1962; Von Wessels, Zumkley and Losse, 1970). An associated reduction in the ouabain-sensitive sodium efflux rate constant (Montari *et al.*, 1980) and abnormalities in other forms of sodium transport have also been found (Meyer and Garay, 1981).

White cells

In essential hypertension the white cell intracellular sodium concentration is raised and the ouabain-sensitive sodium efflux rate constant is decreased (Ambrosioni *et al.*, 1980; Edmondson *et al.*, 1975; Poston *et al.*, 1981b) in whole leukocyte fractions and isolated lymphocytes. These abnormalities which are also present in the white cells of normotensive relatives of hypertensive patients are reversed by the administration of diuretics (Thomas *et al.*, 1975; Poston *et al.*, 1981b; Heagarty *et al.*, 1982).

Vessels

The amount of sodium and water in renal arteries removed at necropsy from hypertensive patients is higher than normal (Tobian and Binion, 1952), consistent with the influence of a sodium transport inhibitor. Overbeck *et al.* (1974) found that the vasodilator response of forearm vessels to an intra-arterial infusion of potassium was less pronounced in patients with essential hypertension and suggested that this phenomenon might be due to reduced $Na^+-K^+-ATPase$ activity in the smooth muscle cell. The calcium entry antagonists, nifedipine and verapamil, cause a greater fall in blood pressure in hypertensive patients than in normotensive subjects (MacGregor *et al.*, 1982). Intra-arterial verapamil also causes a greater increase in forearm blood flow in hypertensive patients than in normotensive subjects, whereas there is an equal increase in blood flow with another vasodilator, nitroprusside (Robinson, Bayley and Dobbs, 1982). This functional abnormality in the response of smooth muscle cells to calcium-entry antagonists in essential hypertension may be related to an abnormality of calcium transport, which may be due to the raised concentration of the sodium-transport inhibitor as the abnormality is reversed by diuretics (Robinson *et al.*, 1981). As discussed in detail in Chapter 4, in spontaneously hypertensive rats rubidium uptake by the tail artery is either normal or high (Overbeck, Ku and Rapp, 1981), and the vasodilatory responses to an arterial infusion of potassium are normal (Overbeck and Clark, 1975). There is also evidence that the $Na^+-K^+-ATPase$ activity of the tail artery of spontaneously hypertensive rats is normal or high (Abel *et al.*, 1981). This finding may be due to the sustained effect of the sodium transport inhibitor, which is manifested only when the artery is removed from the effect of the inhibitor. An analogous mechanism to this apparent adaptive increase in sodium pump activity can be demonstrated in an *in vitro* preparation of red cells from subjects who have been receiving digoxin for several months (Ford *et al.*, 1979). One group has found that the net accumulation of potassium and extrusion of sodium by aortic smooth muscle of spontaneously hypertensive rats are lower than normal (Jones, 1973), and another group has found that the plasma membranes from vascular smooth muscle have abnormally low calcium-binding activity (Posnoff and Orloff, 1984).

Changes in blood volume

In human essential hypertension and in spontaneously hypertensive rats, blood volume is either normal or low (Tarazi, Frolich and Dustan, 1968), but in both forms of hypertension (Safar *et al.*, 1979; Trippodo, Yamamoto and Frolich, 1981) there is a fall in venous compliance and a rise in either the central blood volume or in the ratio of the intrathoracic to the total blood volume (Ellis and Julius, 1973; Lundin, Folkow and Rippe, 1981). These changes have also been demonstrated in several acquired forms of hypertension associated with sodium retention. The proposal that raised peripheral venous tone shifts blood centrally is supported by the increase in pulmonary wedge pressure in human essential hypertension (Safar and London, personal communication) and by increased left atrial pressure in spontaneously hypertensive rats (Noresson, Rickstein and Thoren, 1979). It is possible, therefore, that high circulating inhibition of sodium transport is due to distension of the intrathoracic vascular bed and, in particular, to raised left atrial pressure.

Mechanisms whereby a circulating sodium transport inhibitor might increase vascular smooth muscle tone

Blaustein (1977) suggested that essential hypertension might be due to a circulating sodium transport inhibitor. As there was no evidence of any alteration in vascular smooth muscle contractility in hypertension, it was likely that the increased tone was due to a rise in the concentration of intracellular free calcium, which might be the final common pathway of at least some forms of hypertension. Blaustein pointed out that the intracellular free calcium concentration is linked to the entry of sodium into the cell along its electrochemical gradient and that the energy thereby released moves calcium out of the cell against its electrochemical gradient. Therefore, a rise in intracellular free sodium which diminishes the electrochemical gradient for sodium and reduces the entry of sodium into the cell reduces the movement of calcium out of the cell. According to this concept, an increase in intracellular sodium concentration of vascular smooth muscle is predicted to increase vascular smooth muscle tone. According to existing knowledge it appears that a change of intracellular sodium of only 5% should increase intracellular free calcium concentration in vascular smooth muscle by about 15% and cause a 50% increase in tone! Ouabain, which inhibits $Na^+-K^+-ATPase$ and raises intracellular sodium concentration, increases the tone of vascular smooth muscle. Blaustein (1977) proposed that if the sodium pump is inhibited by an endogenous sodium transport inhibitor, or this inhibitor enhances passive sodium entry into the cell, arterial pressure and venous tone might be influenced. Further, if such a substance were present in excess, it might contribute to or cause hypertension. Such a hypothesis would explain the hypotensive effect of a natriuretic drug in hypertension. As the body stores of sodium are depleted, the production of the sodium transport inhibitor would fall, reducing its effect on vascular smooth muscle, resulting in a decrease in intracellular sodium and calcium concentration. Consequently, the smooth muscle tone and the arterial pressure would fall.

Haddy (1981), on the other hand, has suggested that the circulating sodium-transport inhibitor reduces Na^+ pump current, thus decreasing the pump's contribution to the resting membrane potential. Consequently, membrane depolarization increases the influx of calcium and raises the intracellular concentration of free calcium.

Hypothetical sequence of events in essential hypertension

As shown in *Figure 5.12*, the underlying genetic lesion may be expressed as a deficiency of sodium excretion, which becomes more apparent at higher sodium intake. The reduction in sodium excretion may cause initially a transient increase in total blood volume with a rise in intrathoracic blood volume. This change

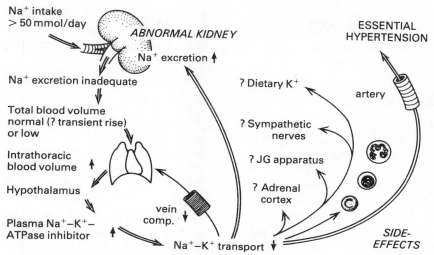

Figure 5.12 Sequence of events to explain a postulated inherited defect in the kidney's ability to secrete sodium, the observed rise in the concentration of a circulating sodium transport inhibitor and the rise in peripheral resistance in essential hypertension

stimulates the hypothalamus to secrete a circulating sodium transport inhibitor, which adjusts renal sodium excretion, returning sodium balance to normal. Normal sodium balance is sustained only by continuously high circulating sodium transport inhibitor, which raises the tone and reactivity of vascular smooth muscle. As a result, arterial pressure rises and venous compliance is diminished. The increased venous tone causes a shift of blood from the periphery to the central vascular bed which raises the intrathoracic pressure and perpetuates the stimulus for greater secretion of the sodium transport inhibitor. Total blood volume may be normal or low.

OTHER POSSIBLE CONSEQUENCES OF A RAISED CONCENTRATION OF A CIRCULATING SODIUM TRANSPORT INHIBITOR

Ouabain inhibits Na$^+$–K$^+$–ATPase in isolated membrane or microsomal fragments and in intact cells. As the effects of ouabain on various intact cells are known, it is possible by extrapolation to suggest some of the consequences of a rise in the concentration of an endogenous inhibitor of Na$^+$–K$^+$–ATPase in essential hypertension.

Plasma renin activity

Many patients with essential hypertension have low plasma renin activity, and those with the lowest renin activity have the highest concentrations of the circulating sodium transport inhibitor as judged by both the G6PD assay (MacGregor *et al.*, 1981) and the sodium efflux rate constant in white cells (Edmondson and MacGregor, 1981). *In vitro*, ouabain diminishes renin secretion in rat cortical slices, isolated glomeruli, and isolated perfused kidneys (Churchill and Churchill, 1980). The low plasma renin activity in essential hypertension may therefore be due partly to the direct effect of the circulating sodium transport inhibitor on the juxtaglomerular cells.

Aldosterone

Though in some forms of essential hypertension the plasma renin activity tends to be low, that of aldosterone is inappropriately high for the plasma renin activity (McAreavey *et al.,* 1983). Exogenous administration of angiotensin II into patients with essential hypertension causes an abnormally steep rise in plasma aldosterone. Saline administration, however, fails to lower circulating aldosterone in the normal manner (Collins *et al.,* 1970).

In vitro adrenal zona glomerulosa cells exposed to ouabain 10^{-5} M have an increased output of aldosterone and the response to exposure to angiotensin II is also greater than without ouabain (Fakunding and Catt, 1980). Exposure to higher concentrations of ouabain 10^{-4} and 10^{-3} M depresses aldosterone secretion and diminishes the aldosterone response to angiotensin II. Thus, in spite of low plasma renin activity inappropriately raised circulating aldosterone may be due to an increase of the circulating sodium transport inhibitor at the adrenal cortex.

Sympathetic activity

As hypertension develops in children of parents with established hypertension (Falkner, Onesti and Angelakos, 1981) and in young rats of the spontaneously hypertensive strains, sympathetic nervous system activity increases (Hallback, 1976) and is further raised by salt loading (Falkner, Onesti and Angelakos, 1981; Schöming *et al.,* 1978). *In vitro,* ouabain increases norepinephrine output from the sympathetic nerve terminal (Nakazato, Ohga and Onoda, 1978) and reduces norepinephrine re-uptake (Leitz and Stefano, 1970), thus raising the amount of norepinephrine available to bind to noradrenergic receptors of target tissues. The re-uptake of norepinephrine in the isolated perfused heart is much reduced in hearts obtained from spontaneously hypertensive rats on high sodium diets (Dietz *et al.,* 1982). Platelets accumulate and store norepinephrine in subcellular granules in a similar way to sympathetic neurons (Pletcher and Laubescher, 1980). Therefore, the high efflux rate of norepinephrine from platelets of hypertensive patients or normotensive first-degree relatives of hypertensive patients could be due to the raised circulating sodium transport inhibitor. Thus, it is possible that some of the changes in sympathetic activity in essential hypertension are related to the circulating sodium transport inhibitor.

Dietary potassium

For approximately 50 years several investigations have shown that the ingestion of potassium reduces the arterial pressure in essential hypertension (Addison, 1928). In addition, a rise in potassium intake lowers the arterial pressure of rats with inherited hypertension (Goto, Tobian and Iwai, 1981). The impaired neuronal re-uptake of norepinephrine induced in spontaneously hypertensive rats by high sodium intake is improved by giving potassium (Dietz *et al., 1981*). In keeping with this observation, feeding potassium reduces hyperactive pressor responses in Dahl salt-sensitive rats (Goto, Tobian and Iwai, 1981).

Potassium at physiological concentrations stimulates the activity of Na^+-K^+-ATPase in red-cell ghosts, an effect opposite to that of ouabain. It is possible that potassium lowers arterial pressure and increases norepinephrine re-uptake in inherited forms of hypertension by counteracting the effect of the raised concentration of a circulating Na^+-K^+-ATPase inhibitor.

References

ABEL, P. W., TRAPANIM, A., MATSUKI, N., INGRAM, M. J. INGRAM, F. D. and HERMSMEYER, K. (1981) Unaltered membrane properties of arterial muscle in Dahl strain genetic hypertension. *American Journal of Physiology,* **241,** 224–227

ALAGHBAND-ZADEH, J., FENTON, S., HANCOCK, K., MILLETT, J. and de WARDENER, H. E. (1983) Evidence that the hypothalamus may be a source of a circulating Na–K-ATPase inhibitor. *Journal of Endocrinology,* **98,** 221–226

AMBROSIONI, E., TARTAGNI, E., MONTEBUGNOLI, L., COSTA, F. V. and MAGNANI, B. (1980) Intralymphocytic sodium in hypertensive patients. In *Intracellular Electrolytes* and *Arterial Hypertension,* edited by H. Zumkley and H. Losse, pp. 78–86. Stuttgart: Georg Thieme Verlag

BAHLMANN, J., McDONALD, S. J., VENTOM, M. G. and de WARDENER, H. E. (1967) The effect on urinary sodium excretion of blood volume expansion without changing the composition of the blood in the dog. *Clinical Science,* **32,** 403–413

BENGELE, H. E., HOUTTUIN, E. and PEARCE, J. W. (1972) Volume natriuresis without renal nerves and renal vascular pressure rise in the dog. *American Journal of Physiology,* **223,** 68–73

BIANCHI, G., FOX, U., DI FRANCESCO, G. F., GIOVANETTI, A. M. and PAGETTI, D. (1974) Blood pressure changes produced by kidney cross transplantation between spontaneously hypertensive rats and normotensive rats. *Clinical Science and Molecular Medicine,* **47,** 435–438

BLAUSTEIN, M. P. (1977) Sodium ions, calcium ions, blood pressure regulation and hypertension: a reassessment and a hypothesis. *American Journal of Physiology,* **232** (3), C165–C173

BLOOM, D. S., STEIN, M. G. and ROSENDORFF, C. (1976) Effects of hypertensive plasma on the responses of isolated artery preparation to noradrenaline. *Cardiovascular Research,* **10,** 268–274

BLYTHE, W. B., D'AVILA, D., GITELMAN, H. J. and WELT, L. G. (1971) Further evidence for a humoral natriuretic factor. *Circulation Research,* **28,** II-21–II-31

BORST, J. G. G. and BORST DE GEUS, A. (1963) Hypertension explained by Starling's theory of circulatory homeostasis. *Lancet,* **1,** 667–682

BRICKER, N. S., KLAHR, S., PUEKERSON, M., SCHULTZE, R. G., AVIOLI, L. V. and BURGE, S. J. (1968) *In vitro* assay for a humoral substance present during volume expansion and uraemia. *Nature (London),* **219,** 1058

CHEN, W. T., BRACE, R. A., SCOTT, J. B., ANDERSON, D. K. and HADDY, F. J. (1972) The mechanism of the vasodilator action of potassium. *Proceedings of the Society of Biological Medicine,* **140,** 820–824

CHURCHILL, M. C. and CHURCHILL, P. C. (1980) Separate and combined effects of ouabain and extracellular potassium on renin secretion from rat renal cortical slices. *Journal of Physiology,* **300,** 105–114

CLARKSON, E. M., KOUTSAIMANIS, K. G., DAVIDMAN, M., DUBOIS, M., PENN, W. P. and DE WARDENER, H. E. (1974) The effect of brain extracts on urinary sodium excretion of the rat and the intracellular sodium concentration of renal tubule fragments. *Clinical Science and Molecular Medicine,* **47,** 201–213

CLARKSON, E. M., RAW, S. M. and DE WARDENER, H. E. (1976) Two natriuretic substances in extracts of urine from normal man when salt-depleted and salt-loaded. *Kidney International,* **10,** 381–394

CLARKSON, E. M., TALNER, L. and DE WARDENER, H. E. (1970) The effect of plasma from blood volume expanded dogs on sodium, potassium and PAH transport of renal tubule fragments. *Clinical Science,* **38,** 617–627

COLLINS, R. D., WEINBERGER, M. H., DOWDY, A. J., NOKES, G. W., GONZALES, C. M. and LUETSCHER, J. A. (1970) Abnormal sustained aldosterone secretion during salt loading in patients with various forms of benign hypertension; relation of plasma renin activity. *Journal of Clinical Investigation,* **49,** 1415–1426

DAHL, L. K. and HEINE, M. (1975) Primary role of renal homografts in setting chronic blood pressure levels in rats. *Circulation Research,* **36,** 692–696

DAHL, L. K., KNUDSEN, K. D. and IWAI, J. (1969) Humoral transmission of hypertension. Evidence from parabiosis. *Circulation Research,* **14** and **15,** I-21–I-133

de WARDENER, H. E. (1977) Natriuretic hormone. *Clinical Science,* **53,** 1–8

de WARDENER, H. E. and CLARKSON, E. M. (1982) The natriuretic hormone: recent developments. *Clinical Science,* **63,** 415–420

de WARDENER, H. E., MACGREGOR, G. A., CLARKSON, E. M., ALAGHBAND-ZADEH, J., BITENSKY, L. and CHAYEN, J. (1981) Effect of sodium intake on ability of human plasma to inhibit renal $Na^+-K^+-ATPase$ adenosine triphosphatase *in vitro.* *Lancet,* **1,** 411–412

de WARDENER, H. E. and MACGREGOR, G. A. (1983) The role of the circulating inhibitor of $Na^+-K^+-ATPase$ in essential hypertension. *American Journal of Nephrology,* **3,** 88–91

de WARDENER, H. E., MILLS, I. H., CLAPHAM, W. F. and HAYTER, C. J. (1961) Studies on the efferent mechanism of the sodium diuresis which follows the administration of intravenous saline in the dog. *Clinical Science,* **21,** 249–258

DIETZ, R., SCHÖMING, A., HAEBARA, A., MAIN, J. F. E., RASELIER, W. and LUTH, J. B. *et al.* (1978) Studies on the pathogenesis of spontaneous hypertension of rats. *Circulation Research,* **43** (Suppl. I), I-98–I-106

DIETZ, R., SCHÖMING, A., RASCHER, W. *et al.* (1982) Contribution of the sympathetic nervous system and the hypertensive effect of a high sodium diet in stroke prone spontaneously hypertensive rats (SHR-sp). *Hypertension,* **4** (6), 773–781

DIETZ, R., SCHÖMING, A., RASCHER, W., STRASSER, R., GANTEN, U. and KIMBER, W. (1981) Partial replacement of sodium by potassium in the diet restores impaired noradrenaline inactivation and lowers blood pressure in SHR-sp. *Clinical Science,* **61** (Suppl. 7), 69S–71S

DIKSTEIN, S. (1971) Stimulability, adenosine, triphosphatases, and their control by cellular redox processes. *Naturwissenchaften,* **58**, 439–443

EDMONDSON, R. P. S. and MACGREGOR, G. A. (1981) Leucocyte cation transport. Its relationship to the renin angiotensin system in essential hypertension. *British Medical Journal,* **282**, 1267–1269

EDMONDSON, R. P. S., THOMAS, R. D., HILTON, P. J., PATRICK, J. and JONES, N. F. (1975) Abnormal leucocyte composition and sodium transport in essential hypertension. *Lancet,* **1**, 1003–1005

ELLIS, C. N. and JULIUS, S. (1973) Role of central blood volume in hyperkinetic borderline hypertension. *British Heart Journal,* **35**, 450–455

EPSTEIN, M., BRICKER, N. S. and BOURGOIGNIE, J. J. (1978) Presence of a natriuretic factor in urine of normal men undergoing water immersion. *Kidney International,* **13**, 152–158

FAKUNDING, J. L. and CATT, K. J. (1980) Dependence of aldosterone stimulation in adrenal glomerulosa cells on calcium uptake: effects of lanthanum and verapamil. *Endocrinology,* **107**, 1345–1353

FALKNER, B., ONESTI, G. and ANGELAKOS, E. (1981) Effect of salt loading on the cardiovascular response to stress in adolescents. *Hypertension,* **3** (6) (Suppl. II), 195–199

FENTON, S., CLARKSON, E. M., MACGREGOR, G. A., ALAGHBAND-ZADEH, J. and de WARDENER, H. E. (1982) An assay of the capacity of biological fluids to stimulate renal glucose-6-phosphate dehydrogenase (G6PD) activity *in vitro* as a marker of their ability to inhibit sodium–potassium dependent adenosine triphosphatase (Na^+–K^+–ATPase) activity. *Journal of Endocrinology,* **94**, 99–110

FISHMAN, M. E. (1979) Endogenous digitalis-like activity in mammalian brain. *Proceedings of the National Academy of Sciences of the USA,* **76**, 4661–4663

FORD, A. R., ARONSON, J. K., GRAHAME-SMITH, D. G. and CARVER, J. G. (1979) The acute changes in cardiac glycoside receptor sites, [86]rubidium uptake and intracellular sodium concentration in the erythrocytes of patients during the early phases of digoxin therapy are not found during chronic therapy; pharmacological and therapeutic implications in chronic digoxin therapy. *British Journal of Clinical Pharmacology,* **2**, 135–142

GESSLER, VON U. (1962) Intra- und extrazelluläre elektrolytver änderungen bei essentieller hypertonie vor und Nacl behandlung. *Zeitschrift für Kreislaufforschung,* **51**, 117–183

GLEIBERMAN, L. (1973) Blood pressure and dietary salt in human populations. *Ecology of Food Nutrition,* **2**, 143–156

GOTO, A., TOBIAN, L. and IWAI, J. (1981) Potassium feeding rats and hyperactive central nervous system pressor responses in Dahl salt sensitive rats. *Hypertension,* **3** (Suppl. II), 128–134

GREENBERG, S., GAINES, K. and SWEATT, D. (1981) Evidence for circulating factors as a cause of venous hypertrophy in spontaneously hypertensive rats. *American Journal of Physiology,* **241**, H241–H430

GRIM, C. E., LUFT, F. C., FINEBERG, N. S. and WEINBERGER, M. (1979a) Responses to volume expansion and contraction in categorised hypertensive and normotensive man. *Hypertension,* **1,** 476–485

GRIM, C. E., MILLER, J. Z., LUFT, F. C., CHRISTIAN, J. C. and WEINBERGER, M. H. (1979b) Genetic influences of renin, aldosterone and the renal excretion of sodium, potassium following volume expansion and contraction in man. *Hypertension,* **1,** 583–590

GRUBER, K. A., RUDEL, L. L. and BULLOCK, B. C. (1982) Increased circulating levels of an endogenous digoxin-like factor in hypertensive monkeys. *Hypertension,* **4,** 348–354

HADDY, F. J. (1981) What is the link between vascular smooth muscle, sodium pump and hypertension? *Clinical and Experimental Hypertension,* **3,** 179–182

HADDY, F. J. and OVERBECK, H. W. (1976) The role of humoral agents in volume expanded hypertension. *Life Sciences,* **19,** 935–948

HALLBACK, M. (1976) Interaction of autonomic hypersensitivity and environmental stimuli: importance for the development of spontaneously hypertensive rats. In *Regulation of Blood Pressure by Central Nervous System,* edited by G. Onesti, M. Fernandes and K. Kim, p. 129–142. New York: Grune and Stratton

HAMLYN, J. M., RINGEL, R., SCHAEFFER, J. *et al.* (1982) A circulating inhibitor of $(Na^+ + K^+)$ ATPase associated with essential hypertension. *Nature (London),* **100,** 650–652

HAUPERT, G. T. and SANCHO, J. M. (1979) Sodium transport inhibitor from bovine hypothalamus. *Proceedings of the National Academy of Sciences of the USA,* **76,** 4658–4660

HEAGARTY, A. M., BING, R. F., THURSTON, H. and SWALES, J. D. (1982) Changes in leucocyte sodium efflux rates in normotensive relatives of known hypertensive patients and normotensive subjects. *Clinical Science,* **63,** 69

JOHNSTON, C. I. and DAVIES, J. O. (1966) Evidence from circulation studies for a humoral mechanism in the natriuresis of saline loading. *Proceedings of the Society for Experimental Biology and Medicine,* **121,** 1058–1063

JOHNSTON, C. I., DAVIS, J. O., HOWARDS, S. S. and WRIGHT, F. S. (1967) Cross-circulation experiments in the mechanism of the natriuresis during saline loading in the dog. *Circulation Research,* **20,** 1–10

JONES, A. W. (1973) Altered ion transport in vascular smooth muscle from spontaneously hypertensive rats. *Circulation Research,* **33.** 563–572

KALOYANIDES, G. J. and AZER, M. (1971) Evidence of a humoral mechanism in volume expansion natriuresis. *Journal of Clinical Investigation,* **50,** 1603–1612

KALOYANIDES, G. J., COHEN, L. and DI BONA, G. F. (1977) Failure of selected endocrine organ ablation to modify the natriuresis of blood volume expansion in the dog. *Clinical Science and Molecular Medicine,* **52,** 351–356

KAWABE, K., WATANABE, T. X., SHIONO, K. and SOKABE, H. (1979) Influence of blood pressure on renal isografts between spontaneously hypertensive and normotensive rats utilizing the F_1 hybrids. *Japanese Heart Journal,* **20,** 886–894

KNOCK, C. A. (1980) Further evidence *in vivo* for a circulating natriuretic substance after expanding the blood volume in rats. *Clinical Science,* **59,** 423–433

KNOCK, C. A. and DE WARDENER, H. E. (1980) Evidence *in vivo* for a circulating natriuretic substance in rats after expanding the blood volume. *Clinical Science,* **59,** 411–421

KNOX, F. G., HOWARDS, S. S., WRIGHT, F. S., DAVIS, B. B. and BERLINER, R. W. (1968) Effect of dilution and expansion of blood volume on proximal sodium reabsorption. *American Journal of Physiology,* **215,** 1041–1048

LICHARDUS, B. and NIZET, A. (1972) Water and sodium excretion after blood volume expansion under conditions of constant arterial, venous and plasma oncotic pressures and constant haematocrit. *Clinical Science,* **42,** 701–709

LICHARDUS, B. and PONEC, J. (1970) Conditions for biological evidence of a natriuretic hormone in experiments with rat cross-circulation. *Physiologia Bohemoslovenica,* **19,** 330

LICHSTEIN, D. and SAMUELOV, S. (1980) Endogenous 'ouabain-like' activity in rat brain. *Biochemical and Biophysics Research Communications,* **96,** 1518–1523

LEITZ, F. H. and STEFANO, F. J. E. (1970) Effect of ouabain and disipramine on the uptake and storage of epinephrine and meteraminol. *European Journal of Pharmacology,* **2,** 278–285

LOSSE, H., ZIDEK, W., ZUMKLEY, H., WESSELS, F. and VETTER, H. (1981) Intracellular Na^+ as a genetic marker of essential hypertension. *Clinical and Experimental Hypertension,* **3,** 627–640

LUNDIN, S., FOLKOW, B. and RIPPE, B. (1981) Central blood volume in spontaneously hypertensive rat. *Acta Physiologica Scandinavica,* **112,** 257–262

MCAREAVEY, D., MURRAY, G. D., LEVER, A. F. and ROBERTSON, J. I. S. (1983) Similarity of idiopathic aldosteronism and essential hypertension. A statistical comparison. *Hypertension,* **5,** 116–121

MACGREGOR, G. A., FENTON, S., ALAGHBAND-ZADEH, J., MARKANDU, N., ROULSTON, J. E. and DE WARDENER, H. E. (1981) Evidence for a raised concentration of a circulating sodium transport inhibitor in essential hypertension. *British Medical Journal,* **283,** 1355–1357

MACGREGOR, G. A., ROTELLAR, C., MARKANDU, M. D., SMITH, S. J. and SAGNELLA, G. A. (1982) Contrasting effects of nifedipine, captopril, and propranolol in normotensive and hypertensive subjects. *Journal of Cardiovascular Pharmacology,* **4** *(Suppl. 3),* S358–S362

MEYER, P. and GARAY, R. P. (1981) Genetic markers in essential hypertension. *Clinical and Experimental Hypertension,* **3,** 569–895

MICHELAKIS, A. M., MIZUKOSHI, H., HUANG, C., MURAKAMI, K. and INAGAMI, T. (1975) Further studies on the existence of a sensitizing factor to pressor agents in hypertension. *Journal of Clinical Endocrinology and Metabolism,* **41,** 90–96

MONTARI, A., BORGHI, L., CANALI, M. *et al.* (1980) Altered sodium efflux in red blood cells from essential hypertensive subjects. In *Intracellular Electrolytes and Arterial Hypertension,* edited by H. Zumkley and H. Losse, pp. 135–144. New York: G. Thieme

NAKAZATO, Y., OHGA, A. and ONODA, Y. (1978) The effect of ouabain on noradrenaline output from peripheral adrenergic neurones of isolated guinea-pig vas deferens. *Journal of Physiology,* **278,** 45–54

NORESSON, E., RICKSTEIN, S. E. and THOREN, P. (1979) Left atrial pressure in normotensive and spontaneously hypertensive rats. *Acta Physiologica Scandinavica*, **107**, 9–12

NUTBOURNE, D. M., HOWSE, J. D., SCHRIER, R. W. *et al.* (1970) The effect of expanding the blood volume of a dog on the short-circuit current across an isolated frog skin incorporated in the dog's circulation. *Clinical Science*, **38**, 629–648

OVERBECK, H. W. and CLARK, D. W. J. (1975) Vasodilator to K^+ in genetic hypertensive and in renal hypertensive rats. *Journal of Laboratory and Clinical Medicine*, **86**, 973–983

OVERBECK, H. W., DERIFIELD, R. S., PAMNANI, M. B. and SOZEN, T. (1974) Attenuated vasodilator response to K^+ in essential hypertension in man. *Journal of Clinical Investigation*, **53**, 678–686

OVERBECK, H. W., KU, D. D. and RAPP, J. P. (1981) Sodium pump activity in arteries of Dahl salt-sensitive rats. *Hypertension*, **3**, 306–312

OVERBECK, H. W., PAMNANI, M. B., AKERA, T., BRODY, T. M. and HADDY, F. J. (1976) Depressed function of an ouabain-sensitive sodium–potassium pump in blood vessels from renal hypertensive dog. *Circulation Research*, **38**, 48–53

PAMNANI, M. B., HUOT, R., STEFFEN, R. P. and HADDY, F. J. (1980) Evidence for a humoral Na^+ transport inhibiting factor in one-kidney, one-wrapped hypertension. *Physiologist*, **23**, 91

PEARCE, J. W., SONNENBERG, H., VERESS, A. T. and ACKERMAN, V. (1969) Evidence for a humoral factor modifying the renal response to blood volume expansion in the rat. *Canadian Journal of Physiology and Pharmacology*, **47**, 377–386

PEARCE, J. W., VERESS, A. T. and SONNENBERG, H. (1975) Time-course of onset and decay of humoral natriuretic activity in the rat. *Canadian Journal of Physiology and Pharmacology*, **53**, 734–741

PLETCHER, A. and LAUBESCHER, A. (1980) Use and limits of platelets as models for neurons: amine release and shape change regulation. In *Platelets: Cellular Response Mechanisms and their Biological Significance*, edited by A. Rotman, F. A. Meyer, C. Gitler and A. Silberger, pp. 267–275. Chichester: John Wiley

POSNOFF, Y. V. and ORLOFF, S. N. (1984) Cell membrane alterations as a source of primary hypertension. *Journal of Hypertension*, **2**, 1–6

POSTON, L., SEWELL, R. B., WILKINSON, S. P. *et al.* (1981a) Evidence for a circulating sodium transport inhibitor in essential hypertension. *British Medical Journal*, **282**, 847–849

POSTON, L., JONES, R. B., RICHARDSON, P. J. and HILTON, P. J. (1981b) The effect of antihypertensive therapy in abnormal leucocyte transport in essential hypertension. *Clinical and Experimental Hypertension*, **3**, 693–701

POSTON, L., WILKINSON, S., SEWELL, B. and WILLIAMS, R. (1982) Sodium transport during natriuresis of volume expansion: a study using peripheral leucocytes. *Clinical Science*, **63**, 243

ROBINSON, B. F., BAYLEY, D. and DOBBS, R. J. (1982) Response of forearm resistance vessels to verapamil and sodium nitroprusside in normotensive and hypertensive men: evidence for a functional abnormality of vascular smooth muscle in primary hypertension. *Clinical Science*, **63**, 33–42

ROBINSON, B. F., CHIODINI, P., DOBBS, R. J., PHILLIPS, R. J. W. and WILSON, P. (1981) On the mechanism of the abnormal response to verapamil and nitroprusside in the resistance vessels of men with primary hypertension. *Clinical Science*, **62**, 32

ROVNER, D. R., CONN, J. W., KNOPF, R. F., COHEN, E. L. and HSUEK, H. T. (1965) Nature of renal escape from the sodium-retaining effect of aldosterone in primary aldosteronism and in normal subjects. *Journal of Clinical Endocrinology and Metabolism*, **25**, 53–64

SAFAR, M. E., LONDON, G. M., LEVENSON, J. A., SIMON, A. CH. and CHAU, N. P. (1979) Rapid dextran infusion in essential hypertension. *Hypertension*, **1**, 615–623

SCHÖMING, A., DIETZ, R., ROSELER, W. *et al.* (1978) Sympathetic vascular tone in spontaneous hypertension of rats. *Klinische Wochenschrift*, **56** (Suppl. 1), 131–138

SEALEY, J. E., KIRSHMAN, J. D. and LARAGH, J. H. (1969) Natriuretic activity in plasma and urine of salt-loaded man and sheep. *Journal of Clinical Investigation*, **48**, 2210–2224

SONNENBERG, H., VERESS, A. T. and PEARCE, J. W. (1972) A humoral component of the natriuretic mechanism in sustained blood volume expansion. *Journal of Clinical Investigation*, **51**, 2631–2644

TARAZI, R. C., FROLICH, E. D. and DUSTAN, H. P. (1968) Plasma volume in man with essential hypertension. *New England Journal of Medicine*, **278**, 762–765

THOMAS, R. D., EDMONDSON, R. P. S., HILTON, P. H. and JONES, N. F. (1975) Abnormal sodium transport from patients with essential hypertension and the effect of treatment. *Clinical Science and Molecular Medicine*, **48**, 169S

TOBIAN, L. and BINION, J. T. (1952) Tissue cation and water in arterial hypertension. *Circulation*, **5**, 754–758

TOBIAN, L., COFFEE, K. and MC CREA, P. (1967) Evidence for a humoral factor of non-renal and non-adrenal origin which influences renal sodium excretion. *Transactions of the Association of American Physicians*, **80**, 200–206

TOBIAN, L., LANGE, J., AZER, S. *et al.* (1978) Reduction of natriuretic capacity and renin release in isolated, blood perfused kidneys of Dahl hypertension-prone rats. *Circulation Research*, **43**, I-92–I-97

TOBIAN, L., PUMPER, M., JOHNSON, S. and IWAI, J. (1979) A circulating humoral pressor agent in Dahl S rats with NaCl hypertension. *Clinical Science*, **57**, 3455–3475

TRIPPODO, N. C., YAMAMOTO, J. and FROLICH, E. D. (1981) Whole body venous capacity and effective total tissue compliance in SHR. *Hypertension*, **3**, 104–111

VON WESSELS, F., ZUMKLEY, H. and LOSSE, H. (1970) Untersuchungen zur frage des zusammenhanges zwischen kationepermeabilitat der erythrozyten und hochdruckdisposition. *Zeitschrift für Kreislaufforschung*, **59**, 415–426

WILLASSEN, Y. and OFFSTAD, J. (1980) Renal sodium excretion and the peritubular capillary physical factors in essential hypertension. *Hypertension*, **2**, 771–779

WILLIS, L. R. and BAUER, J. H. (1978) Aldosterone in the exaggerated natriuresis of spontaneously hypertensive rats. *American Journal of Physiology*, **234**, F25–F35

6
Role of mineralocorticoids in essential hypertension
R. Fraser and P. L. Padfield

INTRODUCTION

The diagnosis of essential hypertension is made on the failure to detect a definite primary cause for raised blood pressure. It is unlikely to represent a homogeneous group of patients and it is not surprising that there are conflicting hypotheses, with associated evidence, to explain its aetiology. One group of hypotheses invokes the adrenal cortex, in particular the mineralocorticoid hormones, and the purpose of this chapter is to discuss whether these are supported by current evidence.

Adrenocortical hormones

The adrenal cortex secretes several biologically active steroid hormones which affect intermediary (glucocorticoid) and electrolyte (mineralocorticoid) metabolism. Most hormones possess both actions to some degree, but one or other usually predominates. Thus, aldosterone is the most potent mineralocorticoid but is also capable of exerting some glucocorticoid effect: the reverse is true of cortisol. Corticosterone, 11-deoxycorticosterone (DOC) and possibly 18-hydroxydeoxycorticosterone (18-OH-DOC) also possess significant mineralocorticoid activity. Other compounds will be mentioned later. A number of synthetic steroids, notably 9-α-fluorocortisol, are also potent mineralocorticoids.

In common with other steroid hormones, mineralocorticoids are thought to exert their effects by altering the rate of synthesis of specific proteins in target organs, in this case particularly the kidney (Fanestil and Park, 1981). They bind to specific cytoplasmic receptors and the resulting steroid–receptor complex is then bound within the nucleus. Stimulation of RNA and protein synthesis then can be demonstrated but the function of the new protein has not been firmly established. An enzyme component of the tricarboxylic acid cycle, which would increase the availability of energy for electrolyte metabolism (Petty, Kokko and Marver, 1981), or the Na, K-dependent ATPase coupling this energy to ion transport, have been suggested (Edelman, 1979). Another possibility is that cell permeability to electrolytes is altered (Crabbé, 1978). It should be emphasized that at least two types of mineralocorticoid receptors exist – 'high' and 'low' affinity (Fanestil and Park, 1981; Kusch, Farman and Edelman, 1978). The low affinity receptors probably also bind cortisol (Fanestil and Park, 1981; Farman, Kusch and Edelman, 1978). However, intervention in nuclear control of protein synthesis may not be the only mechanism by which aldosterone and related steroids affect electrolyte mechanism. A few studies have claimed to show an effect in erythrocytes at physiological concentrations. In these enucleate cells a conventional mode of action is not tenable, and a direct effect, possibly on the Na, K-dependent ATPase, is postulated (Hamlyn and Duffy, 1978; Stern, Beck and Sowers, 1983).

Mineralocorticoids promote sodium reabsorption in exchange for potassium excretion in the distal convoluted tubule, and in the early collecting duct of the kidney (Fanestil and Park, 1981). In the renal epithelial cell this is accomplished by the 'sodium pump' which expels sodium, which has diffused in from tubular fluid, into the peritubular fluid. Excretion of H^+ is also increased. There may be some redistribution of ions within tissues (Young and Jackson, 1982). Thus, the hallmarks of excess mineralocorticoid secretion are:

(1) increases in total body sodium in the presence of reduced sodium excretion;
(2) decreases in total body and plasma potassium with increased urinary potassium levels;
(3) a metabolic alkalosis (*see* Ferriss *et al.*, 1983).

Whether all of these indices need always be present in states of mineralocorticoid excess will be discussed later.

Mineralocorticoids also affect the composition of sweat and saliva and the electrical properties of mucosal tissues such as that of the colon (Skrabal *et al.*, 1978).

Control of corticosteroid secretion

Examination of the quantitative relationship between a hormone and its trophins is a useful indicator of abnormal secretion (Fraser *et al.*, 1983; Williams and Dluhy, 1983). The factors controlling corticosteroid secretion have been discussed in detail in several recent reviews and only a brief summary will be given here. While a large, and increasing, number of substances have been shown to affect steroid hormone levels, particularly that of aldosterone, the major *in vivo* control is probably exerted by a few, namely ACTH, angiotensin II, potassium and sodium. ACTH secretion from the anterior pituitary follows both a short-term pulsatile pattern and a well-defined nycthemeral variation – high in the early morning and lowest late at night – and since it affects the secretion of all major corticoid hormones these follow the same pattern. ACTH secretion, and therefore that of its dependent hormones, increases in response to stress. However, while long-term ACTH excess sustains increases in the levels of cortisol, corticosterone and their respective 11-deoxy precursors, that of aldosterone increases only temporarily, probably because sodium retention, with consequent low angiotensin II levels, occurs (*see below*).

Within the physiological range angiotensin II, a pressor octapeptide generated in the circulation by the consecutive actions of the renal enzyme, renin, and a converting enzyme on an α_2-globulin substrate, is a specific stimulus to aldosterone biosynthesis. Plasma concentrations of aldosterone and its immediate precursor, 18-hydroxycorticosterone (18-OH-B), alone increase in response to angiotensin II administration. The effects of sodium depletion and loading, which raise and depress aldosterone secretion respectively, are mediated largely by parallel changes in the activity of the renin–angiotensin system. It is possible, however, that other factors may interact in altering adrenal aldosterone responsiveness under such conditions (Dawson-Hughes *et al.*, 1981; McCaa *et al.*, 1981). The stimulating action of increased potassium levels is also specific to aldosterone biosynthesis. Finally, sodium status determines the level of aldosterone response, but not that of DOC, corticosterone or cortisol to ACTH, and also to angiotensin II and potassium; sodium depletion amplifies while sodium loading attenuates the response. The importance of dopamine and serotonin as adrenocortical antagonist and agonist *in vivo* is still being assessed (*see* Edwards *et al.*, 1982) and there are several recently discovered aldosterone-stimulating factors in urine (Sen *et al.*, 1981) and plasma (Mendelsohn and Kachel, 1981) to be considered in the future.

Can mineralocorticoids cause hypertension?

Administration of mineralocorticoids such as DOC, aldosterone or 9-α-fluorocortisol to animals leads to an increase in blood pressure providing that a substantial amount of sodium is taken in the diet (Pan and Young, 1982; Selye, Hall and Rowley, 1943). Similar experiments in normal human subjects produce less consistent results but in some studies definite pressor effects have been observed. For example, Nicholls *et al.* (1979a) treated six normal subjects with daily doses of 9-α-fluorocortisol and showed a rise in blood pressure which was reversed by the mineralocorticoid antagonist, spironolactone. The study also illustrates the phenomenon of 'escape' from the effects of exogenous sodium-retaining hormones. A period of sodium retention and potassium loss over a period of several days is followed by an increase in sodium excretion and a reduction in that of potassium until balance is re-achieved despite continued treatment. At this time, plasma sodium concentration remains higher and plasma potassium lower than in the untreated state.

Endogenous hypersecretion of mineralocorticoids may also be associated with hypertension. Evidence is provided by a number of relatively rare diseases. For example, primary aldosteronism (Ferriss *et al.*, 1983), in which an adrenocortical adenoma or bilateral adrenocortical hyperplasia secrete excess quantities of aldosterone, is characterized by hypertension, sodium retention, hypokalaemia and a metabolic alkalosis. These features can be partially or totally corrected by mineralocorticoid antagonists (such as spironolactone, amiloride) or by excision of the tumour, if present. Excess of DOC or corticosterone (B) from adrenal carcinoma tissue has similar effects (Fraser *et al.*, 1968; Kelly *et al.*, 1982). The hypertensive effects of mineralocorticoids are also illustrated by some types of inborn error of corticosteroid biosynthesis (Fraser, 1983). The features of 11-β-hydroxylase and 17-α-hydroxylase deficiency (*Figure 6.1*) resemble those of primary aldosteronism but arise in a different way. In the former, an inability to transform 11-deoxycortisol to cortisol (and DOC to corticosterone) results in hyperstimulation of the adrenal cortex by ACTH and consequent abnormal increases in the secretion of compounds prior to the enzyme block. Among these is

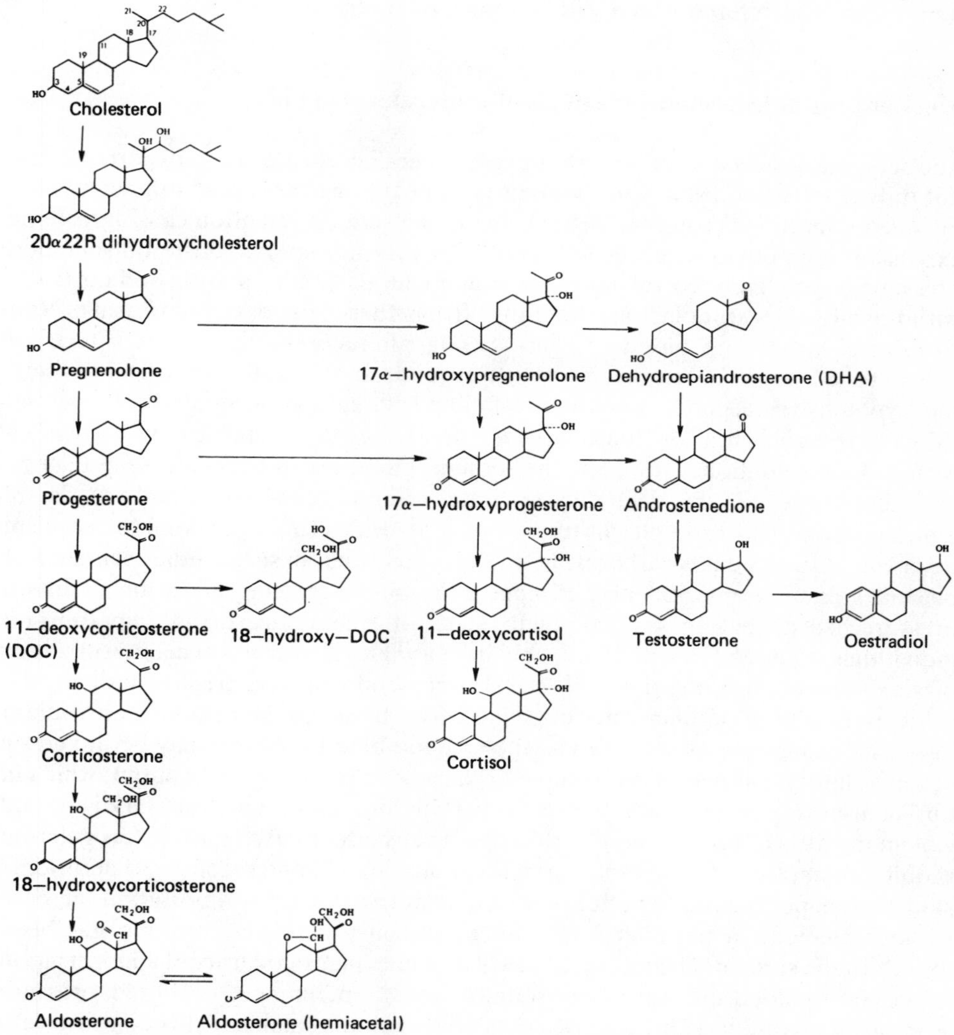

Figure 6.1 Pathway for production of adrenal steroids from the parent compound cholesterol. The 19 carbon atom is indicated in the cholesterol molecule

the mineralocorticoid DOC which could account for the biochemical and blood pressure changes (*see below*). In 17-α-hydroxylase deficiency, there is again cortisol deficiency and increased ACTH secretion raises the biosynthesis of 17-deoxysteroids such as DOC and corticosterone. Aldosterone levels and the activity of the renin–angiotensin system are suppressed in both conditions, probably due to sodium retention. Suppression of ACTH secretion by exogenous glucocorticoids usually corrects the biochemical abnormalities and reduces blood pressure. Therapeutic use of ACTH has also been reported to increase blood pressure in a proportion of recipients (Fraser *et al.*, 1976). This could also be partly due to an increased production of ACTH-dependent mineralocorticoids but other explanations have been offered which will be discussed later.

Mechanisms of hypertensive effects of mineralocorticoids

The sequence of events leading from hypermineralocorticoidism to hypertension is not fully understood. Many mechanisms have been suggested; probably several are involved (Beretta-Piccoli *et al.*, 1983). Increased sodium retention causing volume expansion is an obvious suggestion, particularly as in primary aldosteronism blood pressure is positively correlated with sodium levels (NaE, plasma sodium). On withdrawal of spironolactone therapy from these patients, increasing NaE correlates with rising blood pressure, while after counteracting the effects of aldosterone by spironolactone, amiloride or removal of the adrenocortical tumour, the hypotensive response is related to falling sodium levels. Similarly, in normal subjects treated with 9-α-fluorocortisol, blood pressure increases are associated with sodium retention. However, the sodium–blood pressure relationship may be an indirect one. Several days may separate sodium accumulation and the rise in blood pressure (for example, in treated patients with primary hyperaldosteronism from whom treatment is withdrawn). It is also clear that in such studies evidence of plasma volume expansion may disappear despite increasing elevation in blood pressure, such that in the complete state of mineralocorticoid hypertension individuals do not have a demonstrably increased level of exchangeable sodium or plasma volume (Wenting *et al.*, 1977). Also, mineralocorticoid treatment of normal subjects results in sodium retention, increased blood pressure and then sodium loss. The changes in electrolyte metabolism and blood pressure may be linked by autoregulatory compensation: volume expansion increasing cardiac output which in turn causes raised peripheral resistance (Guyton, 1980; Guyton, Granger and Coleman, 1971). Objections to this hypothesis are firstly, that autoregulation should accomplish a rise in blood pressure more rapidly, and secondly, that in some studies of experimental hypertension cardiac output has been reported to increase without changes in peripheral resistance, and in others the converse has been found. In the study of Nicholls *et al.* (1979a), while mineralocorticoid adminstration raised both blood pressure and sodium levels, increments of blood pressure correlated inversely with those of cumulative sodium balance. This contrast with endogenous mineralocorticoid excess is remarkable, but may have been due to the shorter exposure to steroid or the different compound involved.

Another possibility is that mineralocorticoids exert two independent influences, the first on electrolyte metabolism and the second on blood pressure. Thus, they may have a direct rather than an indirect effect on vascular smooth muscle, possibly altering the distribution of electrolytes across the cell membrane and hence contractility (Garwitz and Jones, 1982; Kornel *et al.*, 1983; Llaurado, Madden and Smith, 1983). Vascular smooth muscle possesses mineralocorticoid receptors.

The responsiveness of the brain or the sympathetic nervous system might also be involved in such a mechanism (Nicholls, Julius and Zweifler, 1981). There has also been a suggestion that an interaction might occur between mineralocorticoids and vasopressin (Berecek *et al.*, 1982), but contrary evidence exists in the rat (Morton, Garcia del Rio and Hughes, 1982). Studies of ACTH-induced hypertension in the sheep suggest that some corticosteroids may be 'hypertensogenic' independently of alterations in electrolyte metabolism (Scoggins *et al.*, 1982), but it is not yet clear whether this applies to hypermineralocorticoidism in general. That the contribution of the direct effect of aldosterone to the hypertension of primary hyperaldosteronism is trivial follows from the finding that blood pressure is reduced to a similar extent by amiloride which raises plasma aldosterone concentration, and removal of the adrenocortical tumour which reduces aldosterone to normal (Beretta-Piccoli *et al.*, 1983). Mineralocorticoids may enhance, or affect, the pressor potency of noradrenaline or angiotensin II, but this is probably indirectly due to their sodium-retaining effects (Beilin and Ziakas, 1972). The potassium loss associated with hypermineralocorticoidism has also been suggested as a contributory factor in hypertension as potassium loading is vasodilatory in animals (Blaustein, Lang and James-Kracke, 1981), but this is probably of little or no importance in primary hyperaldosteronism (Beretta-Piccoli *et al.*, 1983).

Finally, as discussed in detail in Chapters 4 and 5, steroid-dependent sodium retention may trigger the release of a sodium transport inhibitor both to increase sodium excretion and to facilitate sodium redistribution within the body (Briggs *et al.*, 1982; de Wardener, 1982; Hamlyn *et al.*, 1982; Kramer, 1981). In this latter way, intracellular sodium levels may be augmented at the expense of the extracellular compartment without altering external electrolyte balance. The effects of altering vascular smooth muscle electrolyte metabolism were mentioned above. Several inhibitors have been described. One is reported to act like a cardiac glycoside on the membrane Na, K-dependent ATPase and a recent report that antibodies to digitalis may reduce the blood pressure in rats made hypertensive with DOC acetate lends support to this idea (Haddy, Pamnani and Clough, 1978; Kajimi, Yoshihara and Ogata, 1982). These inhibitors may be important in essential hypertension (*see below*).

In summary, in the condition of mineralocorticoid excess, abnormal sodium retention is probably a necessary early step in the development of hypertension but other steps must occur. Direct steroid action and hypokalaemia are relatively unimportant.

Before turning to the situation of essential hypertension it is pertinent to note that not all patients who have subsequently proven primary aldosteronism manifest the characteristic biochemical abnormalities. For example, among 80 patients with proven primary hyperaldosteronism (70 with an adrenocortical tumour) persistent normokalaemia was demonstrated in 27.5%. Apparently this situation persisted in 12.5% despite three days of salt loading (Bravo *et al.*, 1982). It is also clear that in some individuals expanded plasma volume and exchangeable sodium cannot be demonstrated (Ferriss *et al.*, 1983; Wenting *et al.*, 1977) and thus it may not be reasonable to dismiss the possibility of mineralocorticoid excess in the absence of these indices.

Involvement of the adrenal cortex in aetiology of essential hypertension

Mineralocorticoid excess in essential hypertension should reveal itself by the features discussed in previous sections. Increased secretion should be detectable by hormone assays, while increased sensitivity of target cells should be apparent from studies of electrolyte metabolism. Direct pressor effects may be less easy to demonstrate unless tests of sensitivity to steroids are carried out. Again, the effect may be due to a recognized agent such as aldosterone or DOC or it may be necessary to search for other adrenal products or their metabolites. Finally, it is necessary to discover whether primary adrenocortical dysfunction is the cause or whether the excess stimulation by, or sensitivity to, trophic substances such as ACTH, angiotensin II, potassium, sodium, or by the less well-understood factors such as neuramines are responsible.

The adrenal cortex was originally implicated in hypertension by the observation in animal models that adrenalectomy protects against hypertensive manoeuvres and, in man, that inhibitors of corticosteroid biosynthesis, for example aminoglutethimide, reduces blood pressure (Taylor *et al.*, 1978; Woods *et al.*, 1969). There are, of course, alternative explanations of these findings. A given level of blood pressure is achieved by balancing the effects of several biological systems, all of which may be important and of which the adrenal cortex is only one. The hypotensive effect of adrenocortical inhibition in hypertension does not necessarily mean, therefore, that this organ is the primary cause of the disease.

A major feature of mineralocorticoid excess syndromes is the suppression of plasma renin. The observation therefore that approximately 20–30% of patients otherwise labelled as having essential hypertension have low levels of renin (*see* Ganguly and Weinberger, 1979) was taken as indicating the presence of excess mineralocorticoid activity (Melby and Dale, 1979). Controversy still exists as to the meaning of the low renin state in this substantial proportion of patients with hypertension and several reviews on the subject have been written (Dunn and Tannen, 1974; Ganguly and Weinberger, 1979; Gunnels and McGuffin, 1975). The initial study by Woods *et al.* (1969), often quoted as evidence of an expanded exchangeable sodium in patients with low renin hypertension, actually demonstrated that such patients had similar exchangeable sodium levels to normotensive subjects, and it was those with normal renin hypertension who demonstrated somewhat low exchangeable sodium levels. More recently it has been shown that there is no expansion of the exchangeable sodium state or plasma volume in so-called low renin hypertension (Lebel *et al.*, 1974; Schalekamp *et al.*, 1974). For reasons given earlier, however, this does not automatically exclude the possibility of mineralocorticoid excess. Patients with low renin hypertension (as a group) have long been shown to be more sensitive to the hypotensive effect of diuretics (*see* Ganguly and Weinberger, 1979), suggesting at least a more marked dependency upon sodium than other forms of essential hypertension. Most studies have shown that renin levels correlate inversely with age in essential hypertension, suggesting an adaptative process (Meade *et al.*, 1983; Vetter *et al.*, 1980). It is also true, however, that the older hypertensive (often the patient with a low renin state) has a blood pressure more closely related to his sodium status than does the younger patient with essential hypertension (Beretta-Piccoli *et al.*, 1982), lending credence to the view that as hypertension develops it becomes more sodium dependent.

MINERALOCORTICOID LEVELS IN ESSENTIAL HYPERTENSION

Aldosterone

Although plasma aldosterone concentration is by definition within the normal range in essential hypertension, when comparison is made with matched normotensive subjects under carefully controlled conditions levels are significantly higher than in the normal group (Brunner, Sealey and Laragh, 1973; Genest *et al.*, 1978; Grim *et al.*, 1974; Weidmann *et al.*, 1978). Thus, while within the normal range, levels may be inappropriately high for the prevailing level of renin. Furthermore, by integrating plasma concentrations over a 24 h period, Kowarski *et al.* (1978) could distinguish a subgroup of patients with essential hypertension who had abnormally high levels. Plasma aldosterone concentration may also be less readily suppressed by salt loading in patients with essential hypertension than it is in normal subjects, perhaps suggesting a measure of autonomy of secretion (Collins *et al.*, 1970; Helber *et al.*, 1980; Khokhar *et al.*, 1976; Tuck *et al.*, 1976). Also, in addition to patients with essential hypertension and low plasma renin activity, perhaps mistakenly often treated as a discrete subgroup (Padfield *et al.*, 1975), those with normal renin levels show a higher than normal aldosterone:renin or aldosterone:AII ratio (Collins *et al.*, 1970; Fraser *et al.*, 1981; Grim *et al.*, 1974; Re *et al.*, 1978; Safar *et al.*, 1982). Thus there is some evidence of a mild aldosterone excess in essential hypertension. The increment, although statistically significant, is small and it remains to be shown that such an increase in man could result in the rise in blood pressure shown in these patients. The control of aldosterone in the various subgroups of essential hypertension will be discussed below.

Other mineralocorticoids

The demonstration of non-aldosterone mineralocorticoid activity in extracts of urine from patients with hypertension encouraged the continuing search for other steroid hormones or metabolites (Sekihara *et al.*, 1979). A number have been shown to be raised in subgroups of hypertensive patients, but as yet no one compound is raised in all patients. For example, Brown *et al.* (1972) described the occurrence of isolated DOC excess in a small group. The increase over normal was not great and its importance is difficult to assess: increased mineralocorticoid activity due to DOC should be readily compensated for by a small decrease in the production of the more potent aldosterone if normal control mechanisms remain intact but, as mentioned previously, these mechanisms may be less flexible in essential hypertension (*see below*).

Another relatively early steroid candidate was 18-OH-DOC. Again, urinary steroid levels were said to be raised in a small subgroup of patients (Agrin *et al.*, 1978; Melby *et al.*, 1972). The biological importance of 18-OH-DOC in man is less well-documented than that of either aldosterone or DOC. Early studies are reviewed by Melby *et al.* (1972). In the rat, although its mineralocorticoid potency is low compared with that of aldosterone, it is present in much higher concentrations and might, therefore, be biologically significant. In short-term studies, 18-OH-DOC had approximately 0.1% of the sodium-retaining potency of aldosterone and little or no kaliuretic effect (Nicholls *et al.*, 1979b). Its affinity for renal mineralocorticoid receptors is very low compared with aldosterone (Baxter *et al.*, 1976). On longer-term exposure, Carroll, Komanicky and Melby (1981) found blood pressure to rise in rats without detectable changes in electrolyte metabolism and concluded that 18-OH-DOC produces hypertension independently of sodium retention. Other studies have not shown a blood pressure effect. In man, endogenous circulatory levels of 18-OH-DOC are similar to those of aldosterone. It is again much less potent in its effect on electrolyte metabolism and is antinatriuretic with no detectable stimulation of potassium excretion (Nicholls *et al.*, 1977). No hypertensive effect has so far been demonstrated.

Steroid hormones from which the 19-methyl group has been removed have been the subject of renewed interest. This molecular modification has long been known to increase the mineralocorticoid activity *in vivo* in the rat (Kagawa and van Arman, 1957) and more recently has been shown to enhance binding to mineralocorticoid receptors (Funder *et al.*, 1978). The 19-nor-derivative of DOC occurs in the urine of rats with some forms of hypertension (Dale *et al.*, 1982; Funder *et al.*, 1978; Gomez-Sanchez *et al.*, 1979) and is also present in human urine (Dale, Holbrook and Melby, 1981). *In vivo* in the rat it was found to have similar antinatriuretic action to, but less kaliuretic action than, aldosterone (Perrone *et al.*, 1982) but *in vitro*, using a receptor assay, Gomez-Sanchez *et al.* (1979) arrived at a lower, although still significant, potency. It is of interest that 19-norDOC may not be of adrenocortical origin, but produced peripherally, possibly at target sites, from 19-hydroxyDOC (Gomez-Sanchez, 1982) which itself has little or no biological activity (Perrone *et al.*, 1982). The role of this interesting compound in human hypertension is being assessed. Its rate of excretion is said to correlate with blood pressure in 'low renin' essential hypertension (Griffing *et al.*, 1983a) and with aldosterone levels (Griffing *et al.*, 1983b). In this latter correlation the data may not be normally distributed and again only a proportion of the group studied had high excretion rates – many were normal in this respect and a few had low levels. The related compound, 19-norprogesterone, which is also a mineralocorticoid (Komanicky and Melby, 1981; Wynne *et al.*, 1980) has not been extensively studied in man.

Other steroids

In addition to compounds with demonstrable biological activity, several others have been associated with human hypertension but no firm role or mechanism of action has been established. For example, the importance of 16-α-18-hydroxyDOC as an amplifier (in other words, has no intrinsic action but alters the response to other mineralocorticoids) of mineralocorticoid action (Dale and Melby, 1974) requires confirmation while the isolation of the cortisol metabolite 5-α-hydrocortisol from the urine of a case of juvenile hypertension (Ulick, Ramirez and New, 1977) has yet to be repeated in adults. Moreover, in rare cases of possible receptor defects, cortisol itself may act as a potent mineralocorticoid (Oberfield *et al.*, 1983). 18-hydroxycortisol may be a useful diagnostic marker for some forms of mineralocorticoid hypertension (Ulick and Chu, 1982), but is as yet of no known relevance to essential hypertension. Finally, the identity and importance of 'hypersterone', a possible metabolite of aldosterone isolated from the urine of some hypertensive patients, are obscure (Adlerkreutz, Herkali and Wahlroos, 1973).

Perhaps the most interesting recent development has been the suggestion already mentioned that steroids may affect blood pressure independently of electrolyte metabolism and that the screening of putative hypertensive agents by their mineralocorticoid effects or by mineralocorticoid receptor binding may be misleading. The hypothesis arises from studies of the development of ACTH-induced hypertension in the sheep and is discussed in detail by Scoggins *et al.* (1982). It is based on the observation that the hypertensive effects of ACTH could not be repeated by infusing mixtures of ACTH-dependent corticosteroids, but that addition of 17-α-hydroxyprogesterone or 17-α-20-dihydroxyprogesterone to this mixture was rewarded by success. The two compounds appear to have no action when given alone. Further studies have suggested that the electrolyte and hypertensive effects of some mineralocorticoids such as 9-α-fluorocortisol may be distinguishable. Again, application of these findings to human hypertension is an interesting prospect. Some preliminary studies of normal subjects have been published (Whitworth *et al.*, 1983).

Control of aldosterone levels in hypertension

Plasma aldosterone concentration is more sensitive to stimulation in sodium depleted patients with essential hypertension than in normal subjects. This applies to both angiotensin II (Fraser *et al.*, 1981; Honda *et al.*, 1977; Kisch, Dluhy and Williams, 1976; Marks *et al.*, 1979; Wisgerhof and Brown, 1979) and to ACTH (Honda *et al.*, 1977). This also holds true for the concentration of 18-OH-B, a precursor of aldosterone (Fraser *et al.*, 1981). There is some conflict in the literature, however, as to whether such enhanced sensitivity is a general feature of essential hypertension or is confined to the low renin group (*Figures 6.2* and *6.3*). It has been suggested that the hyper-responsiveness of aldosterone to angiotensin II in low renin hypertension is similar to that seen in 'idiopathic hyperaldosteronism'

168

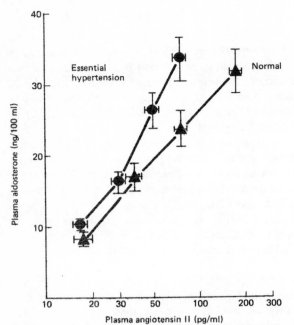

Figure 6.2 Response of plasma aldosterone to angiotensin II infusion in normal subjects and patients with essential hypertension. (Adapted from Fraser *et al.* (1981) and reproduced by kind permission of the Editor of *Hypertension*)

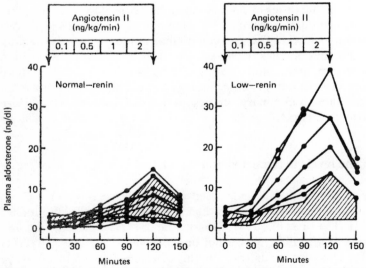

Figure 6.3 Effect of angiotensin II on plasma aldosterone in six patients with low-renin essential hypertension and ten patients with normal renin essential hypertension. Angiotensin II was infused after two days of supplemental sodium and dexamethasone and two hours of supine posture. The hatched area shows the range of plasma aldosterone in 13 normal subjects. (Reproduced from Wisgerhof and Brown (1979) with kind permission of the Authors and the Editor of *Journal of Clinical Investigation*)

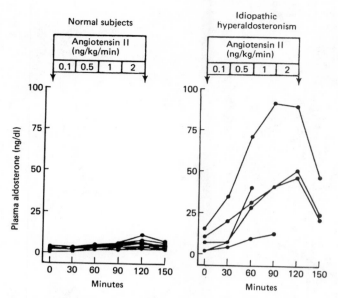

Figure 6.4 Effect of angiotensin II on plasma aldosterone in five patients with idiopathic hyperaldosteronism and 13 normal subjects. Angiotensin II was infused after two days of supplemental sodium and dexamethasone and two hours of supine posture. (Reproduced from Wisgerhof *et al*. (1978) by kind permission of the Authors and the Editor of *Journal of Clinical Endocrinology and Metabolism*)

(*Figure 6.4*), a feature which suggests that this condition (often regarded as a subgroup of primary hyperaldosteronism) has more in common with low reinin essential hypertension (Padfield *et al*., 1981). Certainly, the relationship of renin with aldosterone (negative in patients with adrenocortical adenoma) is positive, suggesting along with other evidence (Padfield *et al*., 1981) that the aldosterone secretion is by no means independent of changes in renin/angiotensin II (*Figure 6.5*). A recent study may indicate that the change in sensitivity occurs during or after the onset of hypertension. In a so-called prehypertensive group of young adults, a blunted response of aldosterone and 18-OH-B to ACTH and to a treadmill exercise is reported (Guthrie, Kotchen and Kotchen, 1983). However, neither renin nor aldosterone respond to sodium depletion as markedly as in normal subjects (Parfrey *et al*., 1981; Padfield *et al*., 1975a) and in some patients increases to subsequent angiotensin II or ACTH infusion are actually subnormal (Dluhy *et al*., 1979). The variation in response between patients can thus be great (Zoccali *et al*., 1983). No explanation is at present available for this imperfect matching of response to changes in electrolyte status but the following are suggestions. It is possible, for example, that there is some increased basal stimulation by factors other than ACTH or AII and that these factors do not increase during sodium depletion. It may be that the newer 'aldosterone-stimulating hormones' mentioned earlier fit into this category. Alternatively, a partial failure of some suppressing factor might explain the supersensitivity to

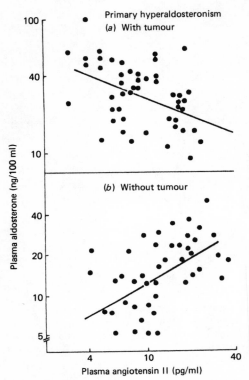

Figure 6.5 Correlation of plasma angiotensin II concentration and plasma aldosterone concentration in (*a*) untreated Conn's syndrome and (*b*) primary hyperaldosteronism without tumour (idiopathic hyperaldosteronism). (Reproduced from Brown *et al.* (1979) by kind permission of the Editor of *Annals of Clinical Biochemistry*)

stimulation and the high basal aldosterone:angiotensin II ratio (Wilson and Carey, 1981). *In vitro* stimulation of aldosterone production by zona glomerulosa cells is certainly less effective in the presence of dopamine (McKenna *et al.*, 1979), but much larger concentrations of the neuramine must be used than occur *in vivo* (Ball *et al.*, 1981). It is of interest that in normal subjects dopamine antagonism prevents the blunting of aldosterone responsiveness to angiotensin II seen on salt loading (Gordon *et al.*, 1983). Another possibility is that in essential hypertension the adrenocortical receptors, for example for angiotensin II, are abnormal. As discussed in detail in Chapter 7, there is evidence that this is true for the adrenal, vascular (Williams *et al.*, 1979, 1982) and renal (Britton, 1981) receptors in a subgroup of patients with normal and/or high renin essential hypertension.

Blood pressure electrolyte relationships in essential hypertension

The characteristic changes in sodium and potassium levels caused by excessive mineralocorticoid activity have been described. Blood pressure could be affected in several ways, by altered sodium and potassium intake, by impairment of renal sodium excretion mechanisms or by a generalized defect in tissue electrolyte transport. The second and third possibilities might occur if mineralocorticoid activity was too high. Whether changes occur in patients with essential hypertension has been studied by Beretta-Piccoli *et al.* (1982). Plasma, exchangeable and total body levels of sodium and potassium were measured and care was taken in the matching of hypertensive patients and control subjects and in correcting for differences in body habitus using a leanness index. No differences were found in absolute values of any of these variables between the normal and hypertensive groups. This does not, however, exclude the possibility that body sodium is increased initially but becomes normal as blood pressure rises but, since body sodium is demonstrably increased in primary hyperaldosteronism after blood pressure has risen, it seems unlikely that an aldosterone excess exists in essential hypertension.

Beretta-Piccoli *et al.* (1982) also showed that the relationship between electrolyte status and blood pressure was quite different from normal in essential hypertension

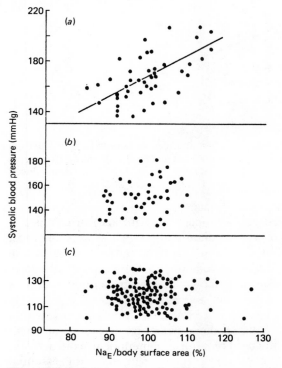

Figure 6.6 Relation of systolic blood pressure and exchangeable sodium (related to body surface area) in (*a*) moderately hypertensive subjects ($r = 0.56$, $P<0.001$); (*b*) mildly hypertensive subjects ($r = 0.25$, $P>0.05$); and in (*c*) normal subjects ($r = 0.04$). The correlation was also significant in the 50 patients who had never received treatment ($r = 0.44$, $P<0.01$). (Reproduced from Beretta-Piccoli *et al.* (1982) by kind permission of the Editor of *Clinical Science*)

(*Figure 6.6*) and the direction of the abnormality is compatible with mineralo-corticoid excess. While neither sodium nor potassium levels, however measured, correlated with blood pressure in normal subjects, significant correlations (positive for sodium, negative for potassium) were found in the hypertensive group (*Figure 6.7*). The sodium–blood pressure relationship was closest in older patients, absent in female patients and, interestingly, younger patients had subnormal exchangeable sodium levels. Statistical analysis of these data suggested that the relationship was

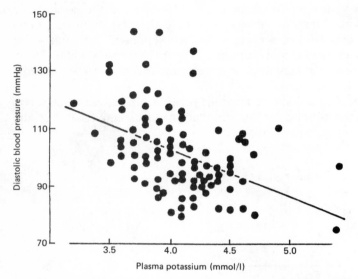

Figure 6.7 Relation of plasma potassium concentration and diastolic blood pressure (BP) in patients with essential hypertension ($r = -0.51$, $P<0.001$). The correlation in the 50 patients who had never received treatment was also significant ($r = -0.33$, $P<0.02$). (Reproduced from Beretta-Piccoli *et al.* by kind permission of the Editor of *Clinical Science*)

not explicable in terms of age (blood pressure increases with age) or changes in renal function as measured by blood urea. Sodium and potassium were the most important determinants of blood pressure in essential hypertension (potassium in young patients) while this role was played by age in normal subjects. Other studies (Brown, Brown and Krishnan, 1971) have shown that when sodium intake is manipulated, changes in exchangeable sodium and blood pressure are positively correlated in patients with hypertension but not in normal subjects. Thus, with a positive relationship of blood pressure with sodium levels and a negative one with potassium, the Na:K ratio, a frequently used monitor of mineralocorticoid activity, also correlated significantly with blood pressure in patients with essential hypertension. However, blood pressure and aldosterone concentration did not correlate and there were no diffferences in sodium, potassium or blood pressure measurements in low renin and normal renin essential hypertension groups. Moreover, the finding that young hypertensive patients have lower than normal exchangeable sodium levels is not in favour of a mineralocorticoid-dependent initial stimulus in the development of essential hypertension. The results so far are therefore inconclusive and one might speculate again that the data are consistent with the suggestion that hypertension becomes more sodium-dependent with age (or duration of hypertension) irrespective of whether or not this is related to a mineralocorticoid effect.

Similarities and differences between essential hypertension and mineralocorticoid hypertension

Studies of the type described above have also been carried out in groups of patients with primary hyperaldosteronism (Beretta-Piccoli *et al.*, 1983) and idiopathic hyperaldosteronism (Lasaridis *et al.*, 1984), a condition in which the involvement of the characteristic adrenal pathology of bilateral micronodular hyperplasia with the development of high blood pressure is less clear (Ferriss *et al.*, 1983). A comparison of these diseases with essential hypertension has been described (Lasaridis *et al.*, 1984). A case has previously been made that idiopathic hyperaldosteronism may be an extreme form of essential hypertension (Brown *et al.*, 1979; Fraser *et al.*, 1981; Padfield, 1975b; Padfield *et al.*, 1981). From this comparison it was clear that electrolyte status was different in essential hypertension from that in either form of hyperaldosteronism, but some similarities in the relationship between sodium and

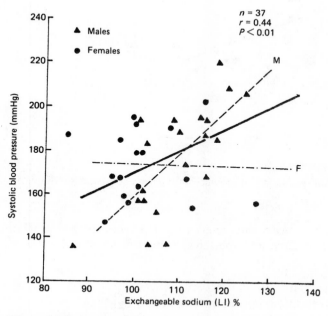

Figure 6.8 Relationship of systolic blood pressure and exchangeable sodium corrected for leanness index in idiopathic hyperaldosteronism. Regressions are shown for the whole group (———) and for males (– – – –) and females (–·–·–·–) separately (Reproduced from Lasaridis *et al.* (in press))

blood pressure were found. For example, both plasma and exchangeable sodium were higher than normal and plasma potassium lower than normal in the groups with hyperaldosteronism, although exchangeable potassium was similar in the groups with essential hypertension and idiopathic hyperaldosteronism. Plasma aldosterone was, of course, raised. However, in all three groups of hypertensive patients the abnormal significant correlation between sodium and blood pressure was apparent (*see above* and *Figure 6.8*). As in essential hypertension, the relationship did not exist in female patients with idiopathic hyperaldosteronism and possible reasons for this are discussed by the authors, including the possibility that changes in sex hormones across the menopause might disturb the relationship. No such sex difference occurred in primary aldosteronism due to aldosterone-producing adenoma. In a similar fashion to essential hypertension there is a negative relationship between plasma potassium and blood pressure (*Figure 6.9*).

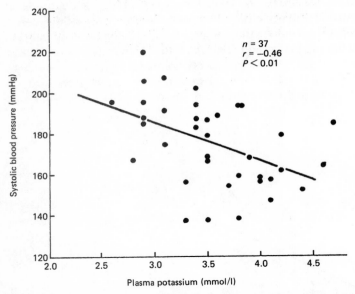

Figure 6.9 Relationship between systolic blood pressure and plasma potassium in idiopathic hyperaldosteronism

Thus, there are both differences and similarities between these forms of hypermineralocorticoidism and essential hypertension, but more study is required to interpret them.

Adrenal function and essential hypertension: 'chicken or egg'

From this account it is clear that there are abnormal features of adrenocortical function in essential hypertension. Evidence of this is observed in slightly raised aldosterone levels, in occasionally raised levels of other corticosteroids and in the altered responsiveness of aldosterone to angiotensin II and ACTH. Renin responses may also be abnormal. However, many of these changes occur only in certain subgroups of the essential hypertensive population. While it is clear that the relationships among sodium, potassium and blood pressure are not normal, electrolyte status is in many ways different from that found in proven mineralocorticoid excess. It is necessary, but as yet impossible, to distinguish those features which are important in and specific to essential hypertension and then to decide whether the changes in adrenal function are implicated in the development and maintenance of hypertension or whether they are merely secondary responses to hypertension or to some other cause of hypertension. For example, cell sodium transport processes may be altered in essential hypertension in a genetically determined manner (Ambrosioni *et al.*, 1981; de Mendonca *et al.* 1981; Walter and Distler, 1982). If this defect affects adrenocortical cells and the renin-producing cells of the juxtaglomerular apparatus, both organs being electrolyte responsive, this might explain the changed responsiveness of each and would make changes in secretion a secondary rather than a primary phenomenon. Certainly, altering sodium transport in the kidney by treatment with the Na, K-dependent ATPase inhibitor, ouabain, reduces renin excretion while leaving renal sodium excretion unaltered (Cruz-Soto *et al.*, 1982). Similar experiments have not been carried out with adrenal tissue.

CONCLUSION

This review has sought to address the evidence for and against a possible role for mineralocorticoids in the genesis of essential hypertension. While it can be shown that certain features of this condition, particularly of that form often described as low-renin essential hypertension, are similar to those of mineralocorticoid hypertension, there are important differences. The evidence for a mineralocorticoid other than aldosterone being secreted in excess in this extremely common condition is lacking, but important abnormalities in aldosterone secretion are clearly demonstrable. Whether these are primary or secondary remains to be discovered.

References

ADLERKREUTZ, H., HERKALI, R. and WAHLROOS, D. (1973) New urinary steroid in hypertension. *British Medical Journal*, **3**, 499

AGRIN, A. J., DALE, S. L., HOLBROOK, M., LaROSSA, J. T. and MELBY, J. C. (1978) Urinary free 18-hydroxy-11-deoxycorticosterone excretion in normal and hypertensive patients. *Journal of Clinical Endocrinology and Metabolism*, **47**, 877–884

AMBROSIONI, E., COSTA, F. V., MONTEBUGNOLI, L., TARTAGNI, E. and MAGNANI, R. (1981) Increased intralymphocytic sodium content in essential hypertension: an index of impaired Na^+ cellular metabolism. *Clinical Science*, **61**, 181–186

BALL, S. G., TREE, M., MORTON, J. J., INGLIS, G. C. and FRASER, R. (1981) Circulating dopamine: its effect on the plasma concentrations of catecholamines, renin, angiotensin, aldosterone and vasopressin in the conscious dog. *Clinical Science*, **61**, 417–722

BAXTER, J. D., SCHAMBERLAN, M., MATULICH, D. T., SPINDLER, B. J., TAYLOR, A. A. and BARTER, F. C. (1976) Aldosterone receptors and the evaluation of plasma mineralocorticoid activity in normal and hypertensive states. *Journal of Clinical Investigation*, **58**, 579–589

BEILIN, L. J. and ZIAKAS, G. (1972) Vascular reactivity in post-deoxycorticosterone hypertension in rats and its relation to 'irreversible' hypertension in man. *Clinical Science*, **42**, 579–590

BERECEK, K. H., MURRAY, R. D., GROSS, F. and BRODY, M. J. (1982) Vasopressin and vascular reactivity in the development of DOCA hypertension in rats with hereditary diabetes insipidus. *Hypertension*, **4**, 3–12

BERETTA-PICCOLI, C., DAVIES, D. L., BODDY, K. et al. (1982) Relation of body sodium, body potassium, plasma potassium with arterial pressure in essential hypertension. *Clinical Science*, **63**, 257–270

BERETTA-PICCOLI, C., DAVIES, D. L., BROWN, J. J. et al. (1983) Relation of blood pressure with body and plasma electrolytes in Conn's syndrome. *Journal of Hypertension*, **1**, 197–205

BLAUSTEIN, M. P., LANG, S. and JAMES-KRACKE, M. (1981) Cellular basis of sodium-induced hypertension. In *Frontiers of Hypertension Research*, edited by J. H. Laragh, F. R. Buhler and D. W. Seldin, pp. 87–90. New York: Springer-Verlag

BRAVO, E. L., TARAZI, R. C., FONAD, F. M. and TEXTOR, S. C. (1982) A reappraisal of the diagnostic criteria for primary aldosteronism. *Clinical Science*, **63**, 97S–100S

BRIGGS, J. P., STEIPE, B., SCHUBERT, G. and SCHNESMANN, J. (1982) Micropuncture studies of the renal effects of atrial natriuresis. *Pflügers Archives European Journal of Physiology*, **395**, 272–276

BRITTON, K. G. (1981) Essential hypertension: a disorder of cortical nephron control. *Lancet*, **2**, 900–902

BROWN, W. J., BROWN, F. K. and KRISHNAN, I. (1971) Exchangeable sodium and blood volume in normotensive and hypertensive humans on high and low sodium intake. *Circulation*, **43**, 508–519

BROWN, J. J., FERRISS, J. B., FRASER, R. et al. (1972) Apparently isolated excess deoxycorticosterone in hypertension. A variant of the mineralocorticoid excess syndrome. *Lancet*, **2**, 243–247

BROWN, J. J., LEVER, A. F., ROBERTSON, J. I. S. et al. (1979) Are idiopathic hyperaldosteronism and low-renin hypertension variants of essential hypertension? *Annals of Clinical Biochemistry*, **16**, 380–388

BRUNNER, H. R., SEALEY, J. E. and LARAGH, J. H. (1973) Renin subgroups in essential hypertension. *Circulation Research*, **32–33** (Suppl. I), I-99–I-109

CARROLL, J., KOMANICKY, P. and MELBY, J. C. (1981) The relationship between plasma 18-hydroxy-11-deoxycorticosterone levels and production of hypertension in the rat. *Journal of Steroid Biochemistry*, **14**, 989–995

COLLINS, R. D., WEINBERGER, M. H., DOWDY, A. J., NOKES, G. W., GONZALES, C. M. and LUETSCHER, J. A. (1970) Abnormally sustained aldosterone secretion during salt loading in patients with various forms of benign hypertension: relation to plasma renin activity. *Journal of Clinical Investigation*, **49**, 1415–1426

CRABBÉ, J. (1978) The sodium-retaining properties of aldosterone. In *The Endocrine Function of the Human Adrenal Cortex*, edited by V. H. T. James, M. Serio, G. Guisti and L. Martini, pp. 351–358. London: Academic Press

CRUZ-SOTO, M. A., BENABE, J. E., LOPEZ-NOVOA, J. M. and MARTINEZ-MALDONADO, M. (1982) Level of ATPase important for renin secretion, ouabain may act on J. G. cells. *American Journal of Physiology*, **243**, F598–F603

DALE, S. L. and MELBY, J. C. (1974) Altered adrenal steroidogenesis in low renin essential hypertension. *Transactions of the Association of American Physicians*, **87**, 248–257

DALE, S. L., HOLBROOK, M. M. and MELBY, J. C. (1981) 19-Nor-deoxycorticosterone in the neutral fraction of human urine. *Steroids*, **37**, 103–110

DALE, S. L., HOLBROOK, M. M., KOMANICKY, P. and MELBY, J. C. (1982) Urinary 19-nor-deoxycorticosterone excretion in the spontaneously hypertensive rat. *Endocrinology*, **110**, 1989–1993

DAWSON-HUGHES, B. F., MOORE, T. J., DLUHY, R. G., HOLLENBERG, N. K. and WILLIAMS, G. H. (1981) Plasma angiotensin II concentration regulates vascular but not adrenal responsiveness to restriction of sodium intake in normal man. *Clinical Science*, **61**, 527–534

DE MENDONCA, M., GARAY, R. P., BEN-ISHAY, D. and MEYER, P. (1981) Abnormal erythrocyte cation transport in primary hypertension. Clinical and experimental studies. *Hypertension*, **3** (Suppl I), I-179–I-183

DE WARDENER, H. E. (1982) The natriuretic hormone. *Annals of Clinical Biochemistry*, **19**, 137–140

DLUHY, R. G., ZAVLI, S. Z., LEUNG, F. K., SOLOMON, H. S. and MOORE, T. J. (1979) Abnormal adrenal responsiveness and angiotensin II dependency in high renin essential hypertension. *Journal of Clinical Investigation*, **64**, 1270–1276

DUNN, M. J. and TANNEN, R. L. (1974) Low renin hypertension. *Kidney International*, **5**, 317–325

EDELMAN, I. S. (1979) Mechanism of action of aldosterone: energetic and permeability factors. *Journal of Endocrinology*, **81**, 49P–53P

EDWARDS, C. R. W., AL-DUJAILI, E. A. S., BOSCARO, M., GOW, I. and WILLIAMS, B. C. (1982) Peptidergic and monoaminergic regulation of aldosterone secretion. In *Endocrinology of Hypertension*, edited by F. Mantero, E. G. Biglieri and C. R. W. Edwards, pp. 11–18. London: Academic Press

FANESTIL, D. D. and PARK, C. S. (1981) Steroid hormones and the kidney. *Annual Review of Physiology*, **43**, 637–649

FARMAN, N., KUSCH, M. and EDELMAN, I. S. (1978) Aldosterone receptor occupancy and sodium transport on the urinary bladder of *Bufo marinus*. *American Journal of Physiology*, **235**, C90–C96

FERRISS, J. B., BROWN, J. J., FRASER, R., LEVER, A. F. and ROBERTSON, J. I. S. (1983) Primary aldosterone excess: Conn's syndrome and related disorders. In *Clinical Aspects of Hypertension (Handbook of Hypertension, Volume 2)*, edited by J. I. S. Robertson, pp. 132–161. Amsterdam: Elsevier

FRASER, R. (1983) Inborn errors of corticosteroid biosynthesis: their effects on electrolyte metabolism and blood pressure. In *Clinical Aspects of Hypertension (Handbook of Hypertension, Volume 2)*, edited by J. I. S. Robertson, pp. 162–188. Amsterdam: Elsevier

FRASER, R., BERETTA-PICCOLI, C., BROWN, J. J. *et al.* (1981) Response of aldosterone and 18-hydroxycorticosterone to angiotensin II in normal subjects and patients with essential hypertension, Conn's syndrome and non-tumorous hyperaldosteronism. *Hypertension*, **3** (Suppl. 1), I-87–I-92

FRASER, R., BROWN, J. J., BROWN, W. C. *et al.* (1976) The adrenal cortex and hypertension: some observations on a possible role for mineralocorticoids other than aldosterone. *Journal of Steroid Biochemistry*, **7**, 963–970

FRASER, R., BROWN, J. J., LEVER, A. F. and ROBERTSON, J. I. S. (1983) Control of aldosterone in hypertension. In *Hypertension (Volume 2)*, edited by J. Genest, O. Kuchel, P. Hamlet and M. Cantin, pp. 338–348. New York: McGraw-Hill

FRASER, R., JAMES, V. H. T., LANDON, J. *et al.* (1968) Clinical and biochemical studies of a patient with a corticosterone-secreting adrenocortical tumour. *Lancet*, **2**, 1116–1120

FUNDER, J. W., MERCER, J., INGRAM, B., FELDMAN, D., WYNNE, K. and ADAM, W. R. (1978) 19-Nor-deoxycorticosterone: mineralocorticoid receptor affinity higher than aldosterone, electrolyte activity lower. *Endocrinology*, **103**, 1514–1517

GANGULY, A. and WEINBERGER, M. H. (1979) Low renin hypertension: a current review of definitions and controversies. *American Heart Journal*, **98**, 642–652

GARWITZ, E. T. and JONES, A. W. (1982) Altered arterial ion transport and its reversal in aldosterone hypertensive rat. *American Journal of Physiology*, **243**, H927–H933

GENEST, J. J., BOUCHER, R., NOWACYZNSKI, W. and KUCHEL, O. (1978) The role of the adrenal cortex in the pathogenesis of essential hypertension. In *The Endocrine Function of the Human Adrenal Cortex*, edited by V. H. T. James, M. Serio, G. Giusti and L. Martini, pp. 389–412. London: Academic Press

GOMEZ-SANCHEZ, C. E. (1982) The role of steroids in human hypertension. *Biochemical Pharmacology*, **31**, 893–898

GOMEZ-SANCHEZ, C. E., HOLLAND, O. B., MURRAY, B. A., LLOYD, H. A. and MILEWICH, L. (1979) 19-Nor-deoxycorticosterone: a potent mineralocorticoid isolated from the urine of rats with regenerating adrenals. *Endocrinology*, **105**, 708–711

GORDON, M. B., MOORE, T. J., DLUHY, R. G. and WILLIAMS, G. H. (1983) Dopaminergic modulation of aldosterone responsiveness to angiotensin II with changing sodium intake. *Journal of Clinical Endocrinology and Metabolism*, **56**, 340–345

GRIFFING, G. T., DALE, S. L., HOLBROOK, M. M. and MELBY, J. C. (1983a) The regulation of urinary free 19-nor-deoxycorticosterone and its relation to systemic arterial blood pressure in normotensive and hypertensive subjects. *Journal of Clinical Endocrinology and Metabolism*, **56**, 99–103

GRIFFING, G. T., DALE, S. L., HOLBROOK, M. M. and MELBY, J. C. (1983b) Relationship of 19-nor-deoxycorticosterone to other mineralocorticoids in low-renin hypertension. *Hypertension*, **5**, 385–389

GRIM, C., WINNACKER, J., PETERS, T. and GILBERT, G. (1974) Low renin 'normal' aldosterone and hypertension: circadian rhythm of renin, aldosterone, cortisol and growth hormone. *Journal of Clinical Endocrinology and Metabolism*, **39**, 247–256

GUNNELS, J. C. and McGUFFIN, W. L. (1975) Low renin hypertension. *Annual Review of Medicine*, **26**, 259–275

GUTHRIE, G. P., KOTCHEN, T. A. and KOTCHEN, J. M. (1983) Suppression of adrenal mineralocorticoid production in pre-hypertensive young adult men. *Journal of Clinical Endocrinology and Metabolism*, **56**, 87–92

GUYTON, A. C., GRANGER, H. J. and COLEMAN, T. G. (1971) Autoregulation of the total systemic circulation and its relation to control of cardiac output and arterial pressure. *Circulation Research*, **28** and **29** (Suppl. I), 93–97

HADDY, F., PAMNANI, M. and CLOUGH, D. (1978) The sodium–potassium pump in volume-expanded hypertension. *Clinical and Experimental Hypertension*, **1**, 295–336

HAMLYN, J. M. and DUFFY, T. (1978) Direct stimulation of human erythrocyte membrane ($Na^+ K^+$) Mg ATPase by physiological concentrations of aldosterone. *Biochemical and Biophysical Research Communications*, **84**, 458

HAMLYN, J., RINGEL, R., SCHAEFFER, J. *et al.* (1982) A circulating inhibitor of ($Na^+ + K^+$) ATPase associated with essential hypertension. *Nature (London)*, **300**, 650–652

HELBER, A., WAMBACH, G., HUMMERICH, W., BONNER, G., MEURER, K. A. and KAUFMANN, W. (1980) Evidence for a subgroup of essential hypertensives with non-suppressible excretion of aldosterone during sodium loading. *Klinische Wochenschrift*, **58**, 439–447

HONDA, M., NOWACZYNSKI, W., GUTHRIE, G. P. *et al.* (1977) Response of several adrenal steroids to ACTH stimulation in essential hypertension. *Journal of Clinical Endocrinology and Metabolism*, **44**, 264–272

KAGAWA, C. M. and VAN ARMAN, C. G. (1957) Sodium retaining activity of 19-norsteroids in adrenalectomised rats. *Proceedings of the Society of Experimental Biology and Medicine*, **94**, 444–448

KELLY, N. F., O'HARE, M. J., LOIZOU, S., DAVIES, D. and LAING, I. (1982) Hypermineralocorticoidism without excessive aldosterone secretion: an adrenal carcinoma producing deoxycorticosterone. *Clinical Endocrinology*, **17**, 353–361

KHOHKAR, A. M., SLATER, J. D. H., JOWETT, T. P. and PAYNE, N. N. (1976) Suppression of the renin–aldosterone system in mild essential hypertension. *Clinical Science and Molecular Medicine*, **50**, 269–276

KISCH, E. S., DLUHY, R. G. and WILLIAMS, G. H. (1976) Enhanced aldosterone response to angiotensin II in human hypertension. *Circulation Research*, **38**, 502–505

KAJIMI, I., YOSHIHARA, S. and OGATA, E. (1982) Involvement of endogenous digitalis-like substance in genesis of deoxycorticosterone–salt hypertension. *Life Sciences*, **30**, 1775–1782

KOMANICKY, P. and MELBY, J. C. (1981) Experimental hypertension induced by 19-nor-progesterone treatment in the rat. *Endocrinology*, **109**, 1164–1167

KORNEL, L., KANAMARLAPUDI, N., RAMSAY, C. *et al.* (1983) Arterial steroid receptors and their putative role in the mechanism of hypertension. *Journal of Steroid Biochemistry*, **19**(1A), 333–344

KOWARSKI, A. A., EDWIN, C. M., AKESODE, A. P., PIOTROWSKI, L. S. and HAMILTON, B. P. (1978) Integrated concentration of plasma renin activity, aldosterone and cortisol in essential hypertension. In *The Endocrine Function of the Human Adrenal Cortex*, edited by V. H. T. James, M. Serio, G. Giusti and L. Martini, pp. 423–430. London: Academic Press

KRAMER, H. J. (1981) Natrium hormone – a circulating inhibitor of sodium – and potassium-activated adenosine triphosphatase. Its potential role in body fluid and blood pressure regulation. *Klinische Wochenschrift*, **59**, 1225–1230

KUSCH, M., FARMAN, N. and EDELMAN, I. S. (1978) Binding of aldosterone to cytoplasmic and nuclear receptors of the urinary bladder epithelium of *Bufo marinus*. *American Journal of Physiology*, **235**, C82–C89

LASARIDIS, A., BROWN, J. J., DAVIES, L., FRASER, R., ROBERTSON, J. I. S. and LEVER, A. S. (1984) Arterial blood pressure and body electrolytes in idiopathic hyperaldosteronism: a comparison with primary hyperaldosteronism and essential hypertension. *Journal of Hypertension* (in press)

LEBEL, M., SCHALEKAMP, M. A., BEEVERS, D. G. *et al.* (1974) Sodium and the renin–angiotensin system in essential hypertension and mineralocorticoid excess. *Lancet*, **2**, 308–309

LLAURADO, J. G., MADDEN, J. A. and SMITH, G. A. (1983) Some effects of aldosterone on sodium kinetics and distribution in porcine arterial wall. *American Journal of Physiology*, **244**, R553–R557

MARKS, A. D., MARKS, D. B., KANEFSKY, T. M., ADLIN, V. E. and CHADWICK, B. J. (1979) Enhanced adrenal responsiveness to angiotensin II in patients with low renin essential hypertension. *Journal of Clinical Endocrinology and Metabolism*, **48**, 266–270

McCAA, R. E., LANGFORD, H. G., MONTALVO, J. M., ANDY, D. J., READ, V. H. and McCAA, C. S. (1981) Regulation of aldosterone biosynthesis during sodium deficiency: evidence for an essential role of the pituitary gland. *Hypertension*, **3** (Suppl. I), I-74–I-80

McKENNA, T. J., ISLAND, D. P., NICHOLSON, W. E. and LIDDLE, G. W. (1979). Dopamine inhibits angiotensin-stimulated aldosterone biosynthesis in bovine adrenal cells. *Journal of Clinical Investigation*, **64**, 287–291

MEADE, T. W., IMESON, J. D., GORDON, D. and PEART, W. S. (1983) The epidemiology of plasma renin. *Clinical Science*, **64**, 273–280

MELBY, J. C. and DALE, S. L. *et al.* (1979) Adrenocorticosteroids in experimental and human hypertension. *Journal of Endocrinology*, **81**, 93P–106P

MELBY, J. C., DALE, S. L., GREKIN, R. J., GAUNT, R. and WILSON, T. G. (1972) 18-Hydroxy-11-deoxycorticosterone secretion in experimental and human hypertension. *Recent Progress in Hormone Research*, **28**, 287–339

MENDELSOHN, F. A. O. and KACHEL, C. D. (1981) Stimulation by serum of aldosterone production from rat adrenal glomerulosa cells: relationship to K^+, serotonin and angiotensin II. *Acta Endocrinologica*, **97**, 231–241

MORTON, J. J., GARCIA DEL RIO, C. and HUGHES, M. J. (1982) Effect of acute infusion of arginine-vasopressin on blood pressure and plasma angiotensin II in normotensive and DOCA–salt hypertensive rats. *Clinical Science*, **62**, 143–149

NICHOLLS, M. G., JULIUS, S. and ZWEIFLER, A. J. (1981) Withdrawal of endogenous sympathetic drive lowers blood pressure in primary aldosteronism. *Clinical Endocrinology*, **15**, 253–258

NICHOLLS, M. G., FRASER, R., HAY, G., MASON, P. and TORSNEY, B. (1977) Urine electrolyte response to 18-hydroxy-11-deoxycorticosterone in normal man. *Clinical Science and Molecular Medicine*, **53**, 493–498

NICHOLLS, M. G., RAMSAY, L. E., BODDY, K., FRASER, R., MORTON, J. J. and ROBERTSON, J. I. S. (1979a) Mineralocorticoid-induced blood pressure, electrolyte and hormone changes and reversal with spironolactone. *Metabolism*, **28**, 584–593

NICHOLLS, M. G., BROWN, W. C. B., HAY, G. D., MASON, P. A. and FRASER, R. (1979b) Arterial levels and mineralocorticoid activity of 18-hydroxy-11-deoxycorticosterone in the rat. *Journal of Steroid Biochemistry*, **10**, 67–70

OBERFIELD, S. E., LEVINE, L. S., CAREY, R. M., GREIG, F., ULICK, S. and NEW, M. I. (1983) Metabolic and blood pressure responses to hydrocortisone and the syndrome of apparent mineralocorticoid excess. *Journal of Clinical Endocrinology and Metabolism*, **56**, 332–339

PADFIELD, P. L., ALLISON, M. E. M., BROWN, J. J. *et al.* (1975a) Effect of intravenous frusemide on plasma renin concentration: suppression of response in hypertension. *Clinical Science and Molecular Medicine*, **49**, 353–358

PADFIELD, P. L., BEEVERS, D. G., BROWN, J. J. *et al.* (1975b) Is low-renin hypertension a state in the development of essential hypertension or a diagnostic entity? *Lancet*, **1**, 548–550

PADFIELD, P. L., BROWN, J. J., DAVIES, D. L. *et al.* (1981) The myth of idiopathic hyperaldosteronism. *Lancet*, **2**, 83–84

PAN, Y.-J. and YOUNG, D. B. (1982) Experimental aldosterone hypertension in the dog. *Hypertension*, **4**, 279–287

PARFREY, P. S., MARKANDU, N. D., ROULSTON, J. E., JONES, B. E., JONES, J. C. and MacGREGOR, G. A. (1981) Relation between arterial pressure, dietary sodium intake and the renin system in essential hypertension. *British Medical Journal*, **283**, 94–97

PERRONE, R. D., BENGELE, H. H., DALE, S. L., MELBY, J. C. and ALEXANDER, E. A. (1982) Mineralocorticoid activity of 19-nor-DOC and 19-OH-DOC in adrenalectomised rats. *American Journal of Physiology*, **242**, E305–E308

PETTY, K. J., KOKKO, J. P. and MARVER, D. (1981) Secondary effect of aldosterone on Na–K-ATPase activity in the rabbit cortical collecting duct. *Journal of Clinical Investigation*, **68**, 1514–1521

RE, R. N., SANCHO, J., KLIMAN, B. and HABER, E. (1978) The characterisation of low renin hypertension by plasma renin activity and plasma aldosterone concentration. *Journal of Clinical Endocrinology and Metabolism*, **46**, 189–195

SAFAR, M. E., SIMON, A. CH., DARD, S. A. *et al.* (1982) Aldosterone in sustained essential hypertension. *Clinical Endocrinology*, **16**, 77–88

SCHALEKAMP, M. A., LEBEL, M., BEEVERS, D. G., FRASER, R., KOLSTERS, G. and BIRKENHAGER, W. H. (1974) Body fluid volume in low renin hypertension. *Lancet*, **2**, 310–311

SCOGGINS, B. A., COGHLAN, J. P., DENTON, D. A., MASON, R. T. and WHITWORTH, J. A. (1982) A review of mechanisms involved in the production of steroid-induced hypertension with particular reference to ACTH-dependent hypertension. In *Endocrinology of Hypertension*, edited by F. Mantero, E. G. Biglieri and C. R. W. Edwards, pp. 41–67. London: Academic Press

SEKIHARA, H., HOLLIFIELD, J. W., ISLAND, D. P., SLATON, P. G. and LIDDLE, G. W. (1979) Evidence for the heterogeneity of mineralocorticoids in the urine of patients with low renin essential hypertension. *Journal of Clinical Endocrinology and Metabolism*, **48**, 143–147

SELYE, H., HALL, C. E. and ROWLEY, E. M. (1943) Malignant hypertension produced by treatment with deoxycorticosterone acetate and sodium chloride. *Canadian Medical Association Journal*, **49**, 88–92

SEN, S., SHAINOFF, J. R., BRAVO, E. L. and BUMPUS, F. M. (1981) Isolation of aldosterone-stimulating factor (ASF) and its effect on rat adrenal glomerulosa cells *in vitro*. *Hypertension*, **3**, 4–10

SKRABAL, F., AUBOCK, J., EDWARDS, C. R. W. and BRAUNSTEIN, H. (1978) Subtraction potential difference: *in vivo* assay for mineralocorticoid activity. *Lancet*, **1**, 298–302

STERN, N., BECK, F. and SOWERS, J. (1983) Effect of aldosterone on the human erythrocyte sodium-potassium pump *in vitro*. *Clinical Science*, **64**, 183–186

TAYLOR, A. A., MITCHELL, J. R., BARTTER, F. C. *et al.* (1978) Effect of aminoglutethimide on blood pressure and steroid secretion in patients with low renin essential hypertension. *Journal of Clinical Investigation*, **62**, 168–172

TUCK, M. L., WILLIAMS, G. H., DLUHY, R. G., GREENFIELD, M. and MOORE, T. J. (1976) A delayed suppression of the renin–aldosterone axis following saline infusion in human hypertension. *Circulation Research*, **39**, 711–717

ULICK, S. and CHU, M. D. (1982) Significance of the secretion of 18-hydroxycortisol by the human adrenal cortex. In *Endocrinology of Hypertension (Serono Symposia 50)*, edited by F. Mantero, E. G. Biglieri and C. R. W. Edwards, pp. 23–28. London: Academic Press

ULICK, S., RAMIREZ, L. and NEW, M. I. (1977) An abnormality in steroid reductive metabolism in the hypertensive syndrome. *Journal of Clinical Endocrinology and Metabolism*, **44**, 799–802

VETTER, H., ZUMKLEY, H., GLANZER, K., WITASSEK, F., WOLLNIK, S. and VETTER, W. (1980) Renin–angiotensin–aldosteron-system bei essentielle Hypertonie. Inadequat hohes plasmaaldosteron bei jungren Patientes mit schwerer Hypertonie sowie bei alteren Hypertonikern. *Schweizerische Medizinische Wochenschrift*, **110**, 1938–1944

WALTER, V. and DISTLER, A. (1982) Abnormal sodium efflux in erythrocyte of patients with essential hypertension. *Hypertension*, **4**, 205–210

WEIDMANN, P., BERETTA-PICCOLI, C., ZIEGLER, W. H., KEUTSCH, G., GLUCK, Z. and REUBI, F. C. (1978) Age versus urinary sodium for judging renin, aldosterone and catecholamine levels: studies in normal subjects and patients with essential hypertension. *Kidney International*, **14**, 619–628

WENTING, G. J. MAN IN'T VELD, A. J., VERHOEVAN, R. P., DERKX, F. H. and SCHALEKAMP, M. A. (1977) Volume–pressure relationships during the development of mineralocorticoid hypertension in man. *Circulation Research*, **40** (Suppl. 1), 163–170

WHITWORTH, J. A., BUKTUS, A., COGHLAN, J. P., DENTON, D. A., SAINES, D. and SCOGGINS, B. A. (1983) Plasma 4-pregnene-17α,20α-diol-3-one (17α20α dihydroxyprogesterone) and 17αhydroxyprogesterone in man. *Acta Endocrinologica (Kbh)*, **102**, 271–276

WILLIAMS, G. H. and DLUHY, R. G. (1983) Control of aldosterone secretion. In *Hypertension* (2nd edition), edited by J. Genest, O. Kuchel, P. Humbt and M. Cantin, pp. 320–338. New York: McGraw-Hill

WILLIAMS, G. H., HOLLENBERG, N. K., MOORE, T. J., SWARTZ, S. L. and DLUHY, R. G. (1979) The adrenal receptor for angiotensin II is altered in essential hypertension. *Journal of Clinical Investigation*, **63**, 419–427

WILLIAMS, G. H., TUCK, M. L., SULLIVAN, J. M., DLUHY, R. G. and HOLLENBERG, N. K. (1982) Parallel adrenal and renal abnormalities in young patients with essential hypertension. *American Journal of Medicine*, **72**, 907–914

WILSON, T. A. and CAREY, R. M. (1981) Low-renin essential hypertension: diminution of aldosterone suppression. In *Frontiers of Hypertension Research*, edited by J. H. Laragh, F. R. Buhler and D. W. Seldin, pp. 199–203. New York: Springer-Verlag

WISGERHOF, M. and BROWN, R. D. (1979) Increased adrenal sensitivity to angiotensin II in low renin essential hypertension. *Journal of Clinical Investigation*, **61**, 1456–1462

WOODS, J. W., LIDDLE, G. W., STANT, E. G., MICHELAKIS, A. M. and BRILL, A. B. (1969) Effect of an adrenal inhibitor on hypertensive patients with suppressed renin. *Archives of Internal Medicine*, **123**, 366–370

WYNNE, K. N., MERCER, J., STOCKIGT, J. R. and FUNDER, J. W. (1980) 19-Nor-analogues of adrenal steroids: mineralocorticoids and glucocorticoid receptor activity. *Endocrinology*, **107**, 1278–1280

YOUNG, D. B. and JACKSON, T. E. (1982) Effects of aldosterone on potassium distribution. *American Journal of Physiology*, **243**, R526–R530

ZOCCALI, C., USHERWOOD, T., BROWN, J. J., LEVER, A. F., ROBERTSON, J. I. S. and FRASER, R. (1983) A comparison of the effects of angiotensin II infusion and variation in salt intake on plasma aldosterone levels in normal subjects, patients with essential hypertension and patients with hyperaldosteronism. *Journal of Steroid Biochemistry*, **19**, 327–331

7

Abnormal adrenal and renal responses to angiotensin II in essential hypertension

Gordon H. Williams and Norman K. Hollenberg

INTRODUCTION

Renin was identified as a potent pressor agent late in the 19th century, in the exciting early days of hormone identification. We have been able to measure renin in plasma for two decades, and angiotensin II, its major biologically active product, for nearly that long. During the same period the factors that determine renin release and its plasma concentration have come into sharp focus (Davis and Freeman, 1976). The structure of angiotensin II was identified almost three decades ago and synthetic angiotensin has been available for administration for 20 years. Despite these advances the precise role played by the renin–angiotensin system in the normal body economy and in the pathogenesis of disease remained obscure, for reasons that also have become more apparent over the same time interval. Why?

First, sensitivity of the kidney, the adrenal gland and blood pressure to angiotensin II is more variable than is the plasma concentration of angiotensin II itself (Hollenberg *et al.*, 1974). For this reason it has been difficult to predict the biological response from the measurement of a plasma concentration of angiotensin II. Second, a key role has been played by glandular ablation as an experimental approach in endocrinology: ablation of the source of the hormone and its replacement have provided the ultimate evidence of a hormone's action (Haber, 1976). In the case of the renin–angiotensin system, where the kidney is both the source of the hormone and a major responding organ, this experimental approach has not been fruitful. For these reasons pharmacological interruption of the system, which is now possible at several levels (Haber, 1976), has been a critical factor in defining angiotensin's contribution to normal physiological processes and to human disease.

That one must define the normal state to understand disease is a truism. In this chapter we shall focus first on the role of the renin–angiotensin–aldosterone system in normal body economy; on lessions learned from pharmacological antagonists; and on accumulating information to indicate that changes in sensitivity to

Table 7.1 Frequency of non-modulating hypertensive patients

Study	Criterion employed	Number studied	Per cent non-modulators	Low renin excluded
1. Christlieb et al. (1969)	Aldo*: diet	2	100	yes
2. Williams et al. (1970)	Aldo: acute volume depletion	16	69	no
3. Hollenberg and Merrill (1970)	RBF†: diet	12	58	no
4. Moore et al. (1977)	Aldo: posture-angiotensin II	64	24	yes
5. Hollenberg, Borucki and Adams (1978)	RBF: diet	103	35	no
6. Williams et al. (1979)	Aldo: saralasin-angiotensin II	70	64	yes
7. Dluhy et al. (1979)	Aldo: posture-angiotensin II	19	37	yes
8. Dawson-Hughes et al. (1981)	Aldo: posture-angiotensin II	15	53	yes
9. Williams et al. (1982)	Aldo: acute volume depletion	18	50	yes
10. Shoback et al. (1983b)	RBF: angiotensin II	18	56	yes
11. Taylor et al. (1983)	Aldo: angiotensin II	31	40	yes
12. Gordon et al. (1983)	RBF: diet	18	44	yes
	Total	386	46% excluding LREH** 44% all EH‡	

* Aldo: aldosterone
† RBF: renal blood flow
** LREH: low renin essential hypertension
‡ EH: essential hypertension

angiotensin II form a critical component in the normal function of this system. To examine renin's contribution to the pathogenesis of hypertension, we shall review renovascular hypertension, perhaps the paradigm of renin-mediated hypertension; review the classification of essential hypertension into the low, normal and high-renin forms, and assess renin's contribution to the pathogenesis in high-renin essential hypertension. Finally, we shall explore accumulating evidence that abnormalities in the modulation of adrenal and renal vascular responsiveness to angiotensin II with changes in sodium balance occur in about 40 per cent of patients with normal renin essential hypertension (*Table 7.1*), and possible mechanisms by which that disordered modulation could contribute to the pathogenesis.

THE ROLE OF RENIN IN THE NORMAL BODY ECONOMY

Recent investigation into the physiological role of the renin–angiotensin–aldosterone system has been focused primarily on its contribution to blood pressure control, ignoring the fact that this system is involved primarily in extracellular fluid volume regulation rather than blood pressure control. Examination of the evolutionary aspects, as these systems adapted during phylogeny, highlights this fact.

In its evolution the kidney, and the control systems that converge on the kidney, have adapted to progressively more difficult challenges in the regulation of body salt as our predecessors shifted from life in salt water to fresh water and to air. The most primitive living vertebrates, the cyclostomes and elasmobranchs, appear not to have had renin activity or juxtaglomerular granules in their kidneys; both appear early, however, first becoming evident in teleosts and tetrapods (Sokabe, 1974). What was the function of this system early in phylogeny? Little is known concerning blood pressure control in primitive organisms, but the lungfish – as a representative example – has an arterial blood pressure of about 15 mmHg, and at this level it would appear that blood pressure is effectively unregulated (Sawyer *et al.*, 1976).

What of the aldosterone response to activation of the renin–angiotensin system? Phylogenetically, the amphibian was the first vertebrate to venture from the protective environment of water to air, where the defence of extracellular fluid volume became substantially more difficult. Capelli, Wesson and Aponte (1970) pointed out that the appearance of the recurrent nephron and the macula densa in the amphibian represents 'the beginnings of a structural element within the nephron to aid electrolyte and volume homeostasis, by sampling fluids reaching the distal segments of the nephron'. It is here that aldosterone first appears on the scene: Berne (1967) concluded that aldosterone was 'an invention of land-living vertebrates', appearing late in phylogeny. Although Vinson *et al.* (1979) have expressed a contrary view, none of the studies they cited of earlier aldosterone synthesis documented significant plasma concentrations of aldosterone, an important role of aldosterone in sodium handling, or responsiveness of the adrenal cortex to angiotensin. What had been documented was the capacity to synthesize aldosterone. However, even in reptiles and amphibia, angiotensin II may have little influence on the adrenal glands.

The simplest interpretation of this overview is that the renin–angiotensin system initially evolved as a primitive extracellular fluid volume control system acting locally on the glomerular circulation by controlling renal plasma flow and thereby modifying pressure delivery to the glomerulus and thus glomerular filtration rate (Sokabe, Mizogame and Sato, 1968). The role of this system broadened with increasingly more ambitious ventures of the organism into new and more hostile environments. Thus, we believe that the primary role of this sytem is control of extracellular fluid volume via sodium homeostasis, and an influence on blood pressure is best seen as incidental to that fundamental process.

Maneuvers that lead to increased renin secretion generally involve a challenge to extracellular fluid volume (Davis and Freeman, 1976). The primary determinant is total body sodium. Certainly an excellent correlation has been widely documented between sodium intake, sodium excretion and the state of this system. A reduction in venous return to the heart in man, for example, by quiet standing results in a rapid burst of renin release. Conversely, a translocation of blood from the lower portion of the body to the thorax by immersion in water to the neck suppresses the system (Epstein, 1978). Clearly, the receptors responsible for volume control and serving as the afferent limb for renin release lie, at least in part, in the thorax, and are sensitive to thoracic blood volume. Both neural and metabolic factors can also influence the renin–angiotensin–aldosterone system. Thus, potassium homeostasis, on the one hand, and neural influences acting via beta-receptors in the juxtaglomerular apparatus also influence renin release (Davis and Freeman, 1976). These influences, are best seen, however, as playing a modulating rather than a dominant role in control of the system.

THE ROLE OF RENIN AND ANGIOTENSIN IN ALDOSTERONE SECRETION

The contribution of aldosterone to sodium handling by the kidney and thus to sodium homeostasis is unequivocal. There is also no doubt that angiotensin II administration increases aldosterone secretion. What had been disputed was the primacy of the renin system in mediating the adrenal response to reduced sodium intake. One major objection was the failure of angiotensin II, when administered to normal subjects ingesting a large sodium intake, to reproduce the increase in aldosterone secretion produced by restriction of sodium intake (Boyd *et al.*, 1972). This observation spurred a response that has been critical to the evolution of our thinking. Two studies answered this objection by documenting an enhanced adrenal response to angiotensin II in normal subjects ingesting a restricted sodium diet (Hollenberg *et al.*, 1974; Oelkers *et al.*, 1974). Both studies demonstrated a virtually identical increase in the slope of the relationship between plasma angiotensin II and plasma aldosterone concentration: at any given plasma angiotensin II concentration individuals on balance on a low sodium intake showed a striking enhancement of adrenal aldosterone release. Because vascular smooth muscle responsiveness to angiotensin was already known to be blunted during reduced sodium intake, it became apparent that there was a reciprocal control of the sensitivity of adrenal steroidogenesis and vascular smooth muscle contraction with changes in sodium intake.

A second objection was based on the inconsistent change in aldosterone secretion with blockade of angiotensin's action. Steele *et al.* (1976) reported that saralasin, an angiotensin antagonist, failed to reduce plasma aldosterone levels in sodium-depleted rabbits. Since that time it has become apparent that the pharmacological probes available are complex: saralasin is not a competitive antagonist, but rather is a partial agonist exerting an angiotensin-like action in settings in which endogenous angiotensin is reduced (Hollenberg *et al.*, 1976). Indeed, even when the renin–angiotensin system is activated, the use of a large dose of saralasin will lead to an agonist response. It is intriguing, and perhaps relevant to the discussion on essential hypertension that follows, that saralasin induces an agonist response at the adrenal cortex, expressed as aldosterone secretion, in about half of an unselected series of patients with essential hypertension, despite the use of saralasin doses that reduce plasma aldosterone in normal subjects, and in patients with renovascular hypertension (Williams *et al.*, 1979). The agonist response to saralasin did not reflect supersensitivity to angiotensin II. Indeed, responsiveness of the adrenal to angiotensin II was reduced in the patient who showed blunted adrenal agonist response.

As converting enzyme inhibitors have become more potent and long-acting it has become clear that angiotensin represents the dominant mediator of adrenal responses to changes in sodium intake in normal man (Swartz *et al.*, 1980; Williams *et al.*, 1978).

THE INFLUENCE OF RENIN AND ANGIOTENSIN ON THE RENAL BLOOD SUPPLY

The major local intrarenal action of angiotensin early in phylogeny has continued in higher vertebrates and in man. In the normal dog (Kimbrough *et al.*, 1977) and man (Hollenberg *et al.*, 1976) ingesting a high salt diet, neither saralasin nor teprotide, the first available converting enzyme inhibitor, increased renal blood flow. When the renin–angiotensin system was activated and renal blood flow reduced by restriction of sodium intake, both classes of inhibitor induced a dose-related increase in renal blood flow, and the magnitude of the increase was consistent with reversal of the effects of sodium restriction. A brisk natriuresis followed blockade of the renal actions of angiotensin II when sodium intake was restricted, suggesting that the local action of angiotensin had contributed to renal sodium handling (Kimbrough *et al.*, 1977; Levens *et al.*, 1981, 1983).

In patients with essential hypertension both teprotide (Williams and Hollenberg, 1977) and captopril (Hollenberg *et al.*, 1981) often induced a supranormal increase in renal blood flow. Moreover, both teprotide and captopril increased glomerular filtration rate in some patients with essential hypertension, a response that did not occur in normal subjects (Hollenberg *et al.*, 1976; Hollenberg, Borucki and Adams, 1978). A contribution of angiotensin to renal sodium handling unrelated to aldosterone was evident in the appearance of a natriuresis within 20 minutes of converting enzyme inhibitor administration, far too quickly to reflect the natriuretic effect of a fall in plasma aldosterone, but parallel to the rise in renal blood flow.

THE INFLUENCE OF RENIN AND ANGIOTENSIN ON BLOOD PRESSURE

In normal recumbent man when the renin–angiotensin system is suppressed by a liberal intake of sodium and potassium, angiotensin antagonists and converting enzyme inhibition reduce arterial blood pressure minimally (Hollenberg *et al.*, 1981; Sancho *et al.*, 1976). Indeed, the modest activation of the renin–angiotensin system induced by quiet standing in that setting does not potentiate markedly the depressor response to either class of agent. When the system is activated further by restriction of sodium intake, however, both classes of agent induce a reproducible reduction in arterial blood pressure despite recumbency in man. The response to interruption of the system remains modest: in our study of 50 normal subjects in balance on a 10 mEq/day sodium intake, for example, the average fall of diastolic blood pressure was 5 mmHg with a standard deviation of 2.5. Thus, a fall exceeding 10 mmHg in diastolic pressure is abnormal (Hollenberg *et al.*, 1979a and b). Increasing degrees of negative sodium balance result in an increasing role for angiotensin in maintaining arterial pressure. Indeed, aggressive depletion of sodium will make even the 'low renin hypertensive' dependent on angiotensin for blood pressure maintenance (Gavras *et al.*, 1976).

Interpretation of the responses to converting enzyme inhibition has been complicated by the likelihood that these agents have actions in addition to blunting angiotensin II formation, including the release of vasodilator prostaglandins (Swartz *et al.*, 1980) and a reduction in bradykinin degradation sufficient to increase plasma bradykinin concentration (Mimran, Targhetta and Laroche, 1980; Williams and Hollenberg, 1977). In general, for these agents too, restriction of sodium intake enhances the depressor response.

Renovascular hypertension represents the paradigm of renin-mediated hypertension. Studies in animal models have documented a central role for renin in its pathogenesis (Brunner *et al.*, 1971; Davis, 1977; Gavras *et al.*, 1973). In man we have shown that 86% of patients with renovascular hypertension, proved by successful surgery, showed a supranormal depressor response to saralasin infused intravenously in graded doses (Hollenberg *et al.*, 1979a). A false-positive, supranormal depressor response occurred in 8.5% of patients with essential hypertension when studied under identical circumstances, including restriction of sodium intake.

Estimates of the frequency with which angiotensin plays a direct role in sustaining an elevated blood pressure in essential hypertension have ranged widely, from 70% of all patients – an estimate based on the frequency of a significant depressor response to converting enzyme inhibition (Case *et al.*, 1977) to a rather more uncommon role – see the 8.5% estimate based on supranormal responses to saralasin described above (Hollenberg *et al.*, 1979a).

The classification of essential hypertension as a function of plasma renin activity into 'low, normal or high renin hypertension' has been the subject of broad interest (Case *et al.*, 1977; Laragh, 1977; Tuck *et al.*, 1973). It is in the patient with high renin hypertension that one might anticipate the largest contribution from a direct pressor action of angiotensin. Case *et al.* (1976), for example, reported depressor responses to saralasin in most patients with high renin values, but their study mixed patients with essential and malignant hypertension and renovascular hypertension. On the other hand, Streeten and Anderson (1977) reported that only about one-half of patients with high renin essential hypertension showed a fall in blood pressure during saralasin infusion. One conclusion from the study of Esler *et al.* (1977) was that an elevated plasma-renin activity could be a marker for other pathophysiological processes, rather than a primary pathogenetic mechanism, perhaps reflecting enhanced sympathetic nervous system activity which produces both the hypertension and the concomitant release of renin.

We undertook a systematic investigation of the factors responsible for renin's participation in blood pressure elevation in 19 patients with high renin essential hypertension (Dluhy *et al.*, 1979). A supranormal depressor response to saralasin occurred in seven, about 37%. As was the case in the abnormal adrenal agonist response to saralasin in normal renin hypertension (Williams *et al.*, 1979), these patients had a blunted adrenal response to angiotensin II. A reasonable speculation was that the mechanism responsible for the elevated renin and blood pressure could be a compensatory activation of the system in response to decreased adrenal responsiveness to angiotensin (Dluhy *et al.*, 1979).

RESPONSIVENESS TO ANGIOTENSIN: VASCULAR SMOOTH MUSCLE AND THE ADRENOCORTICAL

The issue of responsiveness to angiotensin II as a potentially important variable has appeared in several of the preceding sections. The past decade has seen important advances in our understanding of the determinants of responsiveness to angiotensin II, but important areas of controversy still exist.

That pressor responses to angiotensin II varied with the state of sodium balance was long recognized (Kaplan and Silah, 1964), but it was not until 1972 that evidence first appeared to indicate that the variation in the pressor response reflected a change in the vascular smooth muscle, a change that was still evident when isolated arterial smooth muscle strips were placed in tissue bath (Strewler *et al.*, 1972). The fact that the information was located in the smooth muscle strip and the specificity of the influence of sodium intake made it likely that the angiotensin receptor was involved. The blunted response with restriction of sodium intake and the enhanced response on a high sodium intake in animals and in man was specific for angiotensin: no such shift occurred with norepinephrine (Hollenberg *et al.*, 1972; Strewler *et al.*, 1972).

The shifts in responsiveness to angiotensin II of blood pressure and blood flow to an extremity with changes in sodium intake were consistent but substantially smaller than the shift in the responsiveness of the renal blood supply (Hollenberg *et al.*, 1972), where a ten-fold reduction in responsiveness occurred on a low salt diet. The fact that the shift in responsiveness was substantially larger than the change in plasma angiotensin II concentration raised the interesting possibility that free angiotensin concentration in the kidney was increased more than in plasma during restriction of sodium intake.

The development of techniques for assessing tissue binding of radioactively labelled ligands, and their application to the assessment of receptors, has provided a clear indication that the shifts in responsiveness to angiotensin II reflect a reciprocal relationship between plasma angiotensin II concentration and the number of receptors in a wide variety of smooth muscle preparations (Devynck and Meyer, 1976; Gunther, Gimbrone and Alexander, 1980). The radioligand studies, furthermore, are supported by pharmacological evidence favoring a receptor locus for shifts in sensitivity (Williams, Hollenberg and Braley, 1976). To our knowledge no exception to this principle has been reported. The interpretation of the shifts in vascular sensitivity *in vivo*, therefore, was straightforward.

What of the adrenal? Here the underlying mechanism is clearly more complex. In normal man, as indicated above, restriction of sodium intake enhances substantially the adrenal response to angiotensin (Hollenberg *et al.*, 1974; Oelkers *et al.*, 1974). The application of radioligand binding techniques to assessment of the angiotensin receptor on the adrenal, and alternative approaches based on pharmacological principles, have not led to as straightforward an interpretation of the intimate mechanisms. Some studies have suggested a receptor mechanism (Aguilera and Catt, 1978; Bravo, 1977; Douglas and Catt, 1976), whereas others have not (Douglas, 1980; Williams, Hollenberg and Braley, 1976), but rather have favored events beyond the receptor, in the biosynthetic pathway.

What of man? Such direct inquiries, of course, are not possible. An alternative approach to assessing whether the modification in responsiveness of these target tissues reflects changes in circulating angiotensin II, or is linked to other factors dependent on dietary sodium intake, is possible, based on the ability of converting enzyme inhibitors to reduce circulating angiotensin II concentration. With this approach we have shown that reduction in both the pressor response and the renal vascular response to angiotensin in normal man ingesting a low sodium intake is shifted toward the response anticipated on a high salt intake by converting enzyme inhibition (Dawson-Hughes *et al.*, 1981; Shoback *et al.*, 1983a). This response to converting enzyme inhibition is, therefore, precisely that anticipated from the *in vitro* studies.

In the case of the adrenal and aldosterone release in normal man, however, converting enzyme inhibition did nothing to responsiveness to angiotensin II, a finding that favors a different mechanism determining adrenal responsiveness (Dawson-Hughes *et al.*, 1981; Shoback *et al.*, 1983a). The most likely candidate is an alteration in the activity of the late pathway in aldosterone biosynthesis (Haning, Tait and Tait, 1970; Williams, Hollenberg and Braley, 1976).

THE RENAL BLOOD SUPPLY AND ALDOSTERONE SECRETION IN ESSENTIAL HYPERTENSION

During the 1970s it became progressively more clear that the normal control of both the renal blood supply and the adrenal with changes in sodium intake was dominated by angiotensin II, an advance that was heavily dependent on the development of effective means for achieving pharmacological interruption of the renin–angiotensin system. At the same time, evidence for striking variations in the responsiveness to angiotensin of these systems was accumulating. These conceptual advances had implications for two parallel and apparently unrelated lines of investigation on the pathogenesis of essential hypertension in our laboratories.

Abnormal control of the renal circulation was identified in a substantial subgroup of young patients with essential hypertension, and the tentative suggestion was made that the abnormality reflected a subpopulation in whom the renal blood supply was resistant to restriction of sodium intake (Hollenberg and Merrill, 1970). Continued experience confirmed that observation and extended it (Hollenberg, Borucki and Adams, 1978), making it possible to estimate the frequency of the abnormality – about one-third of the patients with essential hypertension studied, without reference to their status in a renin classification. The fact that one or both parents in this subgroup had hypertension in every assessable case provided an intriguing clue: perhaps these individuals inherited the renal abnormality?

At the same time an abnormality in adrenal responsiveness to volume challenge was identified in some patients with essential hypertension (Williams *et al.*, 1970). Because plasma renin activity and plasma angiotensin II concentration in these patients was normal, it was reasonable to suggest that the underlying abnormality was an alteration in the angiotensin–aldosterone relationship, as was subsequently documented (Moore *et al.*, 1977).

SPECTRUM OF ALTERED TISSUE RESPONSIVENESS TO ANGIOTENSIN II IN ESSENTIAL HYPERTENSION

From the foregoing discussion a substantial body of evidence has accumulated which suggests that some patients with essential hypertension have an alteration in their target tissue sensitivity to angiotensin with changes in sodium intake. Indeed, in some of these individuals changing sodium intake has no effect on the sensitivity of these tissues to angiotensin II. Because angiotensin is pivotal to the control of both the renal blood supply and to adrenal secretion of aldosterone as dietary sodium intake varies, it became reasonable to ask whether the abnormality was present in both systems in the same patient. The answer was unequivocal: parallel renal and adrenal abnormalities coexisted in the same patients with essential hypertension (Shoback *et al.*, 1983b; Williams *et al.*, 1982). In the first report 18 patients were studied; all were under the age of 30 in order to minimize the likelihood that the phenomena were secondary to long-standing hypertension. To achieve a wide span of sodium balance, studies were performed during a high (200 mEq) sodium intake, a restricted (10 mEq) sodium intake and a restricted sodium intake supplemented by further short-term diuretic-induced volume deficit (Williams *et al.*, 1982). Renal blood flow was assessed by radioxenon transit while adrenal responsiveness was determined both by plasma aldosterone levels and aldosterone secretion rates. The hypertensive patients were divided into two subgroups based on their aldosterone secretory response to acute volume depletion. Nine of the subjects had an increment in aldosterone secretion in response to acute sodium depletion with at least 300 mEq of sodium deficit in a 24 hour period, similar to what had been previously described in normal subjects (Williams *et al.*, 1970). Nine had minimal or no increment in plasma aldosterone concentration or aldosterone secretion rate, despite an equal increase in plasma renin activity (*Figure 7.1*). Thus, in this study the hypertensive patients were divided into 'normal' and 'abnormal' responders based on their aldosterone secretory response to an increase in endogenous angiotensin II induced by volume depletion. The difference in aldosterone secretory response could not be explained

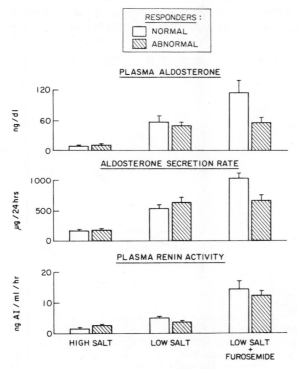

Figure 7.1 Plasma renin activity, plasma aldosterone, and aldosterone secretory rates during three conditions (200 mEq sodium/100 mEq potassium intake; 10 mEq sodium/100 mEq potassium intake; 10 mEq sodium intake with frusemide). The patients have been divided into two groups according to whether their aldosterone secretory rate increased (normal responders) or not (abnormal responders) in response to frusemide administration. There were nine subjects in each group (mean ± SEM). (Reprinted with permission from Williams *et al.*, 1982)

by differences in plasma renin activity in response to volume depletion (which increased in all subjects) nor a change in metabolism of aldosterone since the plasma levels of aldosterone followed a similar pattern to that noted for aldosterone secretion. Therefore, having defined the patients by the absence of a sodium-mediated effect on adrenal responsiveness to angiotensin II, renal blood flow response on a high and low salt diet was assessed. In those who had a normal aldosterone response to volume depletion, sodium restriction appropriately reduced renal blood flow while in those who were abnormal responders changing sodium intake did not modify the basal renal blood flow. The data were compatible with a parallel blunting of responsiveness to angiotensin II in both systems, a testable hypothesis.

In the next study (Shoback *et al.*, 1983b) a second group of 18 hypertensive patients was divided into two subgroups according to the renal vascular response to sodium restriction. In nine normotensive subjects, the normal anticipated 11% increase in renal plasma flow, 63 ± 35 ml/min/1.73 m^2, occurred. Thus, the hypertensive patients were divided into two groups based on whether there was an increment of 10% or greater in basal para-amino hippurate (PAH) clearance from

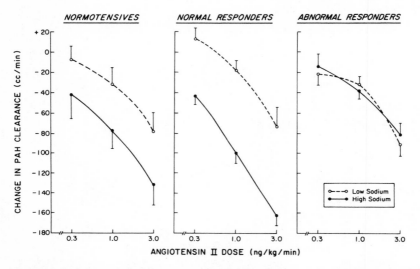

Figure 7.2 Comparison of response in PAH clearance during angiotensin II infusion in normotensive and hypertensives. The decrement in PAH clearance during angiotensin II infusion was significantly ($P<0.01$) greater in the normal responding hypertensive patients (*center panel, n = 9*) on the high compared with the low sodium diet comparable to the normotensive subjects (*left panel, n = 8*). There was no significant difference in the PAH decrement during angiotensin II infusion for the abnormal responders (*right panel*) between the low and high sodium responses (*n = 9*). (Reprinted with permission from Shoback *et al.*, 1983b)

the low to the high sodium diet. In nine of the 18 hypertensive patients the anticipated increase in renal plasma flow occurred with dietary sodium loading. In the other nine hypertensive subjects no significant change occurred (22 ± 12 cc/min/1.73 m^2). In the abnormal responders neither the basal renal blood flow nor the fall with graded angiotensin II infusions (*Figure 7.2*) was statistically different between the low and the high sodium intakes. The response of plasma aldosterone to angiotensin II infusion on the two sodium intakes was then determined in these two subgroups. In the abnormal responders, in this group defined by the renal blood flow response to sodium restriction, aldosterone responsiveness to angiotensin II infusion also did not vary on the high and low sodium intake. On the other hand, those individuals who had an increase in renal blood flow with a sodium load, sodium restriction significantly ($P<0.01$) enhanced the adrenal response to angiotensin II (*Figure 7.3*).

Not only did renal vascular responsiveness to angiotensin II fail to vary with sodium intake in the abnormal responders, but also blood pressure response to angiotensin II was not influenced by sodium intake (*Figure 7.4*). During the infusion of 3 ng/kg/min of angiotensin II, the rise in diastolic blood pressure was significantly greater ($P<0.01$) in the normal responders on a high ($19 \pm 1\,\text{mmHg}$) than on a low ($14 \pm 2\,\text{mmHg}$) sodium intake, similar to the pattern of diastolic blood pressure responses in normotensive individuals. In contrast, the abnormal

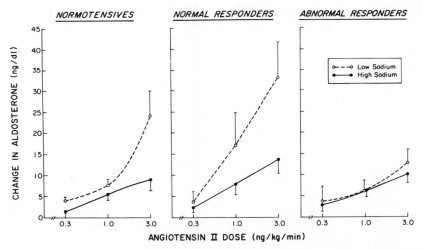

Figure 7.3 Responses of plasma aldosterone to graded infusion of angiotensin II during sodium restriction and loading in normotensives and hypertensives. The aldosterone increment was significantly greater ($P<0.01$) in the normal responders with sodium restriction than with sodium repletion (*center panel*, $n = 8$) comparable to normotensive subjects. The abnormal responders showed no statistical difference between their aldosterone increments during sodium restriction and sodium repletion (*right panel*, $n = 9$). (Reprinted with permission from Shoback *et al.*, 1983b)

responders achieved a similar rise in diastolic blood pressure from control on both diets at all three doses of angiotensin II. The maximum diastolic blood pressure rise at 3 ng/kg/min of angiotensin II was identical ($13 \pm 2\,\text{mmHg}$) for both sodium intakes. Additionally, both groups of hypertensive subjects had a greater maximal blood pressure response ($P<0.03$) than the normotensive subjects to angiotensin II on a low sodium diet but only the normal responders had a greater response on the high sodium intake ($P<0.02$).

Thus, these two studies strongly suggest that there is a subgroup of patients with essential hypertension who fail to modulate their renal blood flow, aldosterone and pressor responses to angiotensin II with changes in dietary sodium intake. The abnormality can be defined either by a failure of sodium-mediated change in responsiveness of the renal vasculature, which becomes apparent on a high sodium intake, or a failure in sodium-mediated change in responsiveness of the adrenal, which becomes apparent on a low sodium intake. Regardless of which technique has been used to define the abnormal responders, abnormalities in angiotensin II target tissues track together.

What could account for the differences in responsiveness to angiotensin II? One possibility is an age difference, since beyond the fourth decade there is a gradual diminution of basal renal blood flow in normotensive subjects (Hollenberg *et al.*, 1974). This seems unlikely since the abnormality was present even in individuals less than 30 years of age (Williams *et al.*, 1982). Furthermore, while basal renal

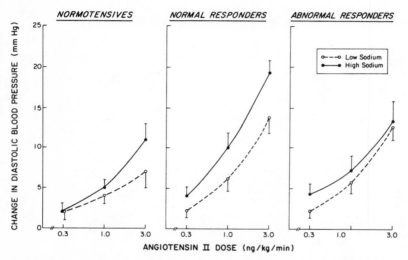

Figure 7.4 Incremental responses of diastolic blood pressure to infused angiotensin II on low and high sodium diets in normotensives and hypertensives. The increment in diastolic blood pressure in the normal responders (*center panel*) was significantly greater ($P<0.01$) at the highest angiotensin II dose on the high compared to the low sodium diet ($n = 9$), and was similar to normotensive subjects (*left panel*, $n = 9$). There was no significant difference between the low and high sodium maximal blood pressure response in the abnormal responders (*right panel*, $n = 9$). (Reprinted with permission from Shoback *et al.*, 1983b)

blood flow tends to decline with age, its responsiveness to infused angiotensin II does not (Hollenberg *et al.*, 1974). Adrenal responsiveness to exogenous angiotensin II is also not modified by age, at least over the age-span of the subjects reported in these two publications (Takeda *et al.*, 1980). The differences between the two subgroups also could not be accounted for by differences in sodium or potassium balance, serum potassium or sodium concentration, renal function, cardiac output or plasma volume (Williams *et al.*, 1982). There is no evidence of intrinsic renal impairment or more severe hypertension in the abnormal responding patient, since there was no easily separable clinical difference in renal function, physical examination, electrocardiograms, duration of hypertension or admission blood pressure between the two groups of patients in either study.

POTENTIAL MECHANISM(S) UNDERLYING THE ALTERED TISSUE RESPONSIVENESS TO ANGIOTENSIN II

There are a number of potential mechanisms which could account for the absence of an effect of sodium intake on tissue responsiveness to angiotensin II. This section briefly reviews four possibilities: a difference in volume status, differences in basal levels of aldosterone and/or renal blood flow, tissue or circulating angiotensin II levels, and/or differences in potassium balance. Either an increased amount of sodium in the body or an error in volume perception could reduce responsiveness of the adrenal to angiotensin II. Indeed, several studies suggested that there is an error in sodium and/or volume perception in at least some patients with essential hypertension (Tarazi, Frohlich and Dustan, 1968; Julius *et al.*, 1971; Tuck *et al.*, 1976). A number of observations suggest that the potential defect does not reside here. In the study of Williams *et al.* (1982) the effect of sodium intake on plasma volume in the two groups of hypertensive patients was assessed. Neither the basal

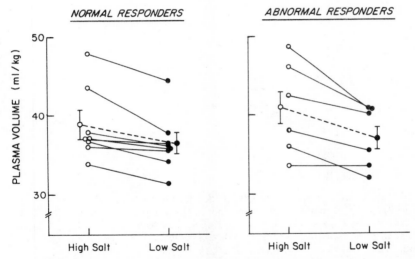

Figure 7.5 Plasma volumes on high and low sodium intakes in patients divided into two groups according to whether their aldosterone secretory rate increased or not in response to frusemide administration. (Reprinted with permission from Williams *et al.*, 1982)

plasma volume nor its response to sodium restriction varied between the two groups (*Figure 7.5*). If anything, the abnormal responders had a greater fall in plasma volume with sodium restriction than did the normal responders. Moreover, the abnormality in aldosterone secretion became more apparent with frusemide-induced volume depletion. Additional support comes from the study of Gordon *et al.* (1982) who infused angiotensin II during three different volume states in a group of patients who had been previously defined as abnormal responders (*Figure 7.6*) The patients were studied on a 200 mEq, 10 mEq, and 10 mEq sodium intake after administration of frusemide in an amount sufficient to produce a

1–1.5 kg weight loss and a deficit of 150–250 mEq of sodium. Tissue responsiveness to angiotensin II did not vary in this group of abnormal responders, despite the fact that the sodium balance varied by more than 350 mEq. Finally, in normal subjects sodium intake reciprocally influences vascular and adrenal responses to angiotensin II, salt restriction blunts the vascular response while salt loading blunts the adrenal response (Hollenberg *et al.*, 1974; Oelkers *et al.*, 1974). If the abnormal responders were volume expanded compared to normal responders and normotensive subjects, then one would anticipate that they would have a blunted adrenal response but an enhanced renal vascular response to angiotensin II. Thus, the

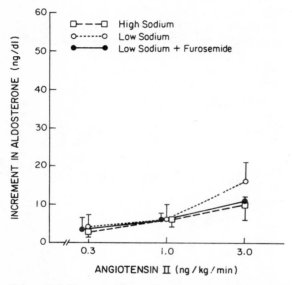

Figure 7.6 Plasma aldosterone response to graded doses of angiotensin II in five patients who were previously defined as abnormal responders. These patients were studied under three different conditions. High sodium intake (200 mEq), low sodium intake (10 mEq) and low sodium intake after administration of frusemide to produce a 1–1.5 kg weight loss over a 24 hour period. There were no significant changes in the adrenal responsiveness to angiotensin II under these three conditions. (Reprinted with permission from Gordon *et al.*, 1982)

subnormal responsiveness of both the adrenal and renal vasculature observed in the abnormal responders would be difficult to account for solely on the basis of an altered sodium space or abnormal volume perception.

In general, both adrenal and renal vascular responsiveness to angiotensin II are directly correlated with their basal levels in normal subjects. Individuals on a high sodium intake have a lower basal aldosterone level and a smaller response to angiotensin II than individuals on a low sodium intake, where the basal levels are higher. Similarly, the basal levels of renal blood flow are lower on the low salt diet, as is the responsiveness to angiotensin II. One possible mechanism for the decreased responsiveness of both target tissues, therefore, is simply a selection of individuals with lower basal values rather than a primary defect in these two systems. The weight of available data would suggest this is not the case. When normal responders and abnormal responders with statistically indistinguishable basal renal blood flow and aldosterone levels are compared, the abnormal responders continue to have a statistically significant reduction in responsiveness to angiotensin II (*Figure 7.7*). The comparisons of renal vascular responses were made in a sodium replete state, and for adrenal response on a 10 mEq sodium intake. Thus, the decreased responsiveness in some patients with essential hypertension is not secondary to their decreased basal aldosterone or renal blood flow *per se*.

One particularly appealing hypothesis to explain the differences in renal vascular responsiveness in the two groups of patients with essential hypertension is an abnormality in the tissue concentration of angiotensin II or the angiotensin II receptor itself. Support for this hypothesis comes from those studies which have

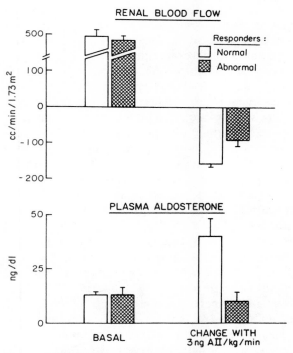

Figure 7.7 Relationship of basal function and responsiveness to angiotensin II in patients with essential hypertension. In the *top panel* patients were selected according to their basal renal blood flow on a high (200 mEq) sodium intake. Even though basal renal blood flow levels were comparable in the two groups, there was a significant (*P*<0.008) difference in the renal blood flow response to angiotensin II in the two subgroups. The *lower panel* depicts similar findings using basal aldosterone levels on a sodium restricted intake. Patients again were selected so that they had comparable basal aldosterone levels and the responses to 3 ng of angiotensin II administration were determined. Again, there was a significant (*P*<0.02) difference in the aldosterone response to angiotensin II in the two subgroups despite the fact they had comparable basal aldosterone levels. (Adapted with permission from Shoback *et al.*, 1983b)

documented an enhanced renal vascular response to converting enzyme inhibitors in patients with essential hypertension (Hollenberg *et al.*, 1981; Williams and Hollenberg, 1977). Since vascular responses to angiotensin II are regulated by local or circulating angiotensin II concentration (Brunner *et al.*, 1972; Gunther, Gimbrone and Alexander, 1980; Williams, Hollenberg and Braley, 1976) one possible explanation for an unresponsive renal vasculature would be an inappropriately high level of angiotensin II in the kidney despite a high sodium intake. Such an inappropriately elevated intrarenal angiotensin II concentration could account for a reduced renal blood flow response to sodium loading, a blunted response to exogenous angiotensin II, and an enhanced renal blood flow response to converting enzyme inhibition. Such a hypothesis would make unnecessary an abnormality in the angiotensin II receptor or a post-receptor event to account for the decreased renal vascular responsiveness with sodium loading. However, such an explanation would not apply to the adrenal.

Clearly, the best explanation would account for abnormalities in both systems on the basis of a single defect. The most plausible candidate is that of the angiotensin II receptor. How would one assess for this possibility *in vivo* in man? Our most recent study provides additional information concerning this possibility (Taylor *et al.*, 1984). Taylor and her colleagues determined the effect of converting enzyme inhibitors on adrenal responses to angiotensin II. Thirty-one patients with normal and high renin essential hypertension and 13 normotensive controls received graded infusions of angiotensin II on a sodium-restricted intake before and after 72 hours of converting enzyme inhibition with either captopril or enalapril. When the converting enzyme inhibitor was administered, no change in adrenal responsiveness to angiotensin II occurred in the normotensive controls or in the hypertensive normal responders (*Figure 7.8*). Yet in the hypertensive abnormal responders both the threshold sensitivity and the entire dose–response relationship was significantly ($P<0.01$) enhanced after converting enzyme inhibition. As in the earlier studies, the increase in sensitivity could not be explained by differences in angiotensin II increments with the angiotensin II infusion, in basal aldosterone levels, or in blood presure or basal angiotensin II response to converting enzyme inhibition. Since both converting enzyme inhibitors were equally effective in producing the increased responsiveness in the abnormal responders, it also appears unlikely that the phenomenon was secondary to a non-specific action of one of the agents, unrelated to converting enzyme inhibition. To date, it is impossible to know whether the change in responsiveness is due to a reduction in angiotensin II, an increase in bradykinin or an increase in prostaglandin levels in response to the converting enzyme inhibitor. However, it is unlikely that either changes in bradykinin or prostaglandin production directly affect aldosterone secretion.

The results of this study raise the intriguing possiblity that angiotensin-mediated aldosterone secretion is not regulated in the same way in the abnormal responding hypertensive patients as in normotensive subjects. As noted earlier, it has been suggested that the major factor regulating the amount of aldosterone produced with changes in angiotensin II concentration is not a change in receptor number or affinity but rather a change in an event distal to that – at the late pathway of aldosterone biosynthesis (Dawson-Hughes *et al.*, 1981; Shoback *et al.*, 1983b).

According to this hypothesis, with sodium loading the late pathway enzymatic activity is modified so that there is a decreased conversion of corticosterone to aldosterone; the opposite occurs with sodium restriction (Haning, Tait and Tait, 1970; Williams and Braley, 1977). If this mechanism were absent in the abnormal responders then one of the ways that the converting enzyme inhibitors could increase adrenal responsiveness is via the same mechanism operating on the vascular smooth muscle, that is, reduction of tissue angiotensin II concentration after converting enzyme inhibition upregulated the adrenal response to angiotensin II.

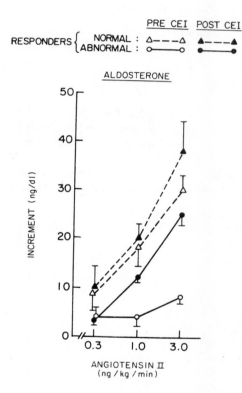

Figure 7.8 Dose–response relationship between dose of angiotensin II infused and increment in plasma aldosterone in hypertensive subjects. The hypertensive subjects were divided into normal and abnormal responders (mean ± SEM). Data are presented for responses both before and after converting enzyme administration ($n = 31$). (Adapted with permission from Taylor *et al.*, 1984)

A final potential mechanism is a change in potassium balance. Hypokalemia and/or a lowering of total body potassium reduces renal vascular and adrenal responses to angiotensin II regardless of the sodium intake (Dluhy, Cain and Williams, 1974; Hollenberg *et al.*, 1975). Thus, if the abnormal responders are relatively potassium-depleted, then one would anticipate a decreased adrenal and renal vascular response to angiotensin II. Furthermore, since converting enzyme inhibitors, consequent to their reduction in aldosterone secretion, favor potassium retention (Gavras *et al.*, 1978) an increase in potassium levels could mediate the increased adrenal responsiveness to angiotensin II following converting enzyme inhibition. While there are no published data directly bearing on this point, several lines of evidence would suggest that this is an unlikely possibility. First, in all the reported studies, serum and urine potassium levels were similar in normal and abnormal responding hypertensive patients (Williams *et al.*, 1970, 1982; Moore *et al.*, 1977; Dluhy *et al.*, 1979; Shoback *et al.*, 1983a and b; Taylor *et al.*, 1984). Secondly, converting enzyme inhibitors had an equivalent effect on serum potassium and potassium balance in the normal and abnormal responders but only the abnormal responders showed an increase in adrenal responses to angiotensin II (Taylor *et al.*, 1984). Finally, in normal subjects, increasing potassium intake is much less potent than decreasing sodium intake in enhancing adrenal responses to angiotensin II (Hollenberg *et al.*, 1975). Thus, while changes in potassium balance could potentially account for part of the abnormalities discussed above, presently there is no evidence to support such a mechanism.

IDENTIFICATION OF THE ABNORMAL RESPONDER

In the past, several specific alterations in endocrine function have been used to classify patients with essential hypertension, for example, low, normal and high renin essential hypertension, normal and high catecholamine essential hypertension. In many cases, after close scrutiny it became apparent that these classifications were in part arbitrary and that instead of being discrete subgroups, the abnormalities may simply be part of a continuum. Does the same *caveat* apply

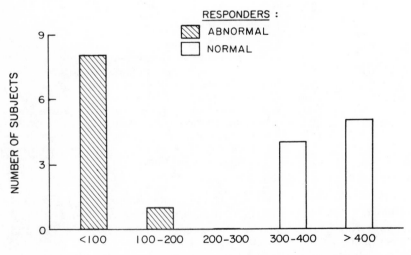

Figure 7.9 Increments in aldosterone secretion induced by frusemide administration in subjects in balance on a low sodium intake (10 mEq Na/100 mEq K). The subjects are divided into two groups (normal responders and abnormal responders) based on previous studies documenting an increment in aldosterone secretion of more than 300 μg/day in normal subjects. Note the distinct bimodal distribution of responses. (Reprinted with permission from Williams *et al.*, 1982)

to the present classification? Several approaches have been used to address this question. Aldosterone secretory response to frusemide administration (*Figure 7.9*) shows a clear bimodal distribution in hypertensive patients. Likewise, renal blood flow responsiveness to angiotensin infusion in sodium deplete hypertensive subjects also appears to be bimodal (*Figure 7.10*). Finally, even the correction of the decreased adrenal response to angiotensin II following converting enzyme inhibition is bimodal. Either the patient's aldosterone response to angiotensin II was increased following converting enzyme inhibition or it was not (*Figure 7.11*). Thus, on the basis of the available evidence there is a high probability that there are

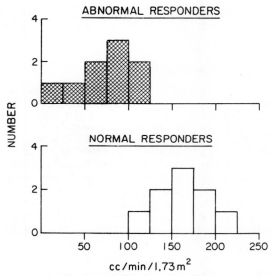

Figure 7.10 Mean renal blood flow response to 3 ng of angiotensin II/kg/min infusion in patients with essential hypertension. The patients were divided into abnormal or normal responders based on their adrenal response to angiotensin II on a low sodium intake. All studies were performed on a 200 mEq sodium intake. (Adapted from Shoback *et al.*, 1983b)

two subgroups of patients with normal or high renin essential hypertension. In one group sodium intake does not influence the vascular or adrenal responsiveness to angiotensin II whereas in the other group it does.

It is also apparent from these studies that there are two approaches to distinguishing these two groups. Either one can examine the adrenal responsiveness to angiotensin II on a low sodium intake (a condition in which the response of aldosterone to angiotensin II is enhanced in normal subjects) or the renal vascular response to angiotensin II on a high sodium intake (a condition in which responsiveness is enhanced in normal subjects). To date, no simple test is available to distinguish the two subgroups of patients since control of sodium intake is of paramount importance.

In normal man the abrupt cessation of sodium intake results in an exponential fall in sodium excretion with a half-time of 24 hours. We have recently completed

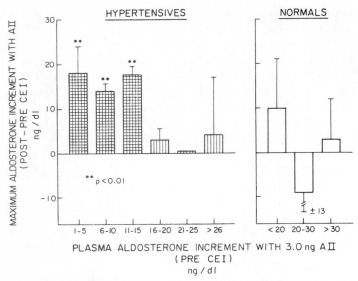

Figure 7.11 The differences in maximum aldosterone response to angiotensin II infusion prior to and after converting enzyme inhibition in 31 hypertensive and 13 normotensive subjects. The subjects are grouped according to their aldosterone increment with 3 ng of angiotensin II kg min prior to converting enzyme inhibitor (CEI) administration (mean SEM). A positive value indicates that the response after CEI was greater than before. Only in the 1–5, 6–10 and 10–15 ng/dl hypertensive subgroups was there a significant difference (*P*<0.01). In the normotensive subjects and the rest of the hypertensive subjects there was no significant difference in the aldosterone response to angiotensin II prior to or after administration of a converting enzyme inhibitor. All subjects were studied on a low sodium intake

an analysis to indicate that the half-time is also 24 hours in the normally modulating essential hypertensive, but is extended to 36 hours in the non-modulating hypertensive. Such an abnormality would result in expansion of sodium space at any sodium intake: moreover, the higher the sodium intake, the larger the difference between the normal and the non-modulating hypertensive.

RELATIONSHIP OF ALTERED TISSUE RESPONSIVENESS TO ANGIOTENSIN II TO THE HYPERTENSION

One of the major conceptual advances of the past decade has been the recognition that the factors responsible for sustaining hypertension vary as conditions change, even in a relatively simple model. In renovascular hypertension, for example, the elevated blood pressure is sustained by the vascular actions of angiotensin II when sodium intake is restricted, but other mechanisms come to the fore when the renin system is suppressed by a high salt intake or sodium retention (Barger, 1979; Brunner *et al.*, 1971; Gavras *et al.*, 1973). This concept is most likely to be applicable to the pathogenesis of essential hypertension in patients in whom the mechanisms for sodium handling are deranged. It is difficult to imagine that a parallel abnormality in adrenal aldosterone release and in the renal blood supply – two systems that are central to sodium homeostasis – does not have implications for how dietary sodium is handled.

The control of both systems is dominated by angiotensin II and both systems normally show changes in sensitivity as sodium intake changes, but the directional changes in sensitivity are reciprocal. Thus, the adrenal abnormality is most evident on a very low sodium intake, and the renal abnormality becomes most evident as sodium intake increases. A setting has been created, therefore, in which the nature of the abnormality at any moment is likely to reflect dietary sodium intake.

In order to assess how these abnormalities in renal blood flow and adrenal responsiveness to angiotensin II could produce hypertension, one needs to examine the conditions under which the function of each is most critical. When the abnormal responders are sodium restricted, on the one hand, the enhanced aldosterone response to angiotensin II which normally facilitates sodium conservation is defective with a resultant lower aldosterone secretion rate. This would lead to increased renin release and angiotensin formation in order to close the renin–angiotensin II–aldosterone–volume feedback loop. On a sodium-restricted intake the abnormal responders would tend to have angiotensin-mediated hypertension. In support of this hypothesis are the following findings: on a sodium-restricted intake the basal aldosterone levels are significantly less and the basal renin and/or angiotensin II levels are significantly greater in the abnormal responders (Shoback *et al.*, 1983a and b; Taylor *et al.*, 1984). Furthermore, this tendency to have increased renin and angiotensin II levels and lowered aldosterone concentrations is accentuated in the upright position, particularly if the subjects are first grouped into normal and high renin subgroups (Dluhy *et al.*, 1979; Moore *et al.*, 1977). Finally, in those high renin hypertensive patients who have a decreased adrenal response to angiotensin II, saralasin (a competitive antagonist of angiotensin II) produces a substantially greater reduction in arterial pressure (similar to what occurs in patients with renal vascular hypertension) than those who have a normal adrenal response (Dluhy *et al.*, 1979).

What occurs as sodium intake increases? The renal blood supply is thought to contribute to normal renal sodium handling via several mechanisms. Glomerular filtration rate is renal plasma flow dependent, and the rate of filtration represents the sodium load presented to the tubules for reabsorption. Peritubular hydrostatic and oncotic pressure are rate limiting for proximal tubular sodium reabsorption, and both are determined by renal hemodynamics. The pattern of intrarenal blood flow distribution may also contribute to renal sodium handling, to the extent, therefore, that the state of the renal blood supply is fixed in these patients (Gordon *et al.*, 1982; Shoback *et al.*, 1983b; Taylor *et al.*, 1984). These factors cannot contribute to renal sodium handling. To handle a sodium load these patients must recruit alternative mechanisms.

There has been substantial interest in the possibility that a natriuretic, or ouabain-like inhibitor of Na–K–ATPase, contributes to the pathogenesis of hypertension in multiple settings (Gruber, Whitaker and Buckalew, 1980; Haddy, Pamnani and Clough, 1979; Overbeck *et al.*, 1976; Poston *et al.*, 1981). Possibly related are abnormalities in membrane sodium handling in some patients with essential hypertension. (Canessa *et al.*, 1980; Garay and Meyer, 1979). None of these hypotheses have dealt with a central issue: what would lead to the abnormal release of the natriuretic factor? An abnormality of the kidney and the adrenal that both varies with sodium intake and can contribute to altered sodium handling obviously represents an outstanding candidate.

CONCLUSIONS

Sodium intake has a profound effect on target tissue responsiveness to angiotensin II. This sodium-mediated modulation of tissue responsiveness appears to be critical in sodium homeostasis and blood pressure. A substantial body of data now suggests that in some patients with essential hypertension this normal sodium-mediated modulation of tissue responsiveness to angiotensin II is absent (*see Table 7.1*). These individuals may have either normal or high renin levels and can be characterized by a decreased adrenal responsiveness to angiotensin II on a low sodium intake and/or decreased vascular, particularly renal vascular responsiveness to angiotensin II on a high sodium intake. While the underlying mechanisms responsible for the abnormality are unclear, it is likely that a defect in the regulation of responsiveness to angiotensin II at the tissue level and/or its receptor is a major factor. The elevated blood pressure may result either from an alteration in renal sodium handling or inappropriate increases in angiotensin II levels, depending on ambient sodium intake. Thus, the patients can have either volume or angiotensin II-dependent hypertension. A most intriguing aspect of the disease process in these patients is that converting enzyme inhibitors appear to correct the underlying abnormality and, thereby, may provide a more specific and more definitive way to treat their hypertension than was anticipated when they were developed.

References

AGUILERA, G. and CATT, K. (1978) Regulation of aldosterone secretion by the renin–angiotensin system during sodium restriction in rats. *Proceedings of the National Academy Sciences of the USA*, **75**, 4057–4061

BARGER, A. C. (1979) The Goldblatt Memorial Lecture Part I: Experimental renovascular hypertension. *Hypertension*, **1**, 447

BERNE, H. A. (1967) Hormones and endocrine glands of fishes. *Science*, **158**, 455–462

BOYD, G. W., ADAMSON, A. R., ARNOLD, M., JAMES, V. H. T. and PEART, W. S. (1972) The role of angiotensin II in the control of aldosterone in man. *Clinical Science*, **42**, 91–104

BRAVO, L. (1977) Regulation of aldosterone secretion: current concepts and newer aspects. *Advances in Nephrology*, **7**, 105–121

BRUNNER, H. R., CHANG, P., WALLACH, R., SEALEY, J. E. and LARAGH, J. H. (1972) Angiotensin II vascular receptors: their avidity in relationship to sodium balance, the autonomic nervous system and hypertension. *Journal of Clinical Investigation*, **51**, 58–67

BRUNNER, H. R., KIRSHMAN, J. D., SEALEY, J. E. and LARAGH, J. H. (1971) Hypertension of renal origin: evidence for two different mechanisms. *Science*, **174**, 1344

CANESSA, M., ADRAGNA, N., SOLOMON, H., CONNOLLY, T. and TOSTESON, D. C. (1980) Increased sodium–lithium countertransport in red cells of patients with essential hypertension. *New England Journal of Medicine*, **302**, 772

CAPELLI, J. P., WESSON, L. G. and APONTE, G. E. (1970) A phylogenetic study of the renin–angiotension system. *American Journal of Physiology*, **218**, 1171–1178

CASE, D. B., WALLACE, J. M., KEIM, H. J., SEALEY, J. E. and LARAGH, J. H. (1976) Usefulness and limitations of saralasin, a partial competitive antagonist of angiotensin II, for evaluating the renin and sodium factors in hypertensive patients. *American Journal of Medicine*, **60**, 825–836

CASE, D. B., WALLACE, J. M., KEIM, H. J., WEBER, M. A., SEALEY, J. E. and LARAGH, J. H. (1977) Possible role of renin in hypertension as suggested by renin-sodium profiling and inhibition of converting enzyme. *New England Journal of Medicine*, **296**, 641–646

CHRISTLIEB, A. R., HICKLER, R. B., LAULER, D. P. and WILLIAMS, G. H. (1969) Hypertension with inappropriate aldosterone stimulation: a syndrome. *New England Journal of Medicine*, **281**, 128–131

DAVIS, J. O. and FREEMAN, R. H. (1976) Mechanisms regulating renin release. *Physiological Review*, **56**, 11–56

DAVIS, J. O. (1977) The pathogenesis of chronic renovascular hypertension. *Circulation Research*, **40**, 439–444

DAWSON-HUGHES, B. F., MOORE, T. J., DLUHY, R. G., HOLLENBERG, N. K. and WILLIAMS, G. H. (1981) Plasma angiotensin concentration regulates vascular but not adrenal responsiveness to restriction of sodium intake in normal man. *Clinical Science*, **61**, 527–534

DEVYNCK, M. A. and MEYER, P. (1976) Angiotensin receptors in vascular tissue. *American Journal of Medicine*, **61**, 758–767

DLUHY, R. G., BAVLI, S. Z., LEUNG, F. K. *et al*. (1979) Abnormal adrenal responsiveness and angiotensin II dependency in high renin essential hypertension. *Journal of Clinical Investigation*, **64**, 1270–1276

DLUHY, R. G., CAIN, J. P. and WILLIAMS, G. H. (1974) Influence of dietary potassium on the renin and aldosterone responses to diuretic-induced volume depletion. *Journal of Laboratory and Clinical Medicine*, **83**, 249–257

DOUGLAS, J. G. and CATT, K. J. (1976) Regulation of angiotensin II receptors in the rat adrenal cortex by dietary electrolytes. *Journal of Clinical Investigation*, **58**, 834–843

DOUGLAS, J. G. (1980) Effects of high potassium diet on angiotensin-induced aldosterone production in rat adrenal glomerulosa cells. *Endocrinology*, **106**, 983–990

EPSTEIN, M. (1978) Studies of volume homeostasis in man utilizing the model of headout water immersion. *Nephron*, **22**, 9–19

ESLER, M., JULIUS, S., ZWEIFLER, A. *et al*. (1977) Mild high-renin essential hypertension. *New England Journal of Medicine*, **296**, 405–411

GARAY, P. and MEYER, P. (1979) A new test showing abnormal net Na and K fluxes in erythrocytes of essential hypertensive patients. *Lancet*, **1**, 349–351

GAVRAS, H., RIBEIRO, A. R., GAVRAS, I. and BRUNNER, H. R. (1976) Reciprocal relation between renin dependency and sodium dependency in essential hypertension. *New England Journal of Medicine*, **295**, 1278–1283

GAVRAS, H., BRUNNER, H. R., TURINI, G. A. *et al*. (1978) Antihypertensive effect of the oral angiotensin converting-enzyme inhibitor SQ 14225 in man. *New England Journal of Medicine*, **298**, 991–995

GAVRAS, H., BRUNNER, H. R., VAUGHAN, E. D. JR and LARAGH, J. H. (1973) Angiotensin–sodium interaction in blood pressure maintenance of renal hypertensive and normotensive rats. *Science*, **180**, 1369

GORDON, M. B., DLUHY, R. G., MOORE, T. J., HOLLENBERG, N. K. and WILLIAMS, G. H. (1982) Abnormal sodium-mediated changes in target tissue responsiveness to angiotensin II in essential hypertensives is not due to differences in total body sodium. Program and Abstracts, The Endocrine Society 64th Annual Meeting. *Endocrinology* (Suppl.), **110**, 185

GRUBER, K. A., WHITAKER, J. M. and BUCKALEW, V. M. JR (1980) Endogenous digitalis-like substance in plasma of volume-expanded dogs. *Nature (London)*, **287**, 743–745

GUNTHER, S., GIMBRONE, M. A. JR and ALEXANDER, R. W. (1980) Regulation by angiotensin II of its receptors in resistance blood vessels. *Nature*, **287**, 230–232

HABER, E. (1976) The role of renin in normal and pathological cardiovascular homeostasis. *Circulation*, **54**, 849–861

HADDY, F. J., PAMNANI, M. B. and CLOUGH, D. L. (1979) Humoral factors and the sodium–potassium pump in volume expanded hypertension. *Life Sciences*, **24**, 2105–2118

HANING, R., TAIT, S. A. S. and TAIT, J. F. (1970) *In vitro* effects of ACTH, angiotensins, serotonin and potassium on steroid output and conversion of corticosterone to aldosterone by isolated adrenal cell. *Endocrinology*, **87**, 1147–1160

HOLLENBERG, N. K. and MERRILL, J. P. (1970) Intrarenal perfusion in the young 'essential' hypertensive: a subpopulation resistant to sodium restriction. *Transactions of the Association of American Physicians*, **83**, 93–101

HOLLENBERG, N. K., SOLOMON, H. S., ADAMS, D. F., ABRAMS, H. L. and MERRILL, J. P. (1972) Renal vascular response to angiotensin and norepinephrine in normal man: effect of salt intake. *Circulation Research*, **31**, 750–757

HOLLENBERG, N. K., CHENITZ, W. R., ADAMS, D. F. and WILLIAMS, G. H. (1974) Reciprocal influence of salt intake on adrenal glomerulosa and renal vascular responses to angiotensin II in normal man. *Journal of Clinical Investigation*, **54**, 34–42

HOLLENBERG, N. K., WILLIAMS, G. H., BURGER, B. and HOOSHMOND, I. (1975) Potassium's influence on the renal vasculature, the adrenal, and their responsiveness to angiotensin II in normal man. *Clinical Science*, **499**, 527–534

HOLLENBERG, N. K., WILLIAMS, G. H., BURGER, B., ISHIKAWA, I. and ADAMS, D. F. (1976) Blockade and stimulation of renal, adrenal, and vascular angiotensin II receptors with 1-sar 8-ala angiotensin II in normal man. *Journal of Clinical Investigation*, **57**, 39–46

HOLLENBERG, N. K., BORUCKI, L. J. and ADAMS, D. F. (1978) The renal vasculature in early essential hypertension: evidence for a pathogenetic role. *Medicine*, **57**, 167–178

HOLLENBERG, N. K., WILLIAMS, G. H., ADAMS, D. F. *et al.* (1979a) Response to saralasin and angiotensin's role in essential and renal hypertension. *Medicine*, **58**, 115–127

HOLLENBERG, N. K., SWARTZ, S. L., PASSAN, D. R. and WILLIAMS, G. H. (1979b) Increased glomerular filtration rate following converting enzyme inhibition in essential hypertension. *New England Journal of Medicine*, **301**, 9–12

HOLLENBERG, N. K., MEGGS, L. G., WILLIAMS, G. H., KATZ, J., GARNIC, J. D. and HARRINGTON, D. P. (1981) Sodium intake and renal responses to captopril in normal man and in essential hypertension. *Kidney International*, **20**, 240–245

JULIUS, S., PASCUAL, A. V., REILLY, K. and LONDON, R. (1971) Abnormalities of plasma volume in borderline hypertension. *Archives of Internal Medicine*, **127**, 116–122

KAPLAN, N. M. and SILAH, J. G. (1964) The effect of angiotensin II on the blood pressure in humans with hypertensive disease. *Journal of Clinical Investigation*, **4**, 659–669

KIMBROUGH, H. M., VAUGHAN, E. D., CAREY, R. M. and AYERS, C. R. (1977) Effect of intrarenal angiotensin II blockade on renal function in conscious dogs. *Circulation Research*, **40**, 174–177

LARAGH, J. H. (1977) Vasoconstriction–volume analysis in treatment of hypertension. In *Hypertension: Mechanisms, Diagnosis and Management*, edited by J. O. Davis, J. H. Laragh and A. Selwyn, Chapter 7, pp. 69–74. New York: HP Publishing Company

LEVENS, N. R., PEACH, M. J. and CAREY, R. M. (1981) Role of intrarenal angiotensin II in the control of renal function. *Circulation Research*, **48**, 157–167

LEVENS, N. R., PEACH, M. J. and CAREY, R. M. (1983) Control of renal function by intrarenal angiotensin II. *Endocrinology*, **112**, 43–49

MIMRAN, A., TARGHETTA, R. and LAROCHE, B. (1980) The antihypertensive effect of captopril – evidence for an influence of kinins. *Hypertension*, **2**, 732–737

MOORE, T. J., WILLIAMS, G. H., DLUHY, R. G., BAVLI, S. Z., HIMATHONGKAM, T. and GREENFIELD, M. (1977) Altered renin–angiotensin–aldosterone relationships in normal renin essential hypertension. *Circulation Research*, **41**, 167–171

OELKERS, W., BROWN, J. J., FRASER, R., LEVER, A. F., MORTON, J. J. and ROBERTSON, J. I. S. (1974) Sensitization of the adrenal cortex to angiotensin II in sodium-deplete man. *Circulation Research*, **34**, 69–77

OVERBECK, H. W., PAMNANI, M. B., AKERA, T., BRODY, T. M. and HADDY, F. J. (1976) Depressed function of an ouabain-sensitive sodium–potassium pump in blood vessels from renal hypertensive dogs. *Circulation Research*, **38** (Suppl.), 48–52

POSTON, L., SEWELL, R. B., WILKINSON, S. P. *et al.* (1981) Evidence for a circulating sodium transport inhibitor in essential hypertension. *British Medical Journal*, **282**, 847–849

SANCHO, J., RE, R., BURTON, J., BARGER, A. C. and HABER, E. (1976) The role of the renin–angiotensin–aldosterone system in cardiovascular homeostasis in normal human subjects. *Circulation*, **53**, 400–405

SAWYER, W. H., BLAIR-WEST, J. R., SIMPSON, P. A. and SAWYER, M. K. (1976) Renal responses of Australian lungfish to vasotocin, angiotensin II and NaCl infusion. *American Journal of Physiology*, **231**, 593–602

SHOBACK, D. M., WILLIAMS, G. H., HOLLENBERG, N. K., DAVIES, R. O., MOORE, T. J. and DLUHY, R. G. (1983a) Endogenous angiotensin II as a determinant of sodium modulated changes in tissue responsiveness to angiotensin II in normal man. *Journal of Clinical Endocrinology and Metabolism*, **57**, 764–770

SHOBACK, D. M., WILLIAMS, G. H., MOORE, T. J., DLUHY, R. G., PODOLSKY, S. and HOLLENBERG, N. K. (1983b) Defect in the sodium-modulated tissue responsiveness to angiotensin II in essential hypertension. *Journal of Clinical Investigation*, **72**, 2115–2124

SOKABE, H. (1974) Physiology of the renal effects of angiotensin. *Kidney International*, **6**, 263–271

SOKABE, H., MIZOGAME, S. and SATO, A. (1968) Role of renin in adaption to sea water in euryhaline fishes. *Japanese Journal of Pharmacology*, **18**, 332–343

STEELE, J. M. JR, NEUSY, A. J. and LOWENSTEIN, J. (1976) The effects of des-Asp[1]–angiotensin II on blood pressure, plasma aldosterone concentration, and plasma renin activity in the rabbit. *Circulation Research*, **38** (Suppl II), II-113–II-116

STREETEN, D. H. P. and ANDERSON, G. H. (1977) Angiotensin blockade in hypertension. *Annals of Internal Medicine*, **86**, 353–354

STREWLER, G. J., HINRICHS, K. J., GUIOD, L. R. and HOLLENBERG, N. K. (1972) Sodium intake and vascular smooth muscle responsiveness to norepinephrine and angiotensin in the rabbit. *Circulation Research*, **31**, 758–766

SWARTZ, S. L., WILLIAMS, G. H., HOLLENBERG, N. K., DLUHY, R. G. and MOORE, T. J. (1980) Primacy of the renin–angiotensin system in mediating the aldosterone response to sodium restriction. *Journal of Clinical Endocrinology and Metabolism*, **50**, 1071–1074

TAKEDA, R., MORIMOTO, S., UCHIDA, K., MIYAMORI, I. and HASHIBA, T. (1980) Effect of age on plasma aldosterone response to exogenous angiotensin II in normotensive subjects. *Acta Endocrinologica*, **94**, 552–558

TARAZI, R. C., FROHLICH, E. D. and DUSTAN, H. P. (1968) Plasma volume in men with hypertension. *New England Journal of Medicine*, **278**, 762–769

TAYLOR, T. T., MOORE, T. J., HOLLENBERG, N. K. and WILLIAMS, G. H. (1984) Converting enzyme inhibition corrects the altered adrenal response to angiotensin II in essential hypertension. *Hypertension*, **6**, 92–99

TUCK, M. L., WILLIAMS, G. H., CAIN, J. P., SULLIVAN, J. M. and DLUHY, R. G. (1973) Relation of age, diastolic pressure and known duration of hypertension to the presence of low renin essential hypertension. *American Journal of Cardiology*, **32**, 637–642

TUCK, M. L., WILLIAMS, G. H., DLUHY R. G. et al. (1976) A delayed suppression of the renin–aldosterone axis following saline infusion in human hypertension. *Circulation Research*, **39**, 711–717

VINSON, G. P., WHITEHOUSE, B. J., GODDARD, C. and SIBLEY, C. P. (1979) Comparative and evolutionary aspects of aldosterone secretion and zona glomerulosa function. *Journal of Endocrinology*, **81**, 5P–24P

WILLIAMS, G. H. and BRALEY, L. M. (1977) Effects of dietary sodium and potassium intake and acute stimulation on aldosterone output by isolated human adrenal cells. *Journal of Clinical Endocrinology and Metabolism*, **45**, 55–64

WILLIAMS, G. H. and HOLLENBERG, N. K. (1977) Accentuated vascular and endocrine response to SQ 20881 in hypertension. *New England Journal of Medicine*, **297**, 184–188

WILLIAMS, G. H., HOLLENBERG, N. K. and BRALEY, L. M. (1976) Influence of sodium intake on vascular and adrenal angiotensin II receptors. *Endocrinology*, **98**, 1343–1350

WILLIAMS, G. H., HOLLENBERG, N. K., BROWN, C. and MERSEY, J. H. (1978) Adrenal responses to pharmacological interruption of the renin–angiotensin system in sodium restricted normal man. *Journal of Clinical Endocrinology and Metabolism*, **47**, 725–731

WILLIAMS, G. H., HOLLENBERG, N. K., MOORE, T. J., SWARTZ, S. L. and DLUHY, R. G. (1979) The adrenal receptor for AII is altered in essential hypertension. *Journal of Clinical Investigation*, **63**, 419–427

WILLIAMS, G. H., ROSE, L. I. and DLUHY, R. G. *et al.* (1970) Abnormal responsiveness of the renin–aldosterone system to acute stimulation in patients with essential hypertension. *Annals of Internal Medicine*, **72**, 317–326

WILLIAMS, G. H., TUCK, M. L., SULLIVAN, J. M., DLUHY, R. G. and HOLLENBERG, N. K. (1982) Parallel adrenal and renal abnormalities in the young patient with essential hypertension. *American Journal of Medicine*, **72**, 907–914

8

The endothelium in hypertension

Michael J. Peach and Harold A. Singer

ENDOTHELIAL CHANGES IN HYPERTENSION

There is extensive evidence of endothelial injury documented by morphological and functional changes in large and small arteries in experimental hypertension. Most of the initial studies on endothelium were based on changes in the permeability of the endothelium in small vessels induced by an acute hypertensive episode during administration of a variety of vasopressor agents. These studies have consistently demonstrated an association between hypertension and increased permeability with evidence of endothelial damage (Giacomelli, Anversa and Wiener, 1976; Giese, 1973; Goldby and Beilin, 1972a and b; Robertson and Khairallah, 1973). Based on the fact that increased endothelial permeability occurred in small arteries and arterioles regardless of the means by which acute hypertension was induced, Goldby and Beilin (1972b) proposed that injury resulted from a pressure load which exceeded the physical limits of endothelial junctions. However, the possibility that the endothelium undergoes myogenic or receptor-mediated contraction does exist. In animals with chronic hypertension, changes in endothelial morphology and permeability have also been extensively documented (Giacomelli, Wiener and Spiro, 1970; Gabbiani, Badonnel and Rona, 1975; Hüttner et al., 1973; Jellinek et al., 1969; Majack and Bhalla, 1980; Still and Dannison, 1974; Wiener et al., 1969). Studies in chronic models of hypertension have focused primarily on large arteries such as the aorta or mesenteric artery.

In the early phases (hours to 7 days) of experimental hypertension induced by aortic ligature (Daniel et al., 1983; Hüttner et al., 1982), renal artery stenosis (Daniel et al., 1982; Hüttner et al., 1982; Schwartz and Benditt, 1977), intravenous angiotensin II (Reidy and Schwartz, 1982), or deoxycorticosterone acetate and sodium chloride (Hüttner et al., 1982), endothelial cell replication is increased several-fold. This hyperplasia of the endothelium is thought to be a response to injury which results from the sudden rise in blood pressure. In vascular areas distal to an experimental stenosis, injury and endothelial proliferation do not occur (Daniel et al., 1983; Hüttner et al., 1982). Schwartz and Lombardi (1982) could not demonstrate increased endothelial replication in the spontaneously hypertensive rat except when pressure rose rapidly after discontinuation of antihypertensive drugs in rats at 6–7 months of age. It is difficult to interpret these results but it is possible that the antihypertensive agents act directly to prevent the production of endothelial growth factors. However, the increase in blood pressure that occurred when drugs were discontinued in the spontaneously hypertensive (SHR) rat would be expected to induce cell replication. Endothelial proliferation in these models of hypertension usually occurred without evidence for desquamation of the endothelium in regions with thymidine labelling.

In established hypertension of several weeks' duration, endothelial cells are not replicating at an accelerated rate (Daniel *et al.*, 1982, 1983; Hüttner *et al.*, 1982; Schwartz and Lombardi, 1982). The data suggest that by the chronic (weeks) stage of hypertension an adaptation has occurred and continued high replication rates for endothelium are no longer required to maintain the endothelial cell population of conduit and muscular arteries. Part of this adaptive change with sustained hypertension appears to be due to hypertrophy of the endothelial cell layer with thickening of the internal elastic lamina (Haudenschild, Prescott and Chobanian, 1980; Hüttner *et al.*, 1982). Hypertension is also associated with an increase in the height of endothelial cells and prominent distortion of the nuclear shape such that cellular protrusions into the lumen are more prevalent (Haudenschild, Prescott and Chobanian, 1980; Svendsen and Tindall, 1981). Accompanying the hypertrophic changes is an increase in endothelial cell volume and an increase in the number of tight junctions among lateral endothelial membrane surfaces (Hüttner *et al.*, 1982). Endothelial gap junction morphology appears to be abnormal in arteries from animals with chronic elevations in blood pressure.

Thus acute hypertension is associated with a change in endothelial permeability and cell proliferation; while chronic hypertension, with hypertrophy of the endothelium, increased the incidence of homocellular tight junctions among endothelial cells and modification of gap junctions. In many cases these changes in the endothelium were shown in the same vessel with all species and in all forms of experimental hypertension. However, several observations remain to be extended to small arteries and arterioles with a variety of species and hypertensive models. As studies proceed in these areas, the problem created by sampling among vascular beds and order (size) of artery or arteriole must be carefully considered.

When the endothelium is removed, arterial smooth muscle cells respond by migrating into the intima and by accelerated replication of muscle cells throughout the vessel wall (Reidy and Schwartz, 1981; Schwartz, Stemerman and Benditt, 1975; Spath *et al.*, 1975). Injury-induced myointimal thickening has been attributed to a variety of growth-promoting factors which are felt to be derived from platelets and monocytes which attach at the site of injury, as well as blood-borne mitogens which evoke cell proliferation (Friedman, Stemerman and Wenz, 1977; Heldin, Westermark and Wasteson, 1979; Ross, 1981). The endothelial cell itself is known to affect growth and proliferation of the smooth muscle in the arterial wall. Studies with co-culture of the endothelium and smooth muscle or the culture of vascular smooth muscle in 'conditioned-medium' from endothelium indicate that the endothelium can promote or inhibit replication of smooth muscle cells (Davies and

Kerr, 1982; Gajdusek and Schwartz, 1982). Further studies are required to determine if growth status of the endothelium determines whether the endothelial cells release factors which promote or arrest smooth muscle growth. Reidy (personal communication) has shown recently that vascular segments with the endothelium removed for long periods of time develop spasm. It is tempting to speculate that comparable situations of endothelial desquamation and repair underlie conditions of arterial spasm (for example, Raynaud's disease, Prinzmetal variant angina, transient cerebral ischemia). Of course, well beyond the scope of this chapter is the enormous amount of research activity which focuses on the role of endothelial injury and arterial smooth muscle proliferation in the development of atherosclerotic lesions (Ross, 1981).

In the face of cellular hypertrophy, altered cell-to-cell contacts, elevated pressure, and altered blood levels of vasoactive substances at the intimal surface, the endothelium is a prime candidate for the modulation of arterial smooth muscle contractile activity. In addition to well-accepted functions relating to hemostasis, thrombosis and atherosclerosis, the endothelial cell may play an important role in modulating or mediating responses to a variety of vasopressor and vasodepressor substances. Consideration of these endothelium-dependent responses is presented in the following sections.

MODULATION OF VASCULAR RESPONSES VIA METABOLIC ACTIVITY

Biogenic amine uptake and metabolism

Uptake and inactivation of biogenic amines was perhaps the first modulatory role described for vascular endothelium. This has been shown most clearly in the pulmonary circulation where serotonin (Gaddum *et al.*, 1953; Junod, 1972) and norepinephrine (Ginn and Vane, 1968; Hughes, Gillis and Bloom, 1979) are partially removed from the circulation and biotransformed. The uptake process has been determined by autoradiography to reside in the endothelium of pulmonary capillaries (Hughes, Gillis and Bloom, 1969; Iwasawa, Gillis and Aghajanian, 1973) as well as endothelial cells of larger arteries (Shepro *et al.*, 1975; Strum and Junod, 1972).

Metabolism of vasoactive peptides

The pulmonary circulation has been shown to inactivate bradykinin (Ferreira and Vane, 1967a) and activate the decapeptide, angiotensin I, by conversion to the octapeptide, angiotensin II (Ng and Vane, 1967; Ryan *et al.*, 1970). Both of these metabolic responses have been shown to be mediated by the same dipeptidyl carboxypeptidase which has been purified from porcine (Dorer *et al.*, 1974) and rabbit (Das and Soffer, 1975; Tsai and Peach, 1977) pulmonary tissue. Similar 'converting enzyme' activities are found in plasma (Skeggs, Kahn and Shumway, 1956), vascular beds such as the mesenteric arcade (DiSalvo and Montefusco,

1971), and isolated vascular tissues such as rabbit aortic strips (Ackerly, Tsai and Peach, 1977; Velletri and Bean, 1982). Since plasma-converting enzyme activity cannot account quantitatively for the rate of angiotensin II production from angiotensin I in blood or buffer perfused lungs (Ng and Vane, 1967; Ryan *et al.*, 1970), and there is no evidence of angiotensin uptake by the lung (Ryan *et al.*, 1970), converting enzyme was hypothesized to be localized on the luminal surface of vascular endothelium. This was proven with pure cultures of pulmonary and umbilical artery endothelium from a number of species (Ryan *et al.*, 1976), including human (Johnson and Erdos, 1977). Converting enzyme was localized to the endothelial cell plasma membrane and alveoli using converting enzyme antibodies with immunohistochemical and immunofluorescent techniques for identification (Ryan *et al.*, 1976). Other cell types such as vascular smooth muscle and fibroblasts were shown to have little enzymatic activity (Johnson and Erdos, 1977). Studies of this type have led to the general acceptance that converting enzyme is a marker protein for endothelial cells.

Adenine nucleotide and adenosine uptake and metabolism

Adenosine triphosphate (ATP) has been shown to be removed from perfusate by the rat lung (Smith and Ryan, 1970). Metabolism of ATP to adenosine (presumably extracellular) has been demonstrated in porcine pulmonary and aortic endothelial cells in culture (Dieterle *et al.*, 1978). Adenosine was taken up by endothelial cells in culture (Dieterle *et al.*, 1978; Pearson *et al.*, 1978). The uptake process was of high affinity ($K_m = 3 \mu M$), saturable, temperature and energy dependent, and inhibited by dipyridamole (Dieterle *et al.*, 1978; Pearson *et al.*, 1978). Pearson and Gordon (1979) have shown that endothelial and smooth muscle cells in culture selectively release adenine nucleotides (ATP, ADP, AMP) in response to mechanical disruption or exposure to trypsin and thrombin. Most of the released nucleotide was apparently degraded by the cells and recovered as adenosine.

HORMONE-REGULATED ENDOTHELIAL RESPONSES

In addition to metabolizing and sequestering circulating vasoactive substances there is evidence that endothelial cells possess specific hormonal receptors which mediate responses that are ultimately capable of stimulating or modulating smooth muscle cell functions. One example of this is the acetylcholine-induced relaxation which is apparently dependent on endothelium (Furchgott and Zawadzki, 1980). Similar observations have subsequently been made with ATP-, bradykinin-, substance P- and thrombin-induced relaxation of isolated arterial segments (Furchgott, 1983).

Acetylcholine

Acetylcholine has been recognized since the early 1900s as a vasodilator when studied *in vivo*. However, when studied on isolated vascular segments, investigators universally found that acetylcholine was a vasoconstrictor substance. This *in vivo* vs. *in vitro* paradox for cholinergic responses remained until 1980. In helically cut rabbit aortic strips, Furchgott (1953) originally observed dose-dependent contractions in response to acetylcholine (10^{-7}–10^{-5} M) which were atropine-sensitive and variable in magnitude among different preparations, eliciting 10–45% of maximum norepinephrine-induced contractile responses. In strips precontracted to a 'moderate' degree with norepinephrine, only additional contractile responses were elicited by acetylcholine administration (10^{-10}–10^{-5} M). Until 1980, with only a single exception, relaxations were never observed in *in vitro* studies of vascular responses to muscarinic agonists. Jeliffe (1962), using a chain of transversely cut rabbit aortic rings, observed that acetylcholine induced both a contraction of rings studied at resting tension and a relaxation of rings which were precontracted by serotonin. The acetylcholine ED_{50} for contraction was approximately $5\,\mu$M whereas the relaxation response was evoked by lower concentrations (5–500 nM). In precontracted rings larger concentrations of acetylcholine (>500 nM) reversed the relaxation and net increments in force development were observed.

The discrepancy between these studies has only recently been addressed by Furchgott and Zawadzki (1980) when it was demonstrated that the vasodilator response in rabbit aorta was indirectly mediated by an action of acetylcholine (muscarinic) which was dependent on an intimal structure, presumably the endothelial cell. Careful preparation of transversely cut rabbit aortic rings, or helically cut strips, resulted in an intact relaxation in response to acetylcholine (10^{-8}–10^{-6} M) when the preparations were precontracted by moderate concentrations of a different contractile agonist such as norepinephrine or elevated extracellular potassium. Higher concentrations of acetylcholine (>10^{-6} M) elicited dose-dependent contractions. Both the constrictor and dilator responses were blocked by atropine. Mechanical (rubbing the intimal surface with filter paper) or enzymatic (collagenase) disruption of the intimal surface abolished only the relaxation component of the acetylcholine response. Thus, the failure to observe relaxation in response to acetylcholine in previous studies (Fuchgott, 1953) was attributed to inadvertent disruption of the endothelium during preparation of the helically cut aortic strips.

This apparent endothelial lability or fragility explained many of the discrepancies in acetylcholine vasoactive effects observed *in vitro* when compared to *in vivo* or *in situ* preparations where the vascular integrity is ensured (Chand and Altura, 1981; DeMey and Vanhoutte, 1981). These studies also demonstrate that in addition to an intact endothelium some degree of active tone must be present in a blood vessel in order to see relaxant effects of acetylcholine. While this seems to be an obvious prerequisite, several investigators have overlooked vascular tone in their attempts to interpret vascular responses to vasoactive substances.

Adenine nucleotides

The potent vasodepressor activity of adenine compounds such as adenosine, ADP and ATP has been recognized for many years (Bennet and Drury, 1931; Folkow,

1949). Both vasodilatation and vasoconstriction in response to ATP have subsequently been observed in a variety of *in vitro* preparations including rabbit aorta (Furchgott, 1966). However, it is generally accepted that the principal action of adenine nucleotides and adenosine is one of vasodilatation in most vascular preparations (Burnstock, 1972; Haddy and Scott, 1968). Following Furchgott's observations on the endothelial dependence of acetylcholine-induced relaxation, DeMey and Vanhoutte (1981) demonstrated that the relaxing properties of ATP and ADP in isolated rings of canine femoral artery are also markedly dependent upon the presence of an intact endothelium. Endothelial disruption in this tissue reduced the potency of ATP and ADP ($ED_{50} = 10^{-5}$ M) for relaxation to a level comparable to that of AMP and adenosine ($ED_{50} = 3 \times 10^{-4}$ M). Adenosine and AMP potencies were independent of endothelial integrity. Since relaxation in response to ATP or ADP was not inhibited by treatment with theophylline, these nucleotides were most likely acting directly on the endothelium to simulate release of factor(s) analogous to those produced following administration of acetylcholine (Furchgott and Zawadzki, 1980). Alternatively, a direct coupling, mediated by cell-to-cell conduction between endothelial and smooth muscle cells, has been hypothesized (DeMey and Vanhoutte, 1981). To date, vasodilation with acetylcholine or ATP and ADP in all species and arteries requires the presence of endothelium.

Other hormones

Bradykinin, angiotensin II, substance P, thrombin and histamine have all been shown to induce endothelium-dependent relaxation of arterial smooth muscle (*see* Furchgott, 1983). The results reported with these hormones are often from studies which were done in a single vessel type obtained from only one or two species. Nevertheless, it is quite obvious that the arterial endothelium plays a major role in the transduction of the signal from circulating vasodilator hormones to arterial smooth muscle. The exceptions to endothelium-dependent vasodilatation appear to represent endogenous compounds which directly activate smooth muscle adenylate cyclase (such as epinephrine and prostacyclin) and adenosine or 5′AMP whose direct mechanisms of action on muscle remain controversial.

Pharmacological agents

Among vasodilating drugs only hydralazine has been shown to demonstrate endothelium-dependent vasodilation (Spokas *et al.*, 1983). In these studies, hydralazine induced relaxation responses which were partially attenuated by removal of the endothelium in the thoracic aorta.

MEDIATORS OF ENDOTHELIUM-DEPENDENT VASODILATATION

It is clear that one important and potentially hormone-regulated endothelial function is the metabolism and production of arachidonic acid derivatives.

Perfusion of prostaglandins E_1, E_2 or $F_{2\alpha}$ (PGE_1, PGE_2, $PGF_{2\alpha}$) through the pulmonary circulation results in their degradation and loss of biological activity (Ferreira and Vane, 1967b; Piper, Vane and Wyllie, 1970). The efficiency of this process (>90% degradation in a single passage) suggests that these prostaglandins are not important as circulating hormones in the regulation of peripheral resistance. On the other hand, angiotensin II-stimulated release of prostaglandins in the renal (McGiff *et al.*, 1970), coronary (Needleman, Marshall and Sobel, 1975) and mesenteric (Blumberg *et al.*, 1977a and b) vascular beds may be important in the local modulation of vasoactive responses. Locally generated prostaglandins in response to bradykinin (Blumberg *et al.*, 1977b) and norepinephrine (Greglewski and Korbut, 1975) seem capable of modulating vascular responses to these agents as well. The vasodilator substances produced in response to these hormones resembled PGE_2 chromatographically and in ability to vasodilate or antagonize the vasoconstriction elicited by these stimuli. The role of endothelium as a potential source of the prostaglandin was not investigated. However, Gimbrone and Alexander (1975) demonstrated release of a PGE-like substance in response to angiotensin II from cultures of human umbilical vein endothelium grown in monolayer culture.

Prostacylin production by endothelium

It seems likely now that much of the PGE-like vasodilator activity released in response to contractile stimuli may actually be prostacyclin (Moncada and Vane, 1978). Prostacyclin (PGI_2) is an arachidonic acid metabolite originally isolated as a product of prostaglandin endoperoxide conversion by segments or homogenates of arteries (Bunting *et al.*, 1976; Moncada *et al.*, 1976). The two principal actions of PGI_2 are potent platelet anti-aggregatory activity (Moncada *et al.*, 1976) and vasodilation (Bunting *et al.*, 1976; Moncada and Vane, 1978). Using assay and chromatographic techniques which distinguished PGE_2 and PGI_2, Dusting, Mullins and Nolan (1981) demonstrated that angiotensin II stimulated release of PGI_2 in the rat mesenteric vasculature. Similarly, bradykinin and angiotensin were found to stimulate release of PGI_2 from blood-perfused vascular beds in the dog (Mullane and Moncada, 1980).

Prostacyclin production by human umbilical vein and bovine aortic endothelial cells in culture was first demonstrated by Weksler, Marcus and Jaffe (1977). This suggested that the PGE-like material released in response to angiotensin II in cultured endothelium, previously observed by Gimbrone and Alexander (1975), was in fact PGI_2 which was established by Puré and Needleman (1979). Subsequently, PGI_2 production was shown to be stimulated by thrombin, trypsin, and the calcium ionophore A23187 in cultured endothelial cells (Weksler, Ley and Jaffe, 1978). Bradykinin (10^{-10}–10^{-8}M), A23187, trypsin, and exogenous arachidonic acid were observed by Hong (1980) to stimulate PGI_2 production in cultures of calf and human endothelial cells. Human umbilical vein fibroblasts (Baenziger, Dillender and Majerus, 1977; Weksler, Ley and Jaffe, 1978) and smooth muscle (Baenziger, Dillender and Majerus, 1977) have also been shown to have the biosynthetic capacity to produce PGI_2.

Production of PGI_2 by fibroblasts and smooth muscle has been confirmed in rat aortic explant cultures (Tansik, Namm and White, 1978) and rabbit aorta (Moncada *et al.*, 1977). However, the relative contribution of the endothelium, which represents only 5% of the total cellular mass in rabbit aorta, to total PGI_2 production by isolated rabbit aorta was estimated to be 40% (Moncada *et al.*, 1977). The concept of the endothelium as a principal source of PGI_2 has been confirmed in rabbit aorta which had been de-endothelialized by *in vivo* balloon catheterization (Eldor *et al.*, 1981). In the hours immediately after catheterization, PGI_2 production by isolated aortic segments was reduced to background. However, over a period of 2–70 days, the ability of the aorta to synthesize PGI_2 recovered, coincident with the proliferation of subendothelial, neo-intimal smooth muscle cells.

Potential mechanisms of acetylcholine-dependent vasodilatation

A potential mechanism of action for acetylcholine as a relaxing agonist in intact arterial tissue involves the Ca^{2+} dependent activation of endothelial phospholipases with subsequent release and metabolism of arachidonic acid. Muscarinic responses such as contraction in smooth muscle (Fay and Singer, 1977) or secretion in exocrine cells (Douglas, 1968; Poulsen and Williams, 1977) are generally accepted as being mediated by increases in intracellular Ca^{2+}. Phospholipases, especially phospholipase A_2, appear in many tissues to be activated in a Ca^{2+}-dependent manner by specific hormonal stimuli (Flower and Blackwell, 1976; Hong and Deykin, 1979; Kennerly, Sullivan and Parker, 1979) or by the Ca^{2+} ionophore A23187 (Borgeat and Samuelsson, 1979; Pickett, Jesse and Cohen, 1977; Weksler, Ley and Jaffe, 1978). There is also evidence that the Ca^{2+} sensitivity of phospholipase A_2 is conferred by the ubiquitous Ca^{2+}-binding protein calmodulin (Cheung, 1980; Walenga, Opas and Feinstein, 1981; Wong and Cheung, 1979). This mechanism of action may explain the stimulation of PGI_2 production by stimuli such as angiotensin (Dusting, Mallins and Nolan, 1981) and A23187 (Hong, 1980; Weksler, Ley and Jaffe, 1978) which are known to be dependent upon Ca^{2+} in other systems (Ackerly, Moore and Peach, 1977; Garrison *et al.*, 1979; Pressman, 1976).

As a first approach to examining the Ca^{2+}-dependence of the endothelium-mediated relaxation, the Ca^{2+} ionophore A23187 was characterized as a pharmacological probe. A23187 was found to initiate relaxations which appeared to be qualitatively similar to acetylcholine-induced relaxations in terms of time-course, magnitude, and endothelial dependence (Singer and Peach, 1982). The A23187 ED_{50} of relaxation was $8 \times 10^{-8} M$, a value comparable to or lower than most other reported A23187-induced biological responses. A23187 exerted negligible contractile activity in intact vascular rings or de-endothelialized rings over the concentration range effective for dilation (10^{-8}–$10^{-6} M$).

We also found that cholinergic vasodilators were not additive to responses induced by A23187, suggesting that both agents work via an identical mechanism. A23187 proved to be a useful probe of the relaxation pathway which bypassed the initial muscarinic agonist–receptor interaction normally required to initiate the response.

The results with A23187 clearly implicated Ca^{2+} in the initiation of the intimal-dependent vasodilation. To confirm this, the effects of Ca^{2+}-deletion from the incubation buffer, and Ca^{2+}-channel blocking agents on both cholinergic-induced and A23187-induced relaxation of intact aortic rings, were determined. Since both contraction and relaxation appeared to be Ca^{2+}-dependent and the production and bioassay of the relaxing factor(s) was in the same tissue, manipulating endothelial Ca^{2+} availability was complicated by simultaneous effects on smooth muscle contractility. Therefore, in the case of Ca^{2+} depletion, exposure to buffers deficient in Ca^{2+} was brief.

It was clear from the results of these experiments that the relaxing activities of both muscarinic agonists and A23187 were markedly dependent upon extracellular calcium. The inhibitory effects of Ca^{2+} removal were observed to be reversible, indicating that the effect of this treatment was not due to damage or loss of endothelium.

Because of difficulties in interpreting the precise cellular events altered by Ca^{2+}-depletion the effects of Ca^{2+}-channel antagonists were assessed under conditions of normal Ca^{2+} concentration. Verapamil and nifedipine are well-known antagonists of voltage-sensitive Ca^{2+} channels in cardiac and vascular smooth muscle tissue (Fleckenstein, 1977; Triggle and Swamy, 1980). Both Ca^{2+} blockers inhibited endothelium-dependent vasodilation responses.

Three lines of evidence directly support a role for Ca^{2+} in mediating or regulating the endothelium-dependent relaxation evoked by acetylcholine:

(1) extracellular Ca^{2+} depletion inhibits the cholinergic-induced relaxation;
(2) the calcium ionophore, A23187, induces similar Ca^{2+}-dependent relaxation;
(3) two Ca^{2+} channel blockers, nifedipine and verapamil, can inhibit both acetylcholine-induced and A23187-induced relaxations.

It should be pointed out that the vasodilation response is much more sensitive to Ca^{2+} blockers than is the contractile activity of vascular smooth muscle. Therefore, low blood concentrations of Ca^{2+} blocker might actually increase peripheral resistance.

Prostacyclin, the cyclo-oxygenase product of arachidonic acid and potent vasodilator, seemed to be a likely candidate as the mediator of acetylcholine-induced or ATP-induced vascular relaxation since it is thought to be principally derived from endothelium. However, the reports by Furchgott and Zawadzki (1980) and DeMey and Vanhoutte (1980) indicated that cyclo-oxygenase inhibitors such as indomethacin and acetylsalicylic acid were without effect on the endothelium-dependent cholinergic-induced and adenine nucleotide-stimulated relaxations. Thus it seems improbable that PGI_2 is the mediator of the cholinergic or ATP response. On the other hand, the acetylenic analog of arachidonic acid, 5,8,11,14-eicosatraynoic acid (ETYA), which is reported to be an irreversible cyclo-oxygense inhibitor (Downing, Ahern and Bachta, 1970; Flower, 1974; Hamberg and Samuelsson, 1974), was effective in reversing the acetylcholine-induced relaxation (Furchgott, 1983; Furchgott and Zawadzki, 1980).

Lipoxygenase metabolites of arachidonic acid

The enzyme lipoxygenase hydroxylates arachidonic acid via unstable hydro-peroxy-intermediates (hydroperoxyeicosatetraenoic acid, HPETE) in a manner analogous to the formation of the endoperoxides PGG_2 and PGH_2 by the cyclo-oxygenase-pathway. The position of the hydroxylation(s) appears to depend upon the source of lipoxygenase.

HETEs and HPETEs have been shown to elicit biological effects. Different isomers of HETE have chemotactic properties for neutrophils and eosinophils (Goetzl and Sun, 1979; Goetzl, Wellar and Sun, 1980). Production of chemotactic agents may account for the attraction of lymphocytes to areas of the intimal surface which have been damaged. HETEs and their HPETE intermediates formed from long-chain unsaturated fatty acids by soybean lipoxidase acted in a dose-dependent manner as contractile agonists in rabbit aortic strips (Asano and Hidaka, 1979). Interestingly, lipoxygenase activity has been detected in isolated rabbit aortic rings on the basis of arachidonic acid conversion to HETE (Greenwald, Bianchine and Wong, 1979). The position of the hydroxyl on the fatty acid was not determined in this study. Recently, a group of lipoxygenase products of arachidonic acid termed 'leukotrienes' has been discovered and seems to represent the slow-reacting substance of anaphylaxis (SRS-A) activity produced and released by various mast cells, basophils, and leukocytes (Borgeat and Samuelsson, 1979; Murphy, Hammarstrom and Samuelsson, 1979; Hammarstrom, Murphy and Samuelsson, 1979). The principal effect of SRS-A on smooth muscle is known to be contractile (Hanna *et al.*, 1981). However, it seems unlikely that the full spectrum of lipoxygenase metabolites and biological activities has been discovered. There is clearly potential for metabolites analogous to the vasodilator products produced via the cyclo-oxygenase pathway.

Cyclo-oxygenase and lipoxygenase inhibition

Confirming earlier reports (Furchgott and Zawadzki, 1980), indomethacin was found to be without inhibitory effect on the relaxation stimulated by methacholine (Singer and Peach, 1983a and b). In addition, A23187-mediated relaxation was not affected by indomethacin pretreatment, confirming the similarity of the two relaxation responses. Since ETYA is known to have both cyclo-oxygenase and lipoxygenase inhibitory activity (Downing, Ahern and Bachta, 1970; Flower, 1974) inhibition by this agent of relaxation in response to both acetylcholine and A23187 implicates involvement of a lipoxygenase-derived product. This was substantiated with another inhibitor, nordihydroguariaretic acid (NDGA), which is reportedly specific for the lipoxygenase pathway (Hamberg, 1976; Goetzl, Wellar and Sun, 1980). Essentially complete blockade of both cholinergic-induced and A23187-induced relaxation was attained with NDGA.

None of the agents used to inhibit arachidonic acid release and metabolism provide convincing evidence of arachidonate involvement in the endothelium-dependent relaxation process when considered individually. The interpretation of these inhibitory effects on relaxation evoked by acetylcholine, A23187, bradykinin, substance P, or thrombin would be simplified if the source and bioassay of the active relaxing material of endothelial origin could be separated. Until this is accomplished, or the material is identified and measured directly, the sites of action of inhibitors such as quinacrine, ETYA or NDGA (in other words, production of, versus sensitivity to, the relaxing factors) cannot be determined with assurance. Though interpretations of the data described above are limited because of this, collectively there is clearly enough evidence to justify the hypothesis that an oxidative metabolite of arachidonic acid mediates the Ca^{2+}-dependent and presumably endothelium-dependent arterial relaxation evoked by a variety of endogenous substances.

Because of the following observations we were not convinced that the formation of the endothelial factor requires phospholipase A_2 activation, arachidonic acid or lipoxygenase:

(1) Steroids known to block phospholipase A_2 do not impair cholinergic vasodilator responses either *in vivo* or *in vitro*.
(2) While arachidonate itself can stimulate endothelium-dependent relaxation (Singer and Peach, 1983a) other unsaturated fatty acids may also elicit this response (Furchgott, 1983).
(3) Not all lipoxygenase inhibitors block cholinergic-induced vascular relaxation.
(4) The doses of ETYA and NDGA required to inhibit vasodilation are in vast excess of the known K_i values for these agents and lipoxygenase.
(5) The production of dilator is exquisitely sensitive to a reduction in Po_2 which suggests the involvement of an oxygenase with a poor K_m for oxygen.

In the search for such an enzyme we were impressed by the cytochrome P_{450} mono-oxygenases. Cytochrome P_{450} has a low affinity for O_2, oxidizes fatty acids (Morrison and Pascoe, 1981; Oliw, Guengerich and Oates, 1982) and is blocked by ETYA but requires high concentrations (Capdevila *et al.*, 1981). While little is known about cytochrome P_{450} in blood vessels, its activity has been detected in homogenates of aorta (Juchau, Bond and Benditt, 1976) and cultured bovine aortic endothelium (Baird *et al.*, 1980). Cytochrome P_{450} isozymes detected by immunocytochemistry have been induced in the endothelium of renal, hepatic and pulmonary arteries of rabbits (Dees *et al.*, 1982). We have recently reported that inhibitors of cytochrome P_{450} block endothelium-dependent vasodilation in rabbit aorta (Singer, Saye and Peach, 1984).

ENDOTHELIUM AND HYPERTENSION

It should be obvious that the metabolic role played by the endothelium directly influences the concentration(s) of blood materials which reach the arterial smooth muscle. As described above, endothelial uptake and enzymatic activities (such as monoamine oxidase, converting enzyme, 5'-nucleotidase, ATPases and cytochrome P_{450}) present a significant barrier between circulating endogenous substances or drugs and the media of the artery. Among these activities one finds that the endothelium protects the vessel wall from low concentrations of most low molecular weight, diffusible substances, regardless of whether or not the hormone or autacoid is a vasopressor or depressor substance. With the exceptions of adenosine and epinephrine, endogenous substances released into the blood stream under physiological circumstances which dictate a reduction in blood pressure or an increase in blood flow appear to act indirectly and rely heavily on the endothelium to produce and/or release either prostacyclin (PGI_2) or endothelium-dependent relaxing factor (EDRF). At the present time, little is known about the role of these substances in hypertension or whether their production (or release) is altered by changes in the intima associated with hypertension. It is known that rapidly dividing endothelial cells in culture do not synthesize PGI_2 but do release PGI_2, upon reaching confluency.

The requisite role played by converting enzyme in the plasma membrane of endothelial cells in the formation of angiotensin II has been well documented. With an increase in plasma renin activity, the efficiency of the conversion of angiotensin I to II depends exclusively on the vascular endothelial enzyme. Reviewing the vast literature on the renin–angiotensin system and primary and secondary hypertension should not be necessary. The renin–angiotensin system is involved in high renin forms of arterial hypertension, and activation of the system by diuretics or vasodilators certainly compromises the antihypertensive efficacy of such agents in the management of high blood pressure.

With regard to *in vitro* studies of vascular segments from hypertensive animals, very few studies have been performed in which the integrity of the endothelium was documented. Without assessment of the endothelium, no comments regarding its role are possible. In fact, variability of the endothelial content may account for the extreme variation of results obtained in *in vitro* studies of vasoactive agents. Konishi and Su (1984) have recently studied a series of vasodilators in rings of arteries with established endothelial integrity from the spontaneously hypertensive (SHR) rat. They found that in general the endothelium played a greater role in drug-induced relaxation of arteries from hypertensive than those from normotensive rats. Denudation of the endothelium also potentiated contractile responses to norepinephrine especially in the SHR rat. The results suggest that the endothelium of the SHR rat may modulate the reactivity of smooth muscle to circulating vasoactive agents.

Numerous studies have been published on isolated vessels, perfused organs and in intact animals which relied on indomethacin or aspirin to block endothelial PGI_2 synthesis. Such studies have reported potentiation of acute pressor responses to angiotensin II (Mullane and Moncada, 1980; Negus, Tannen and Dunn, 1976) as well as an increase in resting blood pressure (Anggard and Larsson, 1973; Colina-Chourio, McGiff and Nasjletti, 1979). Of course, comparable studies would be required with inhibitors of EDRF production (that is, ETYA or NDGA) to fully assess the impact of the endothelium on arterial pressure. We have reported that indomethacin treatment actually potentiates agents which promote the synthesis or release of EDRF (Singer and Peach, 1983b).

It has been proposed that PGI_2 plays a role in hypertension. In the SHR rat, PGI_2 synthesis is increased when compared to WKY normotensive control rats (Limas and Limas, 1977; Pace-Asciak *et al.*, 1978). These data have been the basis for the hypothesis that the increased PGI_2 synthesis in hypertension is secondary to the elevated blood pressure. In such cases PGI_2 synthesis would decrease the severity of the hypertension. Falardeau and Martineau (1983) have reported recently that PGI_2 synthesis was impaired in the salt-sensitive strain of Dahl rats during high sodium intake with associated hypertension. These investigators suggested that the defect in PGI_2 synthesis was causally related to the development of hypertension in the salt-sensitive Dahl rat. Axelrod (1983) has postulated that hypertension associated with glucocorticoid excess is mediated via inhibition of PGI_2 synthesis by the steroid. It is obvious that future studies are needed to understand the role of PGI_2 in arterial hypertension. Assessment of EDRF in arterial hypertension will depend on the identification of this material and on the development of techniques to isolate and quantify this factor.

References

ACKERLY, J. A., MOORE, A. F. and PEACH, M. J. (1977) Demonstration of different contractile mechanisms for angiotensin II and des-Asp[1]–angiotensin II in rabbit aortic strips. *Proceedings of the National Academy of Sciences of the USA*, **74**, 5725–5728

ACKERLY, J. A., TSAI, B. S. and PEACH, M. J. (1977) Role of converting enzyme in the responses of rabbit atria, aortas, and adrenal zona glomerulosa to [des-Asp[1]] angiotensin I. *Circulation Research*, **41**, 231–238

ANGGARD, E. and LARSSON, C. (1973) Arachidonic acid lowers and indomethacin increases the blood pressure of the rabbit. *Journal of Pharmacy and Pharmacology*, **25**, 653–655

ASANO, M. and HIDAKA, H. (1979) Contractile response of isolated rabbit aortic strips to unsaturated fatty acid peroxides. *Journal of Pharmacology and Experimental Therapeutics*, **208**, 347–353

AXELROD, L. (1983) Inhibition of prostacyclin production mediates the permissive effect of glucocorticoids on vascular tone. *Lancet*, **1**, 904–906

BAENZIGER, N. L., DILLENDER, M. J. and MAJERUS, P. W. (1977) Cultured human skin fibroblasts and arterial cells produce a labile platelet–inhibitory prostaglandin. *Biochemical Biophysical Research Communications*, **78**, 294–301

BAIRD, W. M., CHEMERYS, R., GRINSPAN, J. B., MUELLER, S. N. and LEVINE, E. M. (1980) Benzo (a) pyrene metabolism in bovine aortic endothelial and bovine lung fibroblast-like cell cultures. *Cancer Research*, **40**, 1781–1786

BENNET, D. W. and DRURY, A. N. (1931) Further observations relating to the physiologic activity of adenine compounds. *Journal of Physiology*, **72**, 288–320

BLUMBERG, A. L., NISHIKAWA, K., DENNY, S. E., MARSHALL, G. R. and NEEDLEMAN, P. (1977a) Angiotensin (AI, AII, AIII) receptor characterization. Correlation of prostaglandin release with peptide degradation. *Circulation Research*, **41**, 154–158

BLUMBERG, A. L., DENNY, S. E., MARSHALL, G. R. and NEEDLEMAN, P. (1977b) Blood vessel–hormone interactions: angiotensin, bradykinin and prostaglandins. *American Journal of Physiology*, **232**, H305–H310

BORGEAT, P. and SAMUELSSON, B. (1979) Arachidonic acid metabolism in polymorphonuclear leukocytes: effects of ionophore A23187. *Proceedings of the National Academy of Sciences of the USA*, **76**, 2148–2152

BUNTING, S., GRYGLEWSKI, R., MONCADA, S. and VANE, J. R. (1976) Arterial walls generate from prostaglandin endoperoxides a substance (prostaglandin X) which relaxes strips of mesenteric and coeliac arteries and inhibits platelet aggregation. *Prostaglandins*, **12**, 897–915

BURNSTOCK, G. (1972) Purinergic nerves. *Pharmacological Reviews*, **24**, 509–581

CAPDEVILA, J., CHACOS, N., WERRINGLOER, J., PROUGH, R. A. and ESTABROOK, R. W. (1981) Liver microsomal cytochrome P-450 and the oxidative metabolism of arachidonic acid. *Proceedings of the National Academy of Sciences of the USA*, **78**, 5362–5366

CHAND, N. and ALTURA, B. M. (1981) Acetylcholine and bradykinin relax intrapulmonary arteries by acting on endothelial cells: role in lung vascular diseases. *Science*, **213**, 1376–1379

CHEUNG, W. Y. (1980) Calmodulin plays a pivotal role in cellular regulation. *Science*, **207**, 19–27

COLINA-CHOURIO, J., MC GIFF, J. C. and NASJLETTI, A. (1979) Effect of indomethacin on blood pressure in the normotensive unanesthetized rabbit: possible relation to prostaglandin synthesis inhibition. *Clinical Science*, **57**, 359–365

DANIEL, R. E., BIOTNOTT, J. K., BROWN, G. D. and HEPTINSTALL, R. H. (1982) Aortic endothelial cell activity in high renin and normal renin models of hypertension in the rat. *Laboratory Investigation*, **47**, 451–458

DANIEL, R. E., BIOTNOTT, J. K., BROWN, G. D. and HEPINSTALL, R. H. (1983) Endothelial cell activity in experimental hypertension: effects of hemodynamic factors. *Laboratory Investigation*, **48**, 690–697

DAS, M. and SOFFER, R. L. (1975) Pulmonary angiotensin converting enzyme. *Journal of Biological Chemistry*, **250**, 6762–6768

DAVIES, P. F. and KERR, C. (1982) Co-cultivation of vascular endothelial and smooth muscle cells using microcarrier techniques. *Experimental Cell Research*, **141**, 455–459

DEES, J. H., MASTERS, B. S., MULLER-EBERHARD, U. and JOHNSON, E. F. (1982) Effect of 2,3,7,8-tetrachlorodibenzo-p-dioxin and phenobarbital on the occurrence and distribution of four cytochrome P-450 enzymes in rabbit kidney, lung and liver. *Cancer Research*, **42**, 1423–1432

DE MEY, J. G. and VANHOUTTE, P. M. (1980) Interaction between Na^+, K^+ exchanges and the direct inhibitor effect of acetylcholine on canine femoral arteries. *Circulation Research*, **46**, 826–836

DE MEY, J. G. and VANHOUTTE, P. M. (1981) Role of the intima in cholinergic and purinergic relaxation of isolated canine femoral arteries. *Journal of Physiology*, **316**, 347–355

DIETERLE, Y., ODY, C., EHRENSBERGER, A., STADLER, H. and JUNOD, A. F. (1978) Metabolism and uptake of adenosine triphosphate and adenosine by porcine aortic and pulmonary endothelial cells and fibroblasts in culture. *Circulation Research*, **42**, 869–876

DI SALVO, J. and MONTEFUSCO, C. B. (1971) Conversion of angiotensin I to angiotensin II in the canine mesenteric circulation. *American Journal of Physiology*, **221**, 1576–1579

DORER, F. E., KAHN, J. H., LENTZ, K. E., LEVINE, M. and SKEGGS, L. T. (1974) Hydrolysis of bradykinin by angiotensin-converting enzyme. *Circulation Research*, **34**, 824–827

DOUGLAS, W. W. (1968) Stimulus-secretion coupling: the concept and clues from chromaffin and other cells. *British Journal of Pharmacology*, **34**, 451–474

DOWNING, D. T., AHERN, D. G. and BACHTA, M. (1970) Enzyme inhibition by acetylenic compounds. *Biochemical Biophysical Research Communications*, **40**, 218–223

DUSTING, G. J., MULLINS, E. M. and NOLAN, R. D. (1981) Prostacyclin (PGI$_2$) release accompanying angiotensin conversion in rat mesenteric vasculature. *European Journal of Pharmacology*, **70**, 129–137

ELDOR, A., FALCONE, D. J., HAJJAR, D. P., MINICK, C. R. and WEKSLER, B. B. (1981) Recovery of prostacyclin production by de-endothelialized rabbit aorta. *Journal of Clinical Investigation*, **67**, 735–741

FALARDEAU, P. and MARTINEAU, A. (1983) *In vivo* production of prostaglandin I$_2$ in Dahl salt-sensitive and salt-resistant rats. *Hypertension*, **5**, 701–705

FAY, F. S. and SINGER, J. J. (1977) Characteristics of response of isolated smooth muscle cells to cholinergic drugs. *American Journal of Physiology*, **232**, C144–C154

FERREIRA, S. H. and VANE, J. R. (1967a) The disappearance of bradykinin and eledoisin in the circulation and vascular beds of the cat. *British Journal of Pharmacology*, **30**, 417–424

FERREIRA, S. H. and VANE, J. R. (1967b) Prostaglandins: their disappearance from and release into the circulation. *Nature*, **216**, 868–873

FLECKENSTEIN, A. (1977) Specific pharmacology of calcium in myocardium, cardiac pacemakers and vascular smooth muscle. *Annual Review of Pharmacology and Toxicology*, **17**, 149–166

FLOWER, R. J. (1974) Drugs which inhibit prostaglandin biosynthesis. *Pharmacological Reviews*, **26**, 33–65

FLOWER, R. J. and BLACKWELL, G. J. (1976) The importance of phospholipase-A$_2$ in prostaglandin biosynthesis. *Biochemical Pharmacology*, **25**, 285–291

FOLKOW, B. (1949) The vasodilator action of adenosine triphosphate. *Acta Physiologica Scandinavica*, **17**, 311–316

FRIEDMAN, R. J., STEMERMAN, M. B. and WENZ, B. (1977) The effect of thrombocytopenia on experimental atherosclerotic lesion formation in rabbits. Smooth muscle cell proliferation and re-endothelialization. *Journal of Clinical Investigation*, **60**, 1191–1201

FURCHGOTT, R. F. (1953) Reactions of strips of rabbit aorta to epinephrine, isoproterenol, sodium nitrate and other drugs. *Journal of Pharmacology and Experimental Therapeutics*, **108**, 129–143

FURCHGOTT, R. F. (1966) Metabolic factors that influence contractility of vascular smooth muscle. *Bulletin of New York Academy of Medicine*, **42**, 996–1006

FURCHGOTT, R. F. and ZAWADZKI, J. V. (1980) The obligatory role of endothelial cells in the relaxation of arterial smooth muscle by acetylcholine. *Nature*, **288**, 373–376

FURCHGOTT, R. (1983) Role of endothelium in responses of vascular smooth muscle. *Circulation Research*, **53**, 557–573

GABBIANI, G., BADONNEL, M. C. and RONA, G. (1975) Cytoplasmic contractile apparatus in aortic endothelial cells of hypertensive rats. *Laboratory Investigation*, **32**, 227–234

GADDUM, J. H., HEBB, C. D., SILVER, A. and SWAN, A. A. B. (1953) 5-Hydroxytryptamine. Pharmacological action and destruction in perfused lung. *Quarterly Journal of Experimental Physiology*, **38**, 255–262

GAJDUSEK, C. M. and SCHWARTZ, S. M. (1982) Ability of endothelial cells to condition culture medium. *Journal of Cellular Physiology*, **110**, 35–42

GARRISON, J. C., BORLAND, M. K., FLORIO, V. A. and TWIBLE, D. A. (1979) Role of calcium ions as a mediator of the effects of angiotensin, catecholamines, and vasopressin on the phosphorylation and activity of enzymes in isolated hepatocytes. *Journal of Biological Chemistry*, **254**, 7147–7156

GIACOMELLI, F., ANVERSA, P. and WIENER, J. (1976) Effect of angiotensin induced hypertension on rat coronary arteries and myocardium. *American Journal of Pathology*, **84**, 111–138

GIACOMELLI, F., WIENER, J. and SPIRO, D. (1970) The cellular pathology of experimental hypertension. V. Increased permeability of cerebral arterial vessels. *American Journal of Pathology*, **59**, 133–159

GIESE, J. (1973) Renin, angiotensin and hypertensive vascular damage: a review. *American Journal of Medicine*, **55**, 315–331

GIMBRONE, M. A. and ALEXANDER, R. W. (1975) Angiotensin II stimulation of prostaglandin production in cultured human vascular endothelium. *Science*, **189**, 219–220

GINN, R. W. and VANE, J. R. (1968) Disappearance of catecholamines from the circulation. *Nature (London)*, **219**, 740–742

GOETZL, E. J. and SUN, F. F. (1979) Generation of unique mono-hydroxy-eicosatetraenoic acids from arachidonic acid by human neutrophils. *Journal of Experimental Medicine*, **150**, 406–411

GOETZL, E. J., WELLAR, P. F. and SUN, F. F. (1980) The regulation of human eosinophil function by endogenous mono-hydroxy-eicosatetraenoic acids (HETEs). *Journal of Immunology*, **124**, 926–933

GOLDBY, F. S. and BEILIN, L. J. (1972a) Relationship between arterial pressure and the permeability of arterioles to carbon particles in acute hypertension in the rat. *Cardiovascular Research*, **6**, 384–390

GOLDBY, F. S. and BEILIN, L. J. (1972b) How an acute rise in arterial pressure damages arterioles. *Cardiovascular Research*, **6**, 569–584

GREENWALD, J. E., BIANCHINE, J. R. and WONG, L. K. (1979) The production of the arachidonate metabolite HETE in vascular tissue. *Nature (London)*, **281**, 588–589

GREGLEWSKI, R. J. and KORBUT, R. (1975) Prostaglandin feedback mechanism limits vasoconstrictor action of norepinephrine in perfused rabbit ear. *Experientia*, **31**, 89–91

HADDY, F. J. and SCOTT, J. B. (1968) Metabolically linked vasoactive chemicals in local regulation of blood flow. *Physiological Reviews*, **48**, 688–707

HAMBERG, M. (1976) On the formation of thromboxane B_2 and 12L-hydroxy-5,8,10, 14-eicosatetraenoic acid (12 ho-20:4) in tissues from the guinea pig. *Biochimica Biophysica Acta*, **431**, 651–654

HAMBERG, M. and SAMUELSSON, B. (1974) Prostaglandin endoperoxides. Novel transformations of arachidonic acid in human platelets. *Proceedings of the National Academy of Sciences of the USA*, **71**, 3400–3404

HAMMARSTROM, S., MURPHY, R. C. and SAMUELSSON, B. (1979) Structure of leukotriene C. Identification of the amino acid part. *Biochemical Biophysical Research Communications*, **91**, 1266–1272

HANNA, C. J., BACH, M. K., PARE, P. D. and SCHELLENBERG, R. R. (1981) Slow reacting substances (leukotrienes) contract human airway and pulmonary vascular smooth muscle *in vitro. Nature (London)*, **290**, 343–344

HAUDENSCHILD, C. C., PRESCOTT, M. F. and CHOBANIAN, A. V. (1980) Effects of hypertension and its reversal on aortic intima lesions of the rat. *Hypertension*, **2**, 33–44

HELDIN, C. H., WESTERMARK, B. and WASTESON, A. (1979) Platelet derived growth factor, purification and partial characterization. *Proceedings of the National Academy of Sciences of the USA*, **76**, 3722–3726

HONG, S. L. (1980) Effect of bradykinin and thrombin on prostacyclin synthesis in endothelial cells from calf and pig aorta and human umbilical cord vein. *Thrombosis Research*, **18**, 787–795

HONG, S. L. and DEYKIN, D. (1979) Specificity of phospholipases in methylchlor-anthrene-transformed mouse fibroblasts activated by bradykinin, thrombin, serum, and ionophore A23187. *Journal of Biological Chemistry*, **254**, 11463–11466

HUGHES, J., GILLIS, C. N. and BLOOM, F. L. (1969) Uptake and disposition of norepinephrine in perfused rat lung. *Journal of Pharmacology and Experimental Therapeutics*, **169**, 237–248

HÜTTNER, I., BOUTET, M., RONA, G. and MORE, R. H. (1973) Studies on protein passage through arterial endothelium. III. Effect of blood pressure levels on the passage of fine structural protein tracers through rat arterial endothelium. *Laboratory Investigation*, **29**, 536–546

HÜTTNER, I., COSTABELLS, P. M., DECHASTONAY, C. and GABBIANI, G. (1982) Volume, surface, and junctions of rat aortic endothelium during experimental hypertension. *Laboratory Investigation*, **46**, 489–504

IWASAWA, Y., GILLIS, C. N. and AGHAJANIAN, G. (1973). Hypothermic inhibition of 5-hydroxytryptamine and norepinephrine uptake by lung: cellular location of amine uptake. *Journal of Pharmacology and Experimental Therapeutics*, **186**, 498–507

JELIFFE, R. W. (1962) Dilator and constrictor effects of acetylcholine on isolated rabbit aortic chains. *Journal of Pharmacology and Experimental Therapeutics*, **135**, 349–353

JELLINEK, H., NAGY, Z., HÜTTNER, I., BALINT, A., KOCZI, A. and KERENYI, T. (1969) Investigations of the permeability changes of the vascular wall in experimental malignant hypertension by means of a colloidal iron preparation. *British Journal of Experimental Pathology*, **56**, 13–16

JOHNSON, A. R. and ERDOS, E. G. (1977) Metabolism of vasoactive peptides by human endothelial cells in culture. *Journal of Clinical Investigation*, **59**, 684–695

JUCHAU, M. R., BOND, J. A. and BENDITT, E. P. (1976) Aryl-4-monooxygenase and cytochrome P-450 in the aorta: possible role in atherosclerosis. *Proceedings of the National Academy of Sciences of the USA*, **73**, 3723–3725

JUNOD, A. F. (1972) Uptake, metabolism and efflux of ^{14}C-5-hydroxytryptamine in isolated perfused rat lungs. *Journal of Pharmacology and Experimental Therapeutics*, **183**, 341–355

KENNERLY, D. A., SULLIVAN, T. J. and PARKER, C. W. (1979) Activation of phospholipid metabolism during mediator release from stimulated rat mast cells. *Journal of Immunology*, **122**, 152–159

KONISKI, K. and SU, C. (1984) Role of endothelium in dilator responses of spontaneously hypertensive rat arteries. *Hypertension*, **5**, 881–886

LIMAS, C. J. and LIMAS, C. (1977) Vascular prostaglandin synthesis in the spontaneously hypertensive rat. *American Journal of Physiology*, **233**, H493–H499

MAJACK, R. A. and BHALLA, R. C. (1980) Endothelial alterations and colloidal carbon permeability in the peripheral vasculature of the spontaneously hypertensive rat. *Experimental and Molecular Pathology*, **32**, 201–215

MC GIFF, J. C., CROWSHAW, K., TERRANGO, N. A. and LONIGRO, A. J. (1970) Release of a prostaglandin-like substance into renal venous blood in response to angiotensin II. *Circulation Research* **26** and **27** (Suppl. I), I-121–I-130

MONCADA, S., GRYGLEWSKI, R., BUNTING, S. and VANE, J. R. (1976) An enzyme isolated from arteries transforms prostaglandin endoperoxides to an unstable substance that inhibits platelet aggregation. *Nature (London)*, **263**, 633–635

MONCADA, S., HERMAN, A. G., HIGGS, E. A. and VANE, J. R. (1977) Differential formation of prostacyclin (PGX or PGI$_2$) by layers of the arterial wall. An explanation for the antithrombotic properties of vascular endothelium. *Thrombosis Research*, **11**, 323–344

MONCADA, S. and VANE, J. R. (1978) Unstable metabolites of arachidonic acid and their role in haemostasis and thrombosis. *British Medical Bulletin*, **34**, 129–135

MORRISON, A. R. and PASCOE, N. (1981) Metabolism of arachidonate through NADPH-dependent oxygenase of renal cortex. *Proceedings of the National Academy of Sciences of the USA*, **78**, 7375–7378

MULLANE, K. M. and MONCADA, S. (1980) Prostacyclin release and the modulation of some vasoactive hormones. *Prostaglandins*, **20**, 25–49

MURPHY, R. C., HAMMARSTROM, S. and SAMUELSSON, B. (1979) Leukotriene C: a slow-reacting substance from murine mastocytoma cells. *Proceedings of the National Academy of Sciences of the USA*, **76**, 4275–4279

NEEDLEMAN, P., MARSHALL, G. R. and SOBEL, B. E. (1975) Hormone interactions in the isolated rabbit heart: synthesis and coronary vasomotor effects of prostaglandins, angiotensin, and bradykinin. *Circulation Research*, **37**, 802–808

NEGUS, P., TANNEN, R. L. and DUNN, M. J. (1976) Indomethacin potentiates the vasoconstrictor actions of angiotensin II in normal man. *Prostaglandins*, **12**, 175–180

NG, K. K. F. and VANE, J. R. (1967) Conversion of angiotensin I to angiotensin II. *Nature (London)*, **216**, 762–766

OLIW, E. H., GUENGERICH, F. P. and OATES, J. A. (1982) Oxygenation of arachidonic acid by hepatic monoxygenases. *Journal of Biological Chemistry*, **257**, 3771–3781

PACE-ASCIAK, C. R., CARRARA, M. C., RANGARAJ, G. and NICOLAOU, K. C. (1978) Enhanced formation of PGI_2, a potent hypotensive substance, by aortic rings and homogenates of the spontaneously hypertensive rat. *Prostaglandins*, **15**, 1005–1012

PEARSON, J. D., CARLETON, J. S., HUTCHINGS, A. and GORDON, J. L. (1978) Uptake and metabolism by pig aortic endothelial and smooth-muscle cells in culture. *Biochemical Journal*, **170**, 265–271

PEARSON, J. D. and GORDON, J. L. (1979) Vascular endothelial and smooth muscle cells in culture selectively release adenine nucleotides. *Nature (London)*, **281**, 384–386

PICKETT, W. C., JESSE, R. L. and COHEN, P. (1977) Initiation of phospholipase A_2 activity in human platelets by the calcium ionophore A23187. *Biochimica Biophysica Acta*, **486**, 209–213

PIPER, P. J., VANE, J. R. and WYLLIE, J. H. (1970) Inactivation of prostaglandins by the lungs. *Nature (London)*, **255**, 600–604

POULSEN, J. H. and WILLIAMS, J. A. (1977) Effect of the calcium ionophore A23187 on pancreatic acinar cell membrane potentials and amylase release. *Journal of Physiology (London)*, **264**, 323–339

PRESSMAN, B. C. (1976) Biological applications of ionophores. *Annual Review of Biochemistry*, **45**, 501–530

PURÉ, E. and NEEDLEMAN, P. (1979) Effect of endothelial damage on prostaglandin synthesis by isolated perfused rabbit mesenteric artery. *Journal of Cardiovascular Pharmacology*, **1**, 299–309

REIDY, M. A. and SCHWARTZ, S. M. (1982) A technique to investigate surface morphology and endothelial cell replication of small arteries: a study in acute angiotensin-induced hypertensive rats. *Microvascular Research*, **24**, 158–167

REIDY, M. A. and SCHWARTZ, S. M. (1981) Endothelial regeneration. III. Time-course of intimal changes after small defined injury to rat aortic endothelium. *Laboratory Investigation*, **44**, 301–308

ROBERTSON, A. L. and KHAIRALLAH, P. A. (1973) Arterial endothelial permeability and vascular disease: the 'trapdoor' effect. *Experimental and Molecular Pathology*, **18**, 241–260

ROSS, R. (1981) Atherosclerosis: a problem of the biology of arterial wall cells and their interaction with blood components. *Arteriosclerosis*, **1**, 293–311

RYAN, J. W., STEWART, J. M., LEARY, W. P. and LEDINGHAM, J. G. (1970) Metabolism of angiotensin I in the pulmonary circulation. *Biochemistry Journal*, **120**, 221–223

RYAN, U. S., RYAN, J. W., WHITAKER, C. and CHIU, C. (1976) Localization of angiotensin converting enzyme (kininase II). II. Immunocytochemistry and immunofluorescence. *Tissue and Cell*, **8**, 125–145

SCHWARTZ, S. M., STERMERMAN, M. B. and BENDITT, E. P. (1975) The aortic intima. II. Repair of the aortic lining after mechanical denudation. *American Journal of Pathology*, **81**, 15–42

SCHWARTZ, S. M. and BENDITT, E. P. (1977) Aortic endothelial cell replication: 1. Effects of age and hypertension in the rat. *Circulation Research*, **41**, 248–255

SCHWARTZ, S. M. and LOMBARDI, D. M. (1982) Effect of chronic hypertension and antihypertensive therapy on endothelial cell replication in the spontaneously hypertensive rat. *Laboratory Investigation*, **47**, 510–515

SHEPRO, D., BATBOUTA, J. C., ROBBLEE, L. S., CARSON, M. P. and BELAMARICH, F. A. (1975) Serotonin transport by cultured bovine aortic endothelium. *Circulation Research*, **36**, 799–806

SINGER, H. A. and PEACH, M. J. (1982) Calcium- and endothelial-mediated vascular smooth muscle relaxation in rabbit aorta. *Hypertension*, **4** (Suppl. II), II-19–II-25

SINGER, H. A. and PEACH, M. J. (1983a) Endothelium-dependent relaxation of rabbit aorta. I. Relaxation stimulated by arachidonic acid. *Journal of Pharmacology and Experimental Therapeutics*, **226**, 790–795

SINGER, H. A. and PEACH, M. J. (1983b) Endothelium-dependent relaxation of rabbit aorta. II. Inhibition of relaxation stimulated by methacholine and A23187 with antagonists of arachidonic acid metabolism. *Journal of Pharmacology and Experimental Therapeutics*, **226**, 796–801

SINGER, H. A., SAYE, J. A. and PEACH, M. J. (1984) Effects of cytochrome P-450 inhibitors on endothelium-dependent relaxation in rabbit aortia. *Blood Vessels* (in press)

SKEGGS, L. T., KAHN, J. R. and SHUMWAY, N. P. (1956) The preparation and function of the hypertensin-converting enzyme. *Journal of Experimental Medicine*, **103**, 295–299

SMITH, U. and RYAN, J. W. (1970) An electron microscopic study of the vascular endothelium as a site for bradykinin and adenosine-5-triphosphate inactivation in rat lung. *Advances in Experimental Medicine and Biology*, **8**, 249–262

SPATH, T. H., STEMERMAN, M. B., ROWE, J. W., MACIAG, T., FUHRO, R. and GARDNER, R. (1975) Intimal injury and regrowth in the rabbit aorta. Medial smooth muscle cells as a source of neointima. *Circulation Research*, **36**, 58–70

SPOKAS, E. G., FALCO, G., QUILLEY, J., CHANDLER, P. and MCGIFF, J. C. (1983) Endothelial mechanism in the vascular action of hydralazine. *Hypertension*, **5** (Suppl. I), I-107–I-111

STILL, W. S. S. and DANNISON, S. (1974) The arterial endothelium of hyertensive rat. *Archives of Pathology*, **97**, 337–547

STRUM, J. and JUNOD, A. F. (1972) Radioautographic demonstration of 5-hydroxy-tryptamine-^{3}H uptake by pulmonary endothelial cells. *Journal of Cell Biology*, **54**, 456–467

SVENDSEN, E. and TINDALL, A. R. (1981) Raised blood pressure and endothelial cell injury in rabbit aorta. *Acta Pathology Microbiology Scandinavica*, Section A, **89**, 325–334

TANSIK, R. L., NAMM, D. H. and WHITE, H. L. (1978) Synthesis of prostaglandin 6-keto $F_{1\alpha}$ by cultured aortic smooth muscle cells and stimulation of its formation in a coupled system with platelet lysates. *Prostaglandins*, **15**, 399–408

TRIGGLE, D. J. and SWAMY, V. C. (1980) Pharmacology of agents that affect calcium. *Chest*, **78**, 174–179

TSAI, B. S. and PEACH, M. J. (1977) Angiotensin homologs and analogs as inhibitors of rabbit pulmonary angiotensin-converting enzyme. *Journal of Biological Chemistry*, **252**, 4674–4681

VELLETRI, P. and BEAN, B. L. (1982) The effects of captopril on rat aortic angiotensin converting enzyme. *Journal of Cardiovascular Pharmacology*, **4**, 315–325

WALENGA, R. W., OPAS, E. E. and FEINSTEIN, M. B. (1981) Differential effects of calmodulin antagonists on phospholipases A_2 and C in thrombin-stimulated platelets. *Journal of Biological Chemistry*, **256**, 12523–12528

WEKSLER, B. B., MARCUS, A. J. and JAFFE, E. A. (1977) Synthesis of prostaglandin I_2 (prostacyclin) by cultured human and bovine endothelial cells. *Proceedings of the National Academy of Sciences of the USA*, **74**, 3922–3926

WEKSLER, B. B., LEY, C. W. and JAFFE, E. A. (1978) Stimulation of endothelial cell prostacyclin production by thrombin, trypsin, and the ionophore A23187. *Journal of Clinical Investigation*, **62**, 923–930

WIENER, J., LATTES, R. G., MELTZER, B. G. and SPIRO, G. (1969) The cellular pathology of experimental hypertension. IV. Evidence for increased vascular permeability. *American Journal of Pathology*, **54**, 187–207

WONG, P. L. and CHEUNG, W. Y. (1979) Calmodulin stimulates human platelet phospholipase A_2. *Biochemical Biophysical Research Communications*, **90**, 473–480

9

Prostanoids and the development of hypertension

Michael L. Watson

INTRODUCTION

In the last decade there has been a considerable increase in knowledge about the oxygenation products of long-chain fatty acids, particularly with reference to the biological role of prostaglandins, thromboxanes and leukotrienes. This chapter is concerned with the possible role of these compounds in the pathogenesis of essential hypertension. Such a discussion must first review prostanoid synthesis with particular attention to the points at which outside factors may affect their rate of synthesis. Many of the current hypotheses about the role of prostanoids in blood pressure control are based on results of *in vitro* studies. The evidence on which some of these hypotheses are based is examined and attempts to determine the relevance of such studies in whole animals and man described. The influence of prostanoids on both renal and systemic vascular resistance is of particular importance, since any changes may affect systemic blood pressure. However, the most important long-term determinant of systemic blood pressure is the relationship between kidney function and sodium excretion (Guyton *et al.*, 1974, 1981) and therefore particular attention has been directed at the possible roles of prostanoids as determinants of renal function.

PROSTANOID SYNTHESIS

Phospholipase

Most of the prostanoids that are at present thought to have important roles in regulation of vascular tone and renal function are derived from arachidonic acid (C20:4). Substantial amounts of arachidonic acid in the body are esterified to either triglycerides or cholesterol esters, particularly, for example, in the renal medulla (Comai, Farber and Paulsrud, 1975; Nissen and Bojesen, 1969) but in most tissues the major pool of arachidonic acid is in phospholipids (Miller *et al.*, 1976; Morgan,

Tinker and Hannahan, 1963). Synthesis of prostanoids requires initial release of the fatty acid from the phospholipid (Lands and Samuelsson, 1968). Phospholipase A_2, the enzyme most commonly responsible for this process (Flower and Blackwell, 1976), is highly specific, both with regard to the position on the phospholipid of the fatty acid hydrolyzed (2 position only) (Isakson, Raz and Needleman, 1976) and the length of its carbon chain. The metabolic pool of arachidonate available for prostanoid synthesis also does not appear to be a single entity; changes in fatty acid availability, for example by manipulation of dietary intake (Vergroesen *et al.*, 1980), rapidly affect prostanoid synthesis, whilst at the same time causing little change in the fatty acid composition of membrane phospholipids *(see below)*. There are a large number of factors that potentially exert control on phospholipase A_2 activity including peptide hormones such as bradykinin and angiotensin II (Limas and Limas, 1979). Whilst the availability of free arachidonic acid is certainly a major determinant of the rates of prostanoid synthesis, the rate of reacylation of arachidonic acid into phospholipids, by limiting the amount of free arachidonate available, may also be important.

Fatty acid oxygenation

Arachidonic acid is further metabolized to a large range of products after incorporation of molecular oxygen by one of at least three different mechanisms (oxygenase reactions). The monoxygenase (for instance, lipoxygenase) and dioxygenase (for instance, cyclo-oxygenase) reactions are considered by far the

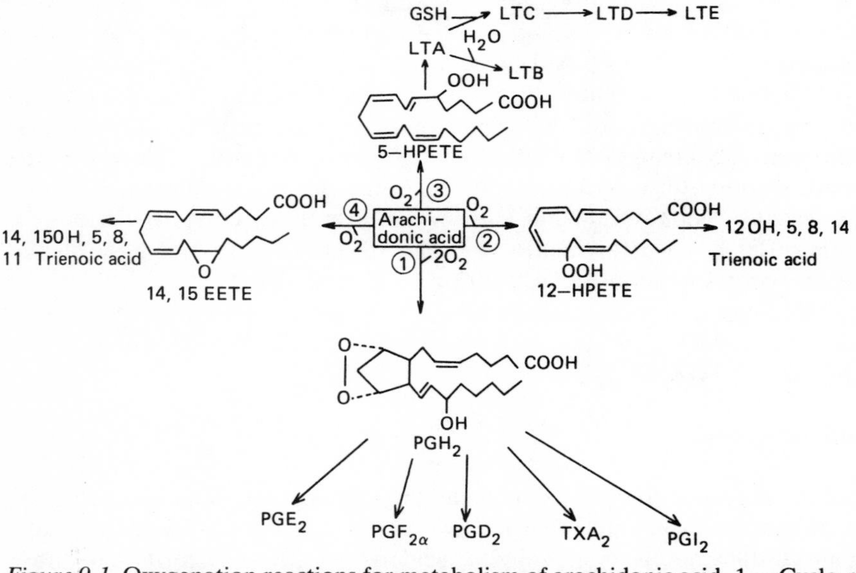

Figure 9.1 Oxygenation reactions for metabolism of arachidonic acid. 1 = Cyclo-oxygenase; 2 = 12-lipoxygenase; 3 = 5-lipoxygenase; 4 = Cytochrome P_{450} mixed function oxidase. HPETE = hydroperoxy-eicosatetraenoic acid; EETE = epoxy-eicosatrienoic acid; LT = leukotriene

most important, but a variety of hydroxylated derivatives of arachidonic acid can also be synthesized by a mixed function oxidase system. Examples of some of the reaction products of each system are shown in *Figure 9.1*.

Cyclo-oxygenase

The products of the arachidonic acid cyclo-oxygenase reaction have been extensively documented. Incorporation of two atoms of molecular oxygen leads to formation of an unstable endoperoxide intermediate which is further metabolized to a variety of products. Until 1976, PGE_2, $PGF_{2\alpha}$ and PGD_2 were regarded as the prostaglandins of most biological significance, but the discovery of thromboxane A_2 and PGI_2 has modified this view. Indeed, on the basis of biological activity there are reasonable grounds to implicate all of these metabolites as potential modulators of blood pressure.

Whilst arachidonate is the major substrate for cyclo-oxygenase, other fatty acids such as dihomo-γ-linolenic acid (C20:3) and eicosapentaenoic acid (C20:5) are also tightly bound to the enzyme, although more varibly metabolized to 1 and 3 series prostanoids respectively (Needleman *et al.*, 1979). Phospholipases also release C20:3 and C20:5 from phospholipids. The relative quantities of these different fatty acids released in response to a given stimulus and therefore competing with arachidonic acid for binding to the cyclo-oxygenase enzyme may serve as an important factor in determining the relative amounts of products formed (Siess *et al.*, 1980).

Lipoxygenase

Molecular oxygen is inserted into the arachidonate molecule by a lipoxygenase system (Borgeat, Hamberg and Samuelsson, 1976). This occurs across the CIS double bond, leading to formation of chemically unstable hydroperoxy intermediates across the C5-6, C11-12, C14-15 double bonds. These hydroperoxides are further metabolized, predominantly to the 5 series leukotrienes (Murphy, Hammarstrom and Samuelsson, 1979), 12 and 15 hydroxyeicosatetraenoic acids (Hamberg, Hedqvist and Radegran, 1980) and 15 series leukotrienes (Maas, Brash and Oates, 1982).

Mixed function oxidase

Incorporation of molecular oxygen via a cytochrome P_{450}-dependent mixed function oxidase system also leads to formation of a range of unstable epoxide intermediates which are further metabolized to a variety of hydroxy fatty acids (Capdevila *et al.*, 1982; Oliw *et al.*, 1981). The biological significance of the lipoxygenase and mixed function oxidase products remains uncertain. Their mere existence serves to confuse the picture since, although under normal circumstances they may have little function, they may become important when the normal metabolic pathways are perturbed. For example, whilst endoperoxides are unstable, they have significant biological activity (Feigen *et al.*, 1978). Inhibition of their metabolism to, for example, thromboxane A_2 may well lead to their accumulation and to occupation of any available thromboxane receptors (Jones and Wilson, 1980). Likewise inhibition of cyclo-oxygenase by non-steroidal anti-inflammatory drugs (NSAID) may cause accumulation of arachidonic acid, and so increase its metabolism by adjacent metabolic pathways such as the lipoxygenase or cytochrome P_{450} systems. These possibilities must always be kept in mind when assessing the evidence for the importance of these compounds in biological systems, where selective inhibitors are the only investigation technique utilized.

Only a limited number of these fatty acid oxygenation products are likely to have a significant role in the control of blood pressure *In vitro* studies that provide evidence of the spectrum of prostanoids synthesized by tissues and organs that are most involved in blood pressure control form the basis for subsequent assessment of the role of individual prostanoids.

LOCALIZATION OF PROSTAGLANDIN SYNTHESIS

PGE_2, $PGF_{2\alpha}$ and PGI_2 are all synthesized by vascular endothelium (Moncada, Higgs and Vane, 1977; Terragno *et al.*, 1975) and by isolated endothelial cells in culture (Gimbrone and Alexander, 1975; Remuzzi *et al.*, 1980; Whorton *et al.*, 1982). The extent to which prostanoids synthesized in endothelial cells can interact with smooth muscle of blood vessels is uncertain. Although platelets are a potent source of thromboxane A_2 very little is synthesized by the vasculature (Hamberg and Samuelsson, 1974). Synthesis of 12 hydroxyeicosatetraenoic acid (Greenwald, Bianchine and Wong, 1979) and leukotriene D_4 (Piper, Letts and Galton, 1983) has also been demonstrated in isolated vascular tissue. The kidney synthesizes many different prostanoids. The distribution of the sites within the kidney is complex. The renal medulla has a massive capacity to synthesize PGE_2 (Daniels *et al.*, 1967; Frolich *et al.*, 1975; Larsson and Anggard, 1973) which is primarily localized in the interstitial cells (Muirhead *et al.*, 1972; Zusman and Keiser, 1977a). Many factors modulate interstitial cell synthesis of PGE_2 including angiotensin II, bradykinin, vasopressin and potassium concentration and osmolarity of the surrounding fluid (Zusman and Keiser, 1977b). Indeed the concept of single hormones or factors stimulating PGE synthesis is unduly simple. For example, aldosterone alters the stimulation of PGE_2 synthesis by vasopressin, giving rise to the potential for extremely complex multifactorial control systems (Zusman, Keiser and Handler, 1978). The renal cortex also synthesizes small amounts of PGE_2 (Larsson and Anggard, 1973) which functionally may be important. Initial reports suggested that PGI_2 in contrast to PGE_2 was primarily synthesized in the renal cortex (Remuzzi *et al.*, 1978; Whorton *et al.*, 1977) with comparatively little being formed in the renal medulla (Whorton *et al.*, 1978). More recent studies, however, suggest that PGI_2 is also synthesized in significant quantities by renal medullary tissue (Okahara, Imanishi and Yamamoto, 1983). Under normal circumstances whole kidneys synthesize very little thromboxane (Morrison, Nishikawa and Needleman, 1977), but there are circumstances, for example after ureteral occlusion, when the renal capacity to synthesize thromboxane appears to be enhanced (Morrison, Nishikawa and Needleman, 1977, 1978). Homogenates of renal cortex can also synthesize epoxide and hydroxylated derivatives of arachidonic acid via the cytochrome P_{450}-dependent system (Oliw et al., 1981).

Most investigators agree that prostanoids are likely to exert their physiological effects at or near their site of synthesis. Studies of prostanoid synthesis in whole tissue homogenates of complex organs such as the kidney therefore provide limited information. Determination of specific cellular sites of prostaglandin synthesis within the kidney is difficult, particularly because of changes in prostanoid synthesis that occur during the tissue separation and fractionation procedures. Isolated glomeruli studied in this fashion have been shown to synthesize a range of arachidonate-derived products, particularly PGE_2, but also PGI_2 (Folkert and Schlondorff, 1979; Hassid, Konieczkowski and Dunn, 1979; Sraer et al., 1979), some thromboxane A_2 (Hassid, Konieczkowski and Dunn, 1979; Petrulis, Aikawa and Dunn, 1981) and to a lesser extent ill-defined lipoxygenase products (Lianos and Dunn, 1983; Petrulis, Aikawa and Dunn, 1981). Isolated segments of renal vasculature have also been shown to synthesize prostaglandins (Terragno, McGiff and Terrangno, 1978). Cell culture studies of renal medullary cells have already been described but more recent studies have also been undertaken using cell lines derived from renal cortical tissue. Mesangial cells appear primarily to synthesize PGE_2, while glomerular epithelial cells synthesize PGI_2 (Kreisberg, Kannovsky and Levine, 1982). This observation may be of considerable functional importance. Mesangial cells are contractile and by this means probably alter the surface area of the glomerulus available for filtration. Recent observations suggest that angiotensin II stimulates PGE_2 release from these mesangial cells (Scharschmidt and Dunn, 1983) which may then modulate the effects of angiotensin on mesangial cell tone. Juxtaglomerular cells which synthesize renin have also been grown in cell culture (Rightsel et al., 1982). Both these cells and mesangial cells are similar smooth muscle derived cells, and like mesangial cells the juxtaglomerular cells also preferentially appear to synthesize PGE_2, in addition to much smaller amounts of PGI_2 (Watson et al., unpublished observations).

An alternative method of identifying sites of prostaglandin synthesis is by using histochemical techniques to localize prostaglandin endoperoxide synthetase, since prostaglandins are not themselves stored in cells. This evidence suggests there is likely to be active synthesis of prostaglandins in the collecting ducts of the renal medulla (Bohman, 1977; Janszen and Nugteren, 1971; Smith and Wilkin, 1977) and in the vascular tissue, and to a lesser extent in the glomeruli of the renal cortex (Smith and Bell, 1978). The kidney is also an important site of prostaglandin catabolism. Large quantities of 15-hydroxy prostaglandin dehydrogenase are present in both the renal cortex (Larsson and Anggard, 1973) and the lungs. This prevents any PGE_2 infused systemically from reaching the urine (Hamberg and Samuelsson, 1971). Beta-oxidation of prostaglandins also occurs in the renal cortex. Ready access of prostanoids to these catabolic enzymes probably limits their action within the kidney to near their site of synthesis. Metabolism of PGE_2

and PGI_2 may also occur at the 9 position. Prostaglandin 9-ketoreductase, an NADH-dependent enzyme, is present within the kidney and promotes conversion of PGE_2 to $PGF_{2\alpha}$ (Stone and Hart, 1975). In rabbits, activity of this enzyme system has been related to the state of sodium balance (Weber, Larsson and Scherer, 1977), and shunting of PGE_2 metabolism through this pathway may provide a further means of controlling the local activity of PGE_2. Also, 6-ketoPGF$_{1\alpha}$ may be metabolized by a similar enzyme 9-hydroxy dehydrogenase to 6-ketoPGE$_1$ (Wong *et al.*, 1980). In view of the potent activity of 6-ketoPGE$_1$ (*see below*) this reaction could be of considerable significance. However, although there is the potential for 6-ketoPGE$_1$ synthesis it remains to be proved whether significant quantities of the compound are actually synthesized *in vivo*.

POTENTIAL ACTIONS OF PROSTANOIDS IN RELATION TO BLOOD PRESSURE CONTROL

Anaesthetized animal and *in vitro* studies provide the main source of knowledge concerning the possible actions of prostaglandins in modulating blood pressure. These have given rise to hypotheses which have then been tested in whole animals and in man. Although useful, the value of this approach is limited by the fact that actions of compounds infused into isolated tissues and organs in substantial doses do not necessarily bear any relationship to their actions in small concentrations at local sites in the intact animal.

Prostaglandins

Infusion of PGE_2, PGI_2, PGD_2 and 6-ketoPGE$_1$ into the renal artery increases renal blood flow, sodium and potassium excretion and to a variable extent renin release (Fitzgerald *et al.*, 1981; Gerber *et al.*, 1978; Jackson *et al.*, 1982; Jones, Watson and Ungar, 1981; Martinez-Maldonado *et al.*, 1972; Schwertschlag, Stahl and Hackenthal, 1982). This type of study suggests that 6-ketoPGE$_1$ is the most potent prostaglandin at stimulating renin release (Jackson *et al.*, 1981). Evidence from renal cortical incubation studies suggests that PGI_2 and to a lesser extent endoperoxides also stimulate renin release (Weber *et al.*, 1976; Whorton *et al.*, 1977). Most of the evidence implicating prostaglandins in the control of renin release *in vivo* is based on studies using prostaglandin synthetase inhibitors. Such studies (Berl *et al.*, 1979; Blackshear *et al.*, 1979; Campbell, Graham and Jackson, 1979; Data *et al.*, 1978; Frolich *et al.*, 1979; Gerber, Olson and Nies, 1981; Henrich, 1981) have implicated prostaglandins as mediators of renin release as a result of baroreceptor and macula densa stimulation. Release as a result of stimulation of sympathetic nervous activity is more likely to be a direct effect that does not involve prostaglandins as intermediates. (Berl *et al.*, 1979; Kopp and Dibona, 1983). Potential action of prostaglandins as both vasodilators and mediators of renin release raises the question of their possible role in mediating tubuloglomerular feedback. The most cogent evidence in favour of prostaglandins as intermediaries in this process stems from the micropuncture study by Schnerman and Briggs (1981) who demonstrated that indomethacin inhibited tubuloglomerular feedback responses in rabbit kidneys, but that these were normal after infusion of PGI_2.

Clearly prostaglandins have the potential to modulate a variety of different physiological functions in the kidney. The question then arises as to what stimuli invoke the release of prostaglandins *in vivo*. The available evidence, derived mostly from studies on anaesthetized animals, suggests that prostaglandins have an important role in modulating the renal response to a number of vasoconstrictive stimuli. For example, infusion of angiotensin II into the renal artery releases both PGE_2 (McGiff *et al.*, 1970) and PGI_2 (Shebuski and Aiken, 1980). Moreover the renal vascular effects of infused angiotensin are ehanced by pretreatment with indomethacin (Aiken and Vane, 1973). Similarly, stimulation of renal nerves promotes release of PGE_2 from the kidney (Davis and Horton, 1972), providing evidence from a whole organ that prostaglandins modulate adrenergic responses at the nerve terminal (Hedqvist, 1976). In anaesthetized, traumatized animals indomethacin and meclofenamate decrease renal blood flow (Lonigro *et al.*, 1973; Terragno, Terragno and McGiff, 1979) apparently confirming an important role for prostaglandins in the maintenance of renal blood flow. However, in conscious animals inhibition of prostaglandin synthesis has little effect on renal blood flow (Swain *et al.*, 1975; Terragno, Terragno and McGiff, 1977). It seems that under normal conditions prostaglandins have comparatively little effect on renal blood flow, but under conditions of stress such as during sodium depletion or after significant blood loss they assume a more important role in maintaining renal blood flow.

Involvement of prostaglandins in control of sodium balance is even more controversial. PGE_2 and PGI_2 cause natriuresis (Jones, Watson and Ungar, 1981) when infused into the kidney, but renal blood flow increases at the same time. It is therefore difficult to be certain whether the natriuresis is the result of renal vasodilatation or direct inhibition of tubular sodium transport. Micropuncture studies indicate that the latter is a distinct possibility (Stokes, 1979; Stokes and Kokko, 1977; Wilson, Honrath and Sonnenberg, 1982). However, Weber, Larsson and Scherer (1977) reported that a high sodium intake in rabbits stimulates conversion of PGE_2 to $PGF_{2\alpha}$ via a prostaglandin 9-ketoreductase. The resulting reduction in PGE_2 during sodium loading argues against a direct role for PGE_2 in promoting sodium excretion (Watson *et al.*, 1982). Perhaps the decrease in PGE_2 levels represents a means by which renal renin release is suppressed in response to a high sodium intake, in view of the known ability of PGE_2 to stimulate renin release. Other studies in conscious dogs have demonstrated that a low sodium intake increases efflux of PGE_2 in the renal venous blood (Oliver *et al.*, 1980). While this may reflect a direct effect of the changes in extracellular fluid volume, it is more likely to be due to the increased adrenergic nervous stimulation and/or renin–angiotensin activity. However, there must be some doubt as to the importance of increased prostaglandin synthesis in this model since it has previously been demonstrated that changes in renovascular responses to angiotensin II can be entirely accounted for by changes in levels of endogenous angiotensin (Oliver and Cannon, 1978). The apparently contrasting actions of PGE_2 under different conditions emphasize that its actions on the kidney are likely to depend on the exact site of synthesis.

Thromboxanes

Thromoxane A_2 is a potent vasoconstrictor which also constricts the renal vasculature (Sakr and Dunham, 1982; Shibouta *et al.*, 1981). Under normal circumstances kidneys have little capacity to synthesize thromboxane A_2, but this is substantially enhanced by ureteral obstruction (Morrison, Nishikawa and Needleman, 1977; Yarger, Schocken and Harris, 1980). Thus isolated perfused normal rabbit kidneys show no increase in synthesis of thromboxane in response to infusion of bradykinin, but the same experiment performed in kidneys with ureters occluded for the previous 48 hours resulted in significant thromboxane synthesis in response to bradykinin. Enhanced thromboxane synthesis may also contribute to the increased vascular resistance in such kidneys (Yarger, Schocken and Harris, 1980).

Leukotrienes

Wide-ranging effects of leukotrienes on vascular tone have only recently become evident. Systemic infusion of LTC_1 and LTD_4 into anaesthetized guinea-pigs and monkeys results, after a transient phase of hypertension, in prolonged hypotension, although the calculated peripheral vascular resistance remains high (Drazen *et al.*, 1980; Smedgard *et al.*, 1982). LTD_4 is a potent coronary vasoconstrictor and negative inotropic agent (Michelassi, 1982) and it seems likely that the systemic hypotension in whole animals results from the latter effect. Interestingly, in spontaneously hypertensive rats LTD_4 caused both a larger initial increase and subsequent decrease in blood pressure than in the Wistar–Kyoto controls (Feuerstein, Zukowska–Grojec and Kopin, 1981; Zukowska–Grojec *et al.*, 1983). There is also a suggestion that some of the cardiovascular effects of leukotrienes may be mediated by secondary stimulation of prostaglandin release. Supportive evidence for this concept has been obtained in studies of inflammatory cells (Williams, 1983), raising the possibility that there is a complex interaction between leukotrienes and prostaglandins, with both sharing the same substrate (arachidonic acid) but having opposing actions. Direct effects of leukotrienes on renal blood vessels have also been observed (Feigen, 1983) but further evidence is required before useful hypotheses can be made about their role in blood pressure control. Leukotrines, like prostaglandins, are unlikely to function as circulating hypotensive agents (Piper, 1983).

From this brief account of potential actions of prostanoids it is clear that there are numerous ways in which they may modulate blood pressure and, in particular, participate in the genesis of essential hypertension. Three main approaches have been used in assessing their importance in whole animals and man. Firstly, measurement of relevant plasma and urinary metabolites allows the calculation of their systemic and/or renal synthesis. Secondly, the effects of various inhibitors of prostanoid synthesis may be examined, and thirdly, the effect of changes in substrate availability, for example by changes in the composition of dietary fatty acids, can be observed.

USE OF INHIBITORS OF PROSTANOID SYNTHESIS TO ASSESS THEIR ROLE IN HYPERTENSION

Specific inhbitors of synthesis of compounds of biological interest have always provided a useful means of assessing their possible function. Prostaglandins are no exception, and the discovery that non-steroidal anti-inflammatory drugs (NSAIDs) inhibit prostaglandin synthesis (Vane, 1971) proved a stimulus to determination of the biological function of prostaglandins. Inhibition of prostaglandin synthesis in animals with different forms of hypertension has resulted in conflicting results. For example, in conscious dogs with one-clip, two-kidney renovascular hypertension, treatment with indomethacin had no effect on systemic blood pressure (Yun, Kelly and Bartter, 1979). Moreover in the same study there were no observed changes in renal haemodynamics and sodium excretion during indomethacin treatment. However, the elevation of blood pressure in this model is comparatively small. The effect of indomethacin on blood pressure in one-clip, two-kidney and one-clip, one-kidney hypertensive rabbits is rather different (Romero and Strong, 1977). Most of the one-clip, two-kidney animals showed the same response to inhibition of prostaglandin synthesis as normal subjects, but a small proportion of these animals developed malignant hypertension during treatment with indomethacin. In these animals renal blood flow was consistently decreased by indomethacin. The one-clip, one-kidney animals consistently developed more severe hypertension during inhibition of prostaglandin synthesis. It seemed that sensitivity of blood pressure to inhibition of prostaglandin synthesis could be directly related to induced changes in renal function. In both spontaneously hypertensive rats (Levy, 1977) and normal man (Negus, Tannen and Dunn, 1976; Vierhapper, Waldhausl and Nowotny, 1981) indomethacin had no effect on systemic blood pressure, although some increase in renal plasma flow has been observed after indomethacin in 6-week-old spontaneously hypertensive rats (SHR) (Shibouta, 1982). This would be consistent with excessive renal synthesis of a vasoconstrictor such as thromboxane A_2 (*see below*). Most of these studies rely on inhibition of prostanoid synthesis by non-steroidal anti-inflammatory drugs (NSAIDs), but these are not specific compounds, (Flower, 1974). Moreover, inhibition of prostaglandin synthesis may at the same time lead to an increase in substrate availability (that is, arachidonic acid) for the lipoxygenase pathway which may further complicate the effects of apparent inhibition of prostaglandin synthesis (*see above*). More recently both thromboxane synthetase inhibitors and thromboxane A_2 receptor antagonists have been developed (Jones, Peesapati and Wilson, 1982; Tai and Yuan, 1978) and these compounds are now providing useful insights into the role of thromboxane A_2 in hypertension. Pinane-thromboxane A_2, a thromboxane A_2 receptor antagonist, caused a large increase in both renal plasma flow and glomerular filtration rate in the 6-week-old spontaneously hypertensive rat, but had no effect on these parameters by 18 weeks. There was no significant effect of the inhibitor in the Wistar–Kyoto normotensive control. There was also no discernible effect on systemic blood pressure, but the inhibitor was only given over 30 minutes (Shibouta *et al.*, 1982). An alternative approach has involved the use of a thromboxane synthetase inhibitor 4'-(imidazol-1-yl) acetophenone. Daily injections of this compound into spontaneously hypertensive rats between the ages of 4 and 10 weeks resulted in significant attenuation of the rise in blood pressure (Uderman, Workman and Jackson, 1982). Another thromboxane synthetase inhibitor, UK38, 485, also decreased blood pressure when given for four days to spontaneously hypertensive rats with established hypertension (Uderman, personal communication). In these latter studies neither the plasma level of 6-ketoPGF$_{1\alpha}$, nor urinary excretion of dinor 6-ketoPGF$_{1\alpha}$, was altered by the inhibitor. Both of these compounds are metabolites of PGI$_2$, thus suggesting that the hypotensive response to the thromboxane synthetase inhibitor was not the result of shunting of endoperoxide metabolism towards increased synthesis of PGI$_2$. There is as yet no data on the effect of a thromboxane synthetase inhibitor on renal haemodynamics in the spontaneously hypertensive rat, but in view of the results of the experiments with pinane-thromboxane A$_2$ (Shibouta *et al.*, 1982) it is attractive to speculate that the primary effect of renal thromboxane A$_2$ is to increase renal vascular resistance. Removal of this effect would then modify renal function so as to favour a decrease in systemic blood pressure.

MEASUREMENT OF PROSTANOID SYNTHESIS IN HYPERTENSION

Methodological considerations

At first sight measurement of prostanoid synthesis in various phases of development of hypertension provides the obvious means of determining the role of prostanoids in this process. However, there are many limitations to the current methods available to assess prostanoid synthesis.

Much of the initial work on prostanoids was based on superfusion bioassay systems (Vane, 1964). While these methods are extremely versatile and have been the basis for discovery of many new compounds in the prostaglandin field, they have neither the specificity nor sensitivity to provide useful quantitative data on changes in prostaglandin synthesis in *in vivo* animal models and man. Radioimmunoassay is an attractive method in view of the great sensitivity and comparatively high rates of sample throughput that can be achieved. The greatest problem with this method is the effect on the assay of unidentified substances which cross-react with even the most specific antibodies (Granstrom, 1978). Suitable chromatographic separation systems, such as used during analysis of PGE in urine (Dray, Charbonnel and Maclouf, 1975), greatly enhance the reliability of these methods. Difficulties in separating prostanoids from plasma are even greater. Siess and Dray (1982) have demonstrated this by analyzing plasma levels of 6-ketoPGF$_{1\alpha}$ by radioimmunoassay. High performance liquid chromatography (HPLC) was used to purify the sample, but significant amounts of material cross-reacting with their antibody was present in almost all the fractions eluted from the HPLC column, emphasizing the requirement for excellent separation techniques. The alternative technique for prostanoid analysis is combined gas chromatography–mass spectrometry. The disadvantage of this technique has always been its relative insensitivity, and the requirement for preparation of very pure samples (Boeynaems and Herman, 1980). Its major advantage is extremely high specificity. Using this technique it has been demonstrated that urinary PGE_2 excretion provides, under certain conditions, a useful measure of renal PGE_2 synthesis (Frolich *et al.*, 1975). Moreover, provided suitable deuterated internal standards are available the same technique can be used to quantify a whole range of prostanoids and their metabolites (Falardeau, Oates and Brash, 1981; Robertson *et al.*, 1981). Recently, using the method of negative ion chemical ionization instead of the more usual electron-impact ionization method, it has been possible to increase greatly the sensitivity of mass spectrometry of prostaglandins (Blair *et al.*, 1982). This type of mass spectrometry combined with capillary column gas chromatography now provides an excellent means of analyzing a number of different prostanoids and their metabolites in the same biological sample, with a sensitivity comparable to that achieved with radioimmunoassay methods.

Methodological difficulties in analysis are always likely to be the major stumbling block to obtaining adequate insights into the *in vivo* role of prostanoids, but these new technologies do provide some hope of improvement.

Prostanoid synthesis in the spontaneously hypertensive rat

Confusion has surrounded the possible role of prostaglandins in determining renal function in the rat. Initial studies suggested that PGE_2 was a vasoconstrictor in the renal circulation (Baer and McGiff, 1979; Malik and McGiff, 1975), in contrast to virtually all other species studied. If this were the case enhanced levels of PGE_2 in the kidneys might have been responsible for the characteristically increased renal vascular resistance in the spontaneously hypertensive animal (Arendshorst and Beierwaltes, 1979; Azar *et al.*, 1979) and therefore have a significant role in pathogenesis of the underlying hypertension. Such a situation might develop either as a result of excessive PGE_2 synthesis or its impaired catabolism, for example by decreased prostaglandin 15-hydroxydehydrogenase activity. Confirmation of the latter possibility has been obtained in the New Zealand (Armstrong *et al.*, 1975) and Japanese spontaneously hypertensive rats (Limas and Limas, 1977; Pace-Asciak, 1976). However, more recent studies have confirmed that, as in other species, PGE_2 dilates the renal vasculature, provided that the blood vessels have a reasonable degree of tone prior to infusion of PGE_2 (Haylor and Towers, 1982; Jackson *et al.*, 1982). Clearly this makes it unlikely that decreased PGE_2 catabolism is a direct cause of the enhanced renal vascular resistance. An alternative hypothesis would be that increased PGE_2 stimulates renin release in the kidney, which may exert an effect on vascular tone via increased synthesis of angiotensin II.

Increased release of PGE_2 from incubated sections of renal medulla from hypertensive rats has also been reported (Dunn, 1976; Limas and Limas, 1977, 1979) although in other studies normal or impaired release of PGE was observed (Leary, Ledingham and Vane, 1974; Limas *et al.*, 1981; Shibouta *et al.*, 1979; Sirois and Gagnon, 1974; Stygles *et al.*, 1978). Prostaglandin synthesis in isolated glomeruli obtained from normotensive and hypertensive rats has also been compared. While baseline levels of synthesis of PGE_2, $PGF_{2\alpha}$ and 6-ketoPGF$_{1\alpha}$ were no different in the two groups, glomeruli from the spontaneously hypertensive rats showed much enhanced rates of synthesis of all of these prostanoids on stimulation with arachidonate and calcium ionophore, compared with their normotensive controls (Konieczkowski *et al.*, 1983).

More indirect assessment of renal prostaglandin synthesis, by measurement of urinary excretion of prostaglandins or their metabolites, provides further conflicting data. Urinary $PGF_{2\alpha}$ excretion was found to be increased in the spontaneously hypertensive rat compared with age-matched normotensive controls, the peak difference being evident at six weeks (Ahnfelt-Ronne and Arrigoni-Martelli, 1977). However, Dunn (1978) was unable to find any difference in renal excretion of either PGE or $PGF_{2\alpha}$, regardless of whether it was measured in urine or renal venous plasma. Similar results were reported by Shibouta *et al.* (1982) who also found no difference in the excretion rate of 6-ketoPGF$_{1\alpha}$. Different results have been obtained using different models of hypertension. In both the Lyon strain (Benzoni, Vincent and Sassaro, 1982) and the Dahl salt-sensitive rat (Sustarsic, McPartland and Rapp, 1981) decreased urinary PGE_2 excretion has been reported, although in both studies the changes only became evident as the animals grew older.

Much of the diversity in the reported results is likely to reflect the inadequacy of the methods used to assess prostaglandin synthesis. However, as discussed earlier, prostaglandins are synthesized at several different sites within the kidney. Altered prostaglandin synthesis in one particular site may be of considerable physiological significance, but not be reflected in measured overall rates of excretion of the compound. Thus the finding of increased prostaglandin synthesis in glomeruli (a comparatively minor site of prostaglandin synthesis in terms of the whole kidney) could still be of pathogenetic significance (Konieczkowski *et al.*, 1983).

Isolated glomeruli from spontaneously hypertensive rats also produce excessive amounts of thromboxane A_2 compared with the normotensive controls (Konieczkowski *et al.*, 1983). Increased urinary excretion of thromboxane B_2 has been reported in these animals at both 6 and 18 weeks (Shibouta *et al.*, 1982). These findings, when considered in conjunction with the already described effects of thromboxane synthetase inhibitors (Uderman, Workman and Jackson, 1982), suggest that enhanced thromboxane A_2 synthesis, particularly in the kidney, may be of pathogenetic significance in the development of hypertension. There are still a number of inconsistencies between the *in vivo* and *in vitro* data. In particular, enhanced prostaglandin synthesis in the spontaneously hypertensive rat appears to affect all the prostaglandins measured, implying that there is increased phospholipase and/or cyclo-oxygenase activity. However, if the mechanism of increased vascular resistance is related to increased thromboxane synthesis, selective enhancement of thromboxane synthesis might be expected in the *in vitro* studies. It is hard to envisage the role of the associated increase in production of PGI_2, PGE_2 and $PGF_{2\alpha}$

Other adaptive changes involving the prostaglandin system may also be important. Sensitivity of blood vessels to PGE_2 is reportedly enhanced (Simpson, 1974) while PGI_2 is also a more potent vasodilator in the spontaneously hypertensive rat than in its normotensive control (Pace-Asciak, Carrara and Nicolaou, 1978). Enhanced synthesis of PGI_2 might then be important in reducing the degree of hypertension (Pace-Asciak *et al.*, 1978). However, an overall increase in PGI_2 synthesis was not found in the spontaneously hypertensive rat (H. D. Uderman, personal communication) and therefore the significance of such a hypotensive mechanism remains unclear.

Prostanoid synthesis in other models of hypertension

Studies of prostaglandin synthesis in other models of hypertension have not provided any clearer idea of their possible role. Lipophilic granules are present in interstitial cells of the renal medulla and their number may be inversely related to the rate of prostaglandin synthesis by these cells. In the desoxycorticosterone acetate (DOCA)-treated, sodium-loaded rat the renal interstitial cell granularity is decreased compared with controls (Muehrcke *et al.*, 1969; Tobian, Ishii and Duke, 1969), suggesting that prostaglandin synthesis is decreased. Pugsley, Mullins and Beilin, (1976) have also demonstrated that renal medullary PGE synthesis is decreased in the period immediately after DOCA–salt treatment, when the animals are still hypertensive. Paradoxically the medullary capacity for PGE synthesis was not altered during DOCA–salt treatment, despite the animals being hypertensive.

We have studied renal PGE synthesis in the established phase of hypertension in one-clip, two-kidney hypertensive dogs and found it to be increased compared with levels before induction of hypertension (Watson *et al.*, 1984). In a previous study in dogs the number of dark lipophilic granules in renal interstitial cells was decreased in the untouched kidney, but there was an increase in the cell content of a distinct type of lighter staining, lipid-containing granule (Taylor *et al.*, 1981). The presence of these granules may reflect increased prostaglandin synthesis, and be part of the mechanism by which this kidney is protected from the effects of even small, but sustained increases in activity of the renin–angiotensin system.

Animal models of hypertension remain a comparatively unsatisfactory alternative for elucidating the possible role of prostanoids in the development of essential hypertension in man. Their clear advantage is that they permit more detailed assessment of changes in cell function; thus, for example, studies of prostaglandin synthesis and thromboxane synthesis in isolated glomeruli can be undertaken with comparative ease, whereas such studies would be extremely difficult in man. It is quite conceivable that small differences in prostanoid synthesis at local sites, such as in glomeruli, will prove to be important in the pathogenesis of hypertension. Demonstration of such defects in animals will at least permit a rational assessment of their possible role in man.

Prostanoid synthesis in essential hypertension

One of the consistent abnormalities in essential hypertension is the finding of increased renal vascular resistance (Fagard *et al.*, 1977; Hollenberg *et al.*, 1975). Taken in conjunction with the strong possibility that the kidney plays a pivotal role in the long-term regulation of blood pressure (Guyton *et al.*, 1974) this implies that changes in activity of factors determining renal vascular resistance may be important in the genesis of hypertension. The experimental evidence implicating prostanoids in this process has already been discussed; what of the evidence from studies in man?

Renal PGE_2 synthesis does appear to be decreased in essential hypertension, as reflected in urinary PGE excretion (Sato *et al.*, 1983; Tan, Sweet and Mulrow, 1978). The rate of urinary PGE excretion does not directly relate to the extent of activation of the renin–angiotensin system (Sato *et al.*, 1983), although others report that PGE_2 excretion may be lowest in patients with low renin hypertension (Rathaus, Bauminger and Bernheim, 1980; Weber, Siess and Scherer, 1980).

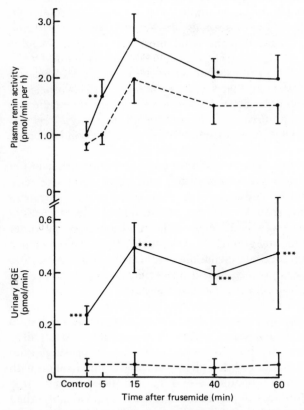

Figure 9.2 Changes in urinary PGE excretion and plasma renin activity in normal subjects after frusemide (30 mg) with (– – –) and without (——) indomethacin. Results are expressed as mean ± SEM. *$P<0.05$; **$P<0.01$; ***$P<0.001$; $n = 8$

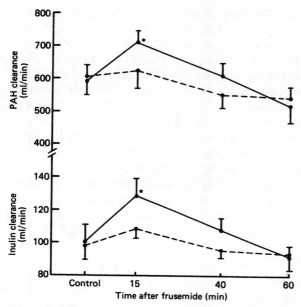

Figure 9.3 Changes in clearance of inulin and para-aminohippuric acid (PAH) in normal subjects after frusemide (30 mg) with (– – –) and without (——) indomethacin. Results are expressed as mean ± SEM. *$P<0.05$; $n = 8$

If renal PGE_2 synthesis is indeed decreased in hypertension, the question to be answered is whether this is a primary aetiological factor in the development of hypertension, or merely a secondary phenomenon. In an attempt to throw further light on this question Scherer and Weber (1979) have studied excretion of PGE_2 and $PGF_{2\alpha}$ in neonates during the first week of life, and correlated these with systolic pressure in both the baby and mother. There was a weak inverse relationship between the babies' systolic pressure and $PGF_{2\alpha}$, but not PGE_2 excretion. While this gives some support to the hypothesis that renal prostaglandin synthesis is decreased in those susceptible to subsequent development of hypertension the significance and function of renal $PGF_{2\alpha}$ is unclear.

An alternative approach has been to determine whether there is any difference in the renal response to stimulation of prostaglandin synthesis in patients with essential hypertension. In animals an intravenous injection of frusemide has been shown to produce an early increase in plasma renin activity and renal blood flow which is dependent on prostaglandin synthesis (Bailie, Barbour and Hook, 1975; Oliw *et al.*, 1976). In man the same early increase in plasma renin activity, renal blood flow and urinary PGE excretion also occurs; moreover, treatment with indomethacin abolishes this effect (*Figures 9.2* and *9.3*) indicating that all three changes are likely to be a result of increased prostaglandin synthesis (Mackay, Muir and Watson, 1984). Urinary 6-ketoPGF$_{1\alpha}$, $PGF_{2\alpha}$ and thromboxane B_2 all increase in a similar fashion after frusemide, suggesting that there is either a transient increase in arachidonic acid release or decrease in prostanoid catabolism.

Using frusemide in this way provides a useful means of assessing the kidneys' capacity to synthesize prostaglandins by measuring both rates of prostaglandin production and the early changes in renal plasma flow and plasma renin activity. Some studies are consistent with the hypothesis that there is a defect in renal capacity to synthesize prostaglandins in hypertension; for example, the early increase in renin release after frusemide was suppressed in patients with essential hypertension (Padfield *et al.*, 1975; Weber, Siess and Scherer, 1980), and there was also less stimulation of PGE_2 excretion after frusemide in such patients (Abe *et al.*, 1977; Rathaus, Korzets and Bernheim, 1983). Others have not confirmed the latter findings (Halushka *et al.*, 1979). Part of the discrepancy in results may be due to differences in the severity of hypertension in the patients studied.

In a study of patients with mild, essential hypertension (mean blood pressure 127 mmHg) we have found that the early frusemide-induced changes in renal plasma flow, plasma renin activity and urinary PGE excretion did not differ significantly from the response in normals (Mackay *et al.*, 1983) (*Figure 9.4*). This

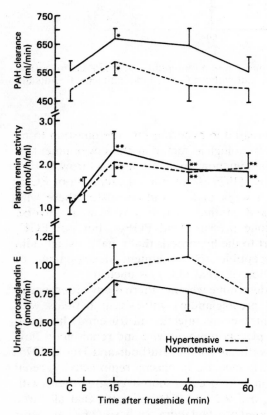

Figure 9.4 Changes in urinary PGE excretion, plasma renin activity and clearance of para-aminohippuric acid (PAH) after frusemide (30 mg) in normotensive and hypertensive subjects. Results expressed as mean ± SEM. Significance values refer to differences relative to the control values in each group. *$P<0.05$; **$P<0.01$

implies that changes in prostaglandin synthesis are secondary to the development of hypertension rather than primary aetiological factors.

Two preliminary reports have appeared of enhanced renal thromboxane A_2 synthesis in essential hypertension (Grose, Lebel and Gbeassor, 1983; Hornych *et al.*, 1983). Furthermore in normal subjects β-adrenoreceptor blockade has been reported to decrease plasma thromboxane B_2 levels, suggesting that thromboxane synthesis may be important in the maintenance of blood pressure (Graham, Campbell and Jackson, 1982). If these findings are confirmed, further developments are likely in this area, particularly in view of the recent data implicating thromboxane in the pathogenesis of hypertension in the spontaneously hypertensive rat (*see above*).

The role of any changes in PGI_2 synthesis in hypertension has not been fully evaluated. Measurement of urinary excretion of one of the metabolites of PGI_2, 2,3-dinor 6-ketoPGF$_{1\alpha}$ provides a useful measure of the rate of entry of PGI_2 into the systemic circulation (Fitzgerald *et al.*, 1981). Although early reports implicated PGI_2 as a modulator of the vasoconstrictor effects of angiotensin II (Dusting, Mullins and Doyle, 1980; Shebuski and Aiken, 1980), no increase in excretion of 2,3-dinor-6-ketoPGF$_{1\alpha}$ was found during infusion of angiotensin II into conscious dogs (Watson, Herzer and Branch, 1983). Moreover, in normal man, stimulation of the renin–angiotensin system by a sodium-restricted diet resulted in a decrease rather than an increase in the urinary excretion of dinor-6-ketoPGF$_{1\alpha}$, indicating that systemic PGI_2 synthesis had also decreased (Watson *et al.*, 1984). In a study of

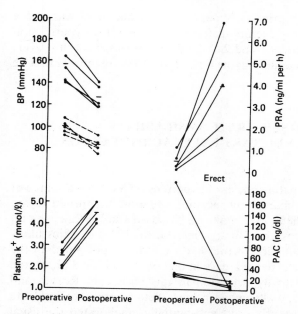

Figure 9.5 Systolic (——) and diastolic (– – –) blood pressure, plasma potassium, plasma renin activity (in erect position) and plasma aldosterone concentration in patients with primary hyperaldosteronism before (preoperative) and after (postoperative) removal of the adenoma. Horizontal bars represent mean values

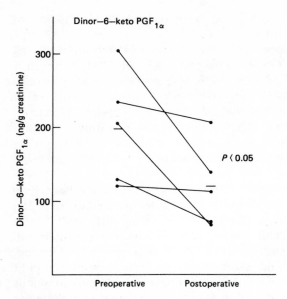

Figure 9.6 Urinary excretion of 2,3-dinor-6-ketoPGF$_{1\alpha}$ in 24-hour urine collections in patients with primary hyperaldosteronism before and after removal of the adenoma. Horizontal bars represent mean values

patients with hypertension due to primary hyperaldosteronism, there was also a small decrease in dinor 6-ketoPGF$_{1\alpha}$ excretion after correction of the hypertension by removal of the adenoma (*Figures 9.5* and *9.6*). The change was small, however, and any role of systemic PGI$_2$ in modulating the high blood pressure must at best be minor.

ALTERATION IN PROSTANOID SUBSTRATE AVAILABILITY — THE EFFECT OF VARIATION IN DIETARY FATTY ACID INTAKE ON BLOOD PRESSURE

The role of dietary sodium in the pathogenesis of hypertension has been a source of controversy for many years. Comparatively recently attention has turned to the possible influence of changes in dietary fat intake on blood pressure. While high fat diets in rabbits increase blood pressure (Burstyn and Furth, 1975) it seems likely that the particular fatty acids contained in the diet are more important than the total fat intake. For example, a selective increase in dietary linoleic acid prevented the development of salt-dependent hypertension in rats (Schoene, Reeves and Ferretti, 1980; Vergroesen *et al.*, 1980) while a high dietary intake of linoleate during the development of hypertensive rats substantially ameliorated the usual progressive rise in blood pressure (Church, Reeves and Schoene, 1977; Tobian *et al.*, 1982). An alternative method of study is to use diets deficient in certain fatty acids. There was no change in basal blood pressure in rats fed a diet deficient in essential fatty acids (EFA) from soon after birth, when sodium intake was also normal. However, feeding of the same fatty acid-deficient diet with an associated high sodium intake resulted in a significantly higher blood pressure (Rosenthal, Simone and Silbergleif, 1974). The essential fatty acids-deficient rats also excreted an acutely administered sodium chloride infusion more slowly than their normal controls. In a similar study the essential fatty acids-deficient animals also showed enhanced renal vasoconstriction in response to infusion of angiotensin II and norepinephrine (Sakr and Dunham, 1982).

Studies in man further support the possibility that dietary fat intake affects blood pressure. A diet containing 25% of the calories as fat (with a ratio of polyunsaturated/saturated fatty acid (P/S) content of 1.0) caused an 8–9% decrease in systemic blood pressure compared with the levels found during a normal diet (16% fat, P/S ratio 0.2) (Iacono, Dougherty and Puska, 1982; Iacono *et al.*, 1981). From these studies there did seem to be an optimum fat intake for lowering blood pressure; increasing the proportion of calories as fat to 35% (P/S ratio 1.0) caused no further significant decrease in blood pressure, an observation that may have some significance in regard to the underlying mechanism (*see below*). Feeding hypertensive males a diet supplemented with linoleic acid (sunflower oil) also significantly decreased blood pressure over a three-week period (Comberg *et al.*, 1978).

Rather than altering dietary fat intake it is possible to obtain a retrospective assessment of dietary fatty acid content by measuring the fatty acid components in adipose tissue (Dayton *et al.*, 1966). Using this technique Oster *et al.* (1980) was able to demonstrate a significant negative correlation between adipose tissue linoleic acid and blood pressure in a study of 650 men. Interestingly, there were also weak correlations between dietary linoleate intake and rates of urine flow and sodium excretion. More carefully controlled studies now further support the preliminary findings. A randomized trial of normal people in Finland has demonstrated that changing from a normal diet to low-fat diet (containing 25% fat calories with a P/S ratio 1.0) was associated with a significant decline in both systolic and diastolic blood pressure (*Table 9.1*) that reversed on return to a normal diet. The decrease in blood pressure was most in subjects whose baseline diastolic blood pressure was greater than 90 mmHg (Puska *et al.*, 1983).

Compelling evidence is therefore accumulating to confirm that dietary fat intake has a significant effect on blood pressure. The question arises as to what is the underlying mechanism of this effect. It might be non-specific, for example as a result of changes in the fatty acid content of phospholipids (Schaeffer and Curtis, 1977). Alternatively the dietary changes may influence the synthesis and/or release of antihypertensive lipids from the kidneys (Muirhead, Chapter 10 of this volume). A third possibility is that changes in dietary linoleate, or other essential fatty acids, might alter substrate availability for synthesis of prostanoids, thereby altering basal or stimulated prostanoid synthesis. Evidence that this may be the case is suggestive, but by no means conclusive. Increasing linoleate intake increases tissue synthesis of PGI_2, PGE_2 and other prostaglandins (Galli *et al.*, 1980; Lagarde, Guichardant and Dechavanne, 1981; Vergroesen *et al.*, 1980; Willis *et al.*, 1981). In spontaneously hypertensive rats an increase in dietary intake of linoleate increased the

Table 9.1 Mean blood pressure ($\pm$ SEM) in last week of each 6-week period in subjects categorized according to diastolic blood pressure

| | Low fat, high P/S diet | | Normal diet | |
	Baseline diastolic blood pressure		Baseline diastolic blood pressure	
	<90 $n = 19$	$\geqslant$90 $n = 16$	<90 $n = 19$	$\geqslant$90 $n = 19$
Baseline				
Systolic	127.2 $\pm$ 2.7	151.7 $\pm$ 3.7	129.5 $\pm$ 1.8	146.1 $\pm$ 2.3
Diastolic	80.1 $\pm$ 1.3	99.4 $\pm$ 1.6	81.3 $\pm$ 1.2	97.3 $\pm$ 1.1
Intervention				
Systolic	121.6 $\pm$ 1.7**	139.0 $\pm$ 3.0*	128.6 $\pm$ 2.0	143.5 $\pm$ 2.9
Diastolic	75.2 $\pm$ 1.3*	88.6 $\pm$ 1.7*	80.9 $\pm$ 1.4	92.8 $\pm$ 1.7**
Switchback				
Systolic	128.9 $\pm$ 2.5**	145.9 $\pm$ 3.6*	129.5 $\pm$ 2.2	145.6 $\pm$ 2.7
Diastolic	79.4 $\pm$ 2.0**	92.3 $\pm$ 1.9†	81.3 $\pm$ 1.6	93.9 $\pm$ 1.4

*$P<0.001$; **$P<0.01$; †$P<0.05$. (After Puska *et al.*, 1983)

prostaglandin content of renal medulla and at the same time systemic blood pressure was lowered. A stimulatory effect of increasing dietary linoleate intake on urinary excretion of tetranorprostanoate and dinorprostanoate metabolites in rats provides more direct evidence of a link between diet and prostaglandin synthesis (Nugteren *et al.*, 1980). Similar changes in excretion of prostanoid metabolites also occurred in man in response to changes in diet (Zollner, Adam and Wolfram, 1979). Also in man, an eight-hour infusion of sunflower oil increased urinary excretion of 6-ketoPGF$_{1\alpha}$ and to a lesser extent PGE$_2$ (Epstein, Lifschitz and Rappaport, 1982). Moreover, essential fatty acids-deficient infants excrete very low levels of the PGE$_2$ metabolite 7-hydroxy 5,11-diketotetranor-1,16-dioic acid (Friedman *et al.*, 1980). In the same study it was noted, however, that feeding Intralipid (very high in linoleate) decreased excretion of the same urinary metabolite of PGE$_2$. As in the study of blood pressure (Iacono *et al.*, 1981) this suggests that excessive linoleate intake may actually decrease prostaglandin synthesis (Spector *et al.*, 1980). Spector noted also that changes in the fatty acid content of cultured endothelial cells altered their ability to synthesize PGI$_2$, in particular high levels of linoleate decreased PGI$_2$ synthesis. One possibility already discussed is that high levels of linoleate may compete with arachidonic acid for binding to prostaglandin synthetase. A similar mechanism may explain the observed decrease in urinary PGE and PGF$_{2\alpha}$ excretion during dietary supplementation with eicosapentaenoic acid (Lorenz *et al.*, 1983).

These findings emphasize the very complex effects that are likely to result from manipulations in dietary fatty acid intake, but also indicate that measurement of certain prostaglandin metabolites in urine may be a useful means of assessing the effects of dietary manipulations. It is certainly attractive to speculate that the changes in blood pressure invoked by alteration of dietary fat intake are in part mediated by changes in prostaglandin synthesis.

CONCLUSIONS

It is an oversimplification to attempt to categorize particular prostaglandins as being prohypertensive and antihypertensive because their individual actions are so dependent on their site of synthesis. However, in general terms PGE_2 and PGI_2 do appear most likely to be vasodepressor, whereas thromboxane A_2 is more likely to be a pressor agent.

If the decrease in blood pressure induced by increased dietary intake of linoleic acid is a result of enhanced prostaglandin synthesis then increased synthesis of PGE_2 or PGI_2 is a likely mechanism. The data suggesting that renal PGE_2 is decreased in essential hypertension would also be consistent with such a mechanism. The hypothesis that such a deficiency in renal prostaglandin synthesis is an important factor in the development of hypertension remains unproven. It may in fact be merely a secondary adaptation to the high blood pressure. The actual mechanism by which such a deficiency of prostaglandin synthesis contributes to the hypertension must at this time be speculative. The simplest explanation would be that deficient prostaglandin synthesis results in increased renal vascular resistance, but this implies that prostaglandins decrease renal vascular resistance in normal kidneys. Most data suggest that prostaglandins have a very minor role in determining renal vascular resistance of the normal kidney. It is attractive to speculate that enhanced renal thromboxane A_2 synthesis contributes to the increased renal vascular resistance. If this were the case it would be reasonable to expect that inhibition of cyclo-oxygenase might decrease renal vascular resistance and lower blood pressure in hypertensive patients. There is no convincing data to support such a hypothesis. Moreover, if enhanced renal thromboxane A_2 synthesis has an important role then increased blood pressure and renal vascular resistance might have been expected to occur during supplementation of dietary linoleic acid.

The wide range of potent effects of many of the prostanoids on renal function and the systemic vasculature has inevitably led to a profusion of hypotheses about their possible role in the development of hypertension. Improvements in the methods available to assess prostanoid synthesis combined with the availability of more selective synthetase inhibitors and receptor antagonists should help to determine which of these hypotheses are more nearly correct.

Acknowledgements

Professor J. S. Robson is thanked for his help in preparation of the manuscript. Part of the work was undertaken during tenure of grants from the Medical Research Council (UK) and the Fogarty International Centre (FO5 TWO 3114-02).

References

ABE, K., YASUJIMA, M., CHIBA, S. *et al.* (1977) Effet of furosemide on urinary excretion of Prostaglandin E in normal volunteers and patients with essential hypertension. *Prostaglandins*, **14**, 513–521

AHNFELT-RONNE, I. and ARRIGONI-MARTELLI, E. (1977) Renal prostaglandin metabolism in spontaneously hypertensive rats. *Biochemical Pharmacology*, **26**, 485–488

AIKEN, J. W. and VANE, J. R. (1973) Intrarenal prostaglandin release attentuates the renal vasoconstrictor activity of angiotensin. *Journal of Pharmacology and Experimental Therapeutics*, **184**, 678–687

ARENDSHORST, W. J. and BEIERWALTES, W. H. (1979) Renal and nephron hemodynamics in spontaneously hypertensive rats. *American Journal of Physiology*, **236**, F246–F251

ARMSTRONG, J. M., BLACKWELL, G. J., FLOWER, R. J., MC GIFF, J. C., MULLANE, K. and VANE, J. R. (1975) Genetic hypertension in rats is accompanied by a defect in renal prostaglandin catabolism. *Nature (London)*, **260**, 582–586

AZAR, S., JOHNSON, M. A., SCHEINMAN, J., BRUNO, L. and TOBIAN, L. (1979) Regulation of glomerular capillary pressure and filtration rate in young Kyoto hypertensive rats. *Clinical Science*, **56**, 203–209

BAER, P. G. and MC GIFF, J. C. (1979) Comparison of effects of prostaglandins E_2 and I_2 on rat renal vascular resistance. *European Journal of Pharmacology*, **54**, 359–363

BAILIE, D., BARBOUR, J. A. and HOOK, J. B. (1975) Effects of indomethacin on frusemide-induced changes in renal blood flow. *Proceedings of the Society for Experimental Biology and Medicine*, **148**, 1173–1176

BENZONI, D., VINCENT, M. and SASSARO, J. (1982) Urinary prostaglandins in the Lyon strains of hypertensive, normotensive and low blood pressure rats. *Hypertension*, **4**, 325–328

BERL, T., HENRICH, W. L., ERICKSON, A. L. and SCHRIER, R. W. (1979) Prostaglandins in the beta-adrenergic and baroreceptor-mediated secretion of renin. *American Journal of Physiology*, **236**, F472–F477

BLACKSHEAR, J. L., SPIELMAN, W. S., KNOX, F. G. and ROMERO, J. C. (1979) Dissociation of renin release and renal vasodilatation by prostaglandin synthesis inhibitors. *American Journal of Physiology*, **237**, F20–F24

BLAIR, I. A., BARROW, S. E., WADDELL, K. A., LEWIS, P. J. and DOLLERY, C. T. (1982) Prostacyclin is not a circulating hormone in man. *Prostaglandins*, **23**, 579–589

BOEYNAEMS, J. M. and HERMAN, A. G. (1980) *Prostaglandins, Prostacyclin and Thromboxanes Measurement*. The Hague: Martius Nijhoff

BOHMAN, S. D. (1977) Demonstration of prostaglandin synthesis in collecting duct cells and other cell types of the rabbit renal medulla. *Prostaglandins*, **14**, 739–744

BORGEAT, P., HAMBERG, M. and SAMUELSSON, B. (1976) Transformation of arachidonic acid and homo-γ-linolenic acid by rabbit polymorphonuclear leukocytes. *Journal of Biological Chemistry*, **251**, 7816–7820

BURSTYN, P. G. and FIRTH, W. R. (1975) Effects of three fat-enriched diets on the arterial pressure of rabbits. *Cardiovascular Research*, **9**, 807–810

CAMPBELL, W. B., GRAHAM, R. M. and JACKSON, E. K. (1979) Role of renal prostaglandins in sympathetically mediated renin release in the rat. *Journal of Clinical Investigation*, **65**, 448–456

CAPDEVILA, J., MARNETT, L. J., CHACOS, N., PROUGH, R. A. and ESTABROOK, R. W. (1982) Cytochrome P-450-dependent oxygenation of arachidonic acid to hydroxyeicosatetraenonic acids. *Proceedings of the National Academy of Sciences of the USA*, **79**, 767–770

CHURCH, J. P., REEVES, V. B. and SCHOENE, N. W. (1977) Effects of essential fatty acid deficiency on blood pressure in the spontaneously hypertensive rat. *Federation Proceedings*, **36**, 1159

COMAI, K., FARBER, S. J. and PAULSRUD, J. R. (1975) Analysis of renal medullary lipid droplets from normal, hydronephrotic and indomethacin treated rabbits. *Lipids*, **10**, 555–561

COMBERG, H. U., HEYDEN, S., HAMES, C. G., VERGROESEN, A. J. and FLEISCHMAN, A. I. (1978) Hypertensive effect of dietary prostaglandin precursor in hypertensive men. *Prostaglandins*, **15**, 193–197

DANIELS, E. G., HINMAN, J. W., LEACH, B. E. and MUIRHEAD, E. E. (1967) Identification of prostaglandin E_2 as the principal vasodepressor lipid of rabbit renal medulla. *Nature (London)*, **215**, 1298–1299

DATA, J. L., GERBER, J. G., CRUMP, W. J., FROLICH, J. C., HOLLIFIELD, J. W. and NIES, A. S. (1978) The prostaglandin system: a role in canine baroreceptor control of renin release. *Circulation Research*, **42**, 454–458

DAVIS, H. A. and HORTON, E. W. (1972) Output of prostaglandins from the rabbit kidney, its increase on renal nerve stimulation and its inhibition by indomethacin. *British Journal of Pharmacology*, **46**, 658–675

DAYTON, S., HASHIMOTO, S., DIXON, W. and PEARCE, M. L. (1966) Composition of lipids in human serum and adipose tissue during prolonged feeding of a diet high in unsaturated fat. *Journal of Lipid Research*, **7**, 103–111

DRAY, F., CHARBONNEL, B. and MACLOUF, J. (1975) Radioimmunoassay of $PGF_{1\alpha}$, PGE and PGE_2 in human plasma. *European Journal of Clinical Investigation*, **5**, 311–318

DRAZEN, J. M., AUSTEN, K. F., LEWIS, R. A. *et al.* (1980) Comparative urinary and vascular activities of leukotrienes C-1 and D *in vivo* and *in vitro*. *Proceedings of the National Academy of Sciences of the USA*, **77**, 4354–4358

DUNN, M. J. (1978) Renal prostaglandin production in the Japanese spontaneously hypertensive rat. *Clinical Science and Molecular Medicine*, **55**, 191S

DUNN, M. J. (1976) Renal prostaglandin synthesis in the spontaneously hypertensive rat. *Journal of Clinical Investigation*, **58**, 862–870

DUSTING, G. J., MULLINS, E. M. and DOYLE A. E. (1980) Angiotensin-induced prostacyclin release may contribute to the hypotensive action of converting enzyme. *Advances in Prostaglandin and Thromboxane Research*, **7**, 815–819

EPSTEIN, M., LIFSCHITZ, M. and RAPPAPORT, K. (1982) Augmentation of prostaglandin production by linoleic acid in man. *Kidney International*, **21**, 260 (Abstract 16)

FAGARD, R., AMERY, A., REYBROUCK, T., LIJNEN, P., BILLIET, L. and JOOSSENS, J. V. (1977) Plasma renin levels and systemic haemodynamics in essential hypertension. *Clinical Science and Molecular Medicine*, **52**, 591–597

FALARDEAU, P., OATES, J. A. and BRASH, A. R. (1981) Quantitative analysis of two dinor urinary metabolites of Prostaglandin I_2. *Analytical Biochemistry*, **115**, 359–367

FEIGEN, L. P., CHAPNICK, B. M., FLEMING, J. E., FLEMING, J. M. and KADOWITZ, P. J. (1978) Renal vascular effects of endoperoxide analogs, prostaglandins and arachidonic acid. *American Journal of Physiology*, **233**, H573–H579

FEIGEN, L. P. (1983) Differential effects of leukotrienes C_4, D_4 and E_4 in the canine renal and mesenteric vascular beds. *Journal of Pharmacology and Experimental Therapeutics*, **225**, 682–687

FEUERSTEIN, G., ZUKOWSKA-GROJEC, Z. and KOPIN, I. J. (1981) Cardiovascular effects of leukotriene D_4 in SHR and WKY rats. *European Journal of Pharmacology*, **76**, 107–110

FITZGERALD, G. A., HOSSMANN, V., HUMMERICH, W. and KONRADS, A. (1981) The renin–kallikrein–prostaglandin system; plasma active and inactive renin and urinary kallikrein during prostacyclin infusion in man. *Prostaglandins in Medicine*, **5**, 445–456

FITZGERALD, G. A., BRASH, A. R., FALARDEAU, P. and OATES, J. A. (1981) Estimated rate of prostacyclin secretion into the circulation of normal man. *Journal of Clinical Investigation*, **68**, 1272–1276

FLOWER, R. J. (1974) Drugs which inhibit prostaglandin biosynthesis. *Pharmacological Reviews*, **26**, 33–67

FLOWER, R. J. and BLACKWELL, G. J. (1976) The importance of phospholipase A_2 in prostaglandin biosynthesis. *Biochemical Pharmacology*, **25**, 285–291

FOLKERT, V. W. and SCHLONDORFF, D. (1979) Prostaglandin synthesis in isolated glomeruli. *Prostaglandins*, **17**, 79–86

FRIEDMAN, Z., SEYBERTH, H., FROLICH, J. C. and OATES, J. A. (1980) Effects of dietary variation in linoleic acid content on the major urinary metabolites of the E prostaglandins (PGE-M) in infants. *Advances in Prostaglandin and Thromboxane Research*, **8**, 1799–1805

FROLICH, J. C., WILSON, T. W., SWEETMAN, B. J. *et al.* (1975) Urinary prostaglandins. Identification and origin. *Journal of Clinical Investigation*, **55**, 763–770

FROLICH, J. C., SWEETMAN, B. J., CARR, K. and OATES, J. A. (1975) Prostaglandin synthesis in rabbit renal medulla. *Life Science*, **17**, 1105–1112

FROLICH, J. C., HOLLIFIELD, J. W., MICHELAKIS, A. M. *et al.* (1979) Reduction of plasma renin activity by inhibition of the fatty acid cycloxygenase in human subjects. Independence of sodium retention. *Circulation Research*, **44**, 781–787

GALLI, C., AGRADI, E., PETRONI, A. and TREMOLI, E. (1980) Dietary essential fatty acids, tissue fatty acids and prostaglandin synthesis. *Progress in Food and Nutritional Science*, **4**, 1–7

GERBER, J. G., BRANCH, R. A., NIES, A. S. *et al.* (1978) Assessment of renin secretion following infusion of PGI_2, PGE_2 and PGD_2 into the renal artery of anesthetised dogs. *Prostaglandins*, **15**, 81–88

GERBER, J. G., OLSON, R. D. and NIES, A. S. (1981) Interrelationship between prostaglandins and renin release. *Kidney International*, **9**, 816–821

GIMBRONE, M. A. and ALEXANDER, R. W. (1975) Angiotensin II stimulation of prostaglandin production in cultured human vascular endothelium. *Science*, **189**, 219–220

GRAHAM, R. M., CAMPBELL, W. B. and JACKSON, E. K. (1982) Effects of short term beta-blockade on blood pressure, plasma thromboxane B_2 and plasma and urinary prostaglandins E_2 and $F_{2\alpha}$ in normal subjects. *Clinical Pharmacology and Therapeutics*, **31**, 324–329

GRANSTROM, E. (1978) Radioimmunoassay of prostaglandins. *Prostaglandins*, **15**, 3–17

GREENWALD, J. E., BIANCHINE, J. R. and WONG, L. K. (1979) The production of the arachidonate metabolite HETE in vascular tissue. *Nature (London)*, **281**, 588–589

GROSE, J. H., LEVEL, M. and GBEASSOR, F. M. (1983) Imbalanced prostacyclin and thromboxane A_2 production in essential hypertension. *Advances in Prostaglandin, Thromboxane and Leukotriene Research*, **11**, 413–415

GUYTON, A. C., COLEMAN, T. G., COWLEY, A. W., MANNING, R. D., NORMAN, R. and FERGUSON, J. D. (1974) A systems analysis approach to understanding long-range arterial blood pressure control and hypertension. *Circulation Research*, **35**, 159–176

GUYTON, A. C., HALL, J. E., LOHMEIR, T. E., JACKSON, T. E. and MANNING, R. D. (1981) The many roles of the kidney in arterial pressure control and hypertension. *Canadian Journal of Physiology and Pharmacology*, **59**, 513–519

HALUSHKA, P. V., MARGOLIUS, H. S., ALLEN, H. and CONRADI, E. C. (1979) Urinary excretion of PGE like material and kallikrein; effects of frusemide. *Prostaglandins*, **18**, 359–369

HAMBERG, M. and SAMUELSSON, B. (1971) On the metabolism of prostaglandin E (1 and 2) in man. *Journal of Biological Chemistry*, **246**, 6713–6721

HAMBERG, M. and SAMUELSSON, B. (1974) Prostaglandin endoperoxides. Novel transformations of arachidonic acid in human platelets. *Proceedings of the National Academy of Sciences of the USA*, **71**, 3400–3404

HAMBERG, M., HEDQVIST, P. and RADEGRAN, K. (1980) Identification of 15-hydroxy-5,8,11,13-eicosatetraenoic acid (15-HETE) as a major metabolite of arachidonic acid in human lung. *Acta Physiologica Scandinavica*, **110**, 219–221

HASSID, A., KONIECZKOWSKI, M. and DUNN, M. J. (1979) Prostaglandin synthesis in isolated rat kidney glomeruli. *Proceedings of the National Academy of Sciences of the USA*, **76**, 1155–1159

HAYLOR, J. and TOWERS, J. (1982) Renal vasodilator activity of prostaglandin E_2 in the rat anesthetised with phenobarbitone. *British Journal of Pharmacology*, **76**, 131–137

HEDQVIST, P. (1976) Prostaglandin action on transmitter release at adrenergic neuroeffector junctions. *Advances in Prostaglandin and Thromboxane Research*, **1**, 357–363

HENRICH, W. L. (1981) Role of prostaglandins in renin secretion. *Kidney International*, **19**, 822–830

HOLLENBERG, N. K., ADAMS, D. F., SOLOMON, H. *et al.* (1975) Renal vascular tone in essential and secondary hypertension. Hemodynamic and angiographic responses to vasodilators. *Medicine (Baltimore)*, **54**, 29–44

HORNYCH, A., SAFAR, M., SIMON, A. and BARIETY, J. (1983) Thromboxane B_2 in borderline and essential hypertension. *Advances in Prostaglandin, Thromboxane and Leukotriene Research*, **11**, 417–422

IACONO, J. M., MARSHALL, M. W., DOUGHERTY, R. M., WHEELER, M. A., MACKIN, J. F. and CANARY, J. J. (1975) Reduction in blood pressure associated with high polyunsaturated fat diets that reduce blood cholesterol in man. *Preventive Medicine*, **4**, 426–443

IACONO, J. M., JUDO, J. T., MARSHALL, M. W. *et al.* (1981) The role of dietary essential fatty acids and prostaglandins in reducing blood pressure. *Progress in Lipid Research*, **20**, 349–364

IACONO, J. M., DOUGHERTY, R. M. and PUSKA, P. (1982) Reduction of blood pressure associated with dietary polyunsaturated fat. *Hypertension*, **4**, 34–42

ISAKSON, P. C., RAZ, A. and NEEDLEMAN, P. (1976) Selective incorporation of ^{14}C arachidonic acid into the phospholipids of intact tissues and subsequent metabolism to ^{14}C prostaglandins. *Prostaglandin*, **12**, 739–748

JACKSON, E. K., HERZER, W. A., ZIMMERMAN, J. B., BRANCH, R. A., OATES, J. A. and GERKENS, J. F. (1981) 6-Keto-prostaglandin E_1 is more potent than prostaglandin I_2 as a renal vasodilator and renin secretogogue. *Journal of Pharmacology and Experimental Therapeutics*, **216**, 24–27

JACKSON, E. K., HEIDEMAN, H. T., BRANCH, R. A. and GERKENS, J. F. (1982) Low dose intrarenal infusions of PGE_2, PGI_2 and 6-keto-PGE_1 vasodilate the *in vivo* rat kidney. *Circulation Research*, **51**, 67–72

JANSZEN, F. H. A. and NUGTEREN, D. H. (1971) Histochemical localisation of prostaglandin synthetase. *Histochemie*, **27**, 159–164

JONES, R. L. and WILSON, N. H. (1980) Partial agonism of prostaglandin H_2 analogs and 11-deoxy-prostaglandin F_2 alpha to thromboxane-sensitive preparation. *Advances in Prostaglandin and Thromboxane Research*, **6**, 467–475

JONES, R. L., WATSON, M. L. and UNGAR, A. (1981) A comparison of the effects of prostaglandins E_2 and I_2 on renal function and renin release in salt-loaded and salt-depleted anaesthetised dogs. *Quarterly Journal of Experimental Physiology*, **66**, 1–15

JONES, R. L., PEESAPATI, V. and WILSON, N. H. (1982) Antagonism of the thromboxane-sensitive contractile systems of the rabbit aorta, dog saphenous vein and guinea-pig trachea. *British Journal of Pharmacology*, **76**, 423–438

KONIECZKOWSKI, M., DUNN, M. J., STORK, J. E. and HASSID, A. (1983) Glomerular synthesis of prostaglandins and thromboxane in spontaneously hypertensive rats. *Hypertension*, **5**, 446–453

KOPP, U. and DIBONA, G. F. (1983) Interaction of renal β_1-adrenoreceptors and prostaglandins in reflex renin release. *American Journal of Physiology*, **245**, F418–F424

KREISBERG, J. I., KARNOVSKY, M. J. and LEVINE, L. (1982) Prostaglandin production by homogenous cultures of rat glomerular epithelial and mesangial cells. *Kidney International*, **22**, 355–359

LAGARDE, M., GUICHARDANT, M. and DECHAVANNE, M. (1981) Human platelet PGE_2 and arachidonic acid. *Progress in Lipid Research*, **20**, 439–443

LANDS, W. E. M. and SAMUELSSON, B. (1968) Phospholipid precursors of prostaglandins *Biochimica Biophysica Acta*, **164**, 426–429

LARSSON, C. and ANGGARD, E. (1973) Regional differences in the formation and metabolism of prostaglandins in rabbit kidney. *European Journal of Pharmacology*, **21**, 30–36

LEARY, W. P., LEDINGHAM, J. F. and VANE, J. R. (1974) Impaired prostaglandin release from the kidneys of salt-loaded and hypertensive rats. *Prostaglandins*, **7**, 425–432

LEVY, J. V. (1977) Changes in systolic arterial blood pressure in normal and spontaneously hypertensive rats produced by acute administration of inhibitors of prostaglandin biosynthesis. *Prostaglandins*, **13**, 153–160

LIANOS, E. and DUNN, M. J. (1983) Glomerular arachidonate lipooxygenation in nephrotoxic serum nephritis. *Clinical Research*, **31**, 550A

LIMAS, C. J. and LIMAS, C. (1977) Prostaglandin metabolism in the kidneys of spontaneously hypertensive rats. *American Journal of Physiology*, **233**, H87–H92

LIMAS, C. and LIMAS, C. J. (1979) Enhanced renomedullary prostaglandin synthesis in spontaneously hypertensive rats – role of a phospholipase A_2. *American Journal of Physiology*, **236**, H65–H72

LIMAS, C., GOLDMAN, P., LIMAS, C. J. and IWAI, J. (1981) Effect of salt on prostaglandin metabolism in hypertension-prone and resistant Dahl rats. *Hypertension*, **3**, 219–224

LONIGRO, A. J., ITSKOVITZ, H. D., CROWSHAW, K. and MCGIFF, J. C. (1973) Dependency of renal blood flow on prostaglandin synthesis in the dog. *Circulation Research*, **32**, 712–717

LORENZ, R., SPENGLER, U., FISCHER, S., DUHM, J. and WEBER, P. C. (1983) Platelet function, thromboxane formation and blood pressure during supplementation of the Western diet with cod liver oil. *Circulation*, **67**, 504–511

MAAS, R. L., BRASH, A. R. and OATES, J. A. (1982) A second pathway of leukotriene biosynthesis in porcine leukocytes. *Proceedings of the National Academy of Sciences of the USA*, **78**, 5523–5527

MACKAY, I. G., MUIR, A. L. and WATSON, M. L. (1984) Contribution of prostaglandins to the systemic and renal vascular response to frusemide in normal man. *British Journal of Clinical Pharmacology*, **17**, 513–519

MACKAY, I. G., WATSON, M. L., NATH, K. A., CUMMING, A. and MUIR, A. L. (1983) Urinary prostaglandin and kallikrein in mild hypertension. *Clinical Science*, **65**, 59

MALIK, K. U. and MCGIFF, J. C. (1975) Modulation by prostaglandins of adrenergic transmission in the isolated perfused rabbit and rat kidney. *Circulation Research*, **36**, 599–609

MARTINEZ-MALDONADO, M., TSAPARAS, N., EKNOYAN, G. and SUKI, W. N. (1972) Renal actions of prostaglandins: comparison with acetylcholine and saline expansion. *American Journal of Physiology*, **222**, 1147–1152

MCGIFF, J. C., CROWSHAW, K., TERAGNO, N. A. and LONIGRO, A. J. (1970) Release of a prostaglandin-like substance into renal venous blood in response to angiotensin II. *Circulation Research*, **27** (Suppl. 1), 121–130

MICHELASSI, F., LANDA, L., HILL, R. D. et al. (1982) Leukotriene D_4: a potent coronary artery vasoconstrictor associated with impaired ventricular contraction. *Science*, **217**, 841–843

MILLER, M. M., KAISER, E., BAVER, P., SCHEIBER, V. and HOHENEGGER, M. (1976) Lipid composition of the rat kidney. *Nephron*, **17**, 41–50

MONCADA, S., HIGGS, E. A. and VANE, J. R. (1977) Human arterial and venous tissues generate prostacyclin (prostaglandin X), a potent inhibitor of platelet aggregation. *Lancet*, **1**, 18–20

MORGAN, T. E., TINKER, D. O. and HANNAHAN, D. J. (1963) Phospholipid metabolism in kidney. 1. Isolation and identification of lipids of rabbit kidney. *Archives of Biochemistry and Biophysics*, **103**, 54–64

MORRISON, A. R., NISHIKAWA, K. and NEEDLEMAN, P. (1977) Unmasking of thromboxane A_2 synthesis by ureter obstruction in the rabbit kidney. *Nature (London)*, **267**, 259–260

MORRISON, R., NISHIKAWA, K. and NEEDLEMAN, P. (1978) Thromboxane A_2 biosynthesis in the ureter obstructed isolated perfused kidney of rabbit. *Journal of Pharmacology and Experimental Therapeutics*, **205**, 1–8

MUEHRCKE, R. C., MANDAL, A. K., EPSTEIN, M. and VOLINI, F. I. (1969) Cytoplasmic granularity of renal medulla interstitial cells in experimental hypertension. *Journal of Laboratory and Clinical Medicine*, **73**, 299–308

MUIRHEAD, E. E., GERMAIN, G., LEACH, B. E. *et al.* (1972) Production of renomedullary prostaglandins by renomedullary intersitial cells grown in tissue culture. *Circulation Research*, **30–31** (Suppl. 2), 161–172

MURPHY, R. C., HAMMARSTROM, S. and SAMUELSSON, B. (1979) Leukotriene C: a slow-reacting substance from murine mastocytoma cells. *Proceedings of the National Academy Sciences of the USA*, **76**, 4275–4279

NEEDLEMAN, P., RAZ, A., MINKES, M. S., FERRENDELLI, J. A. and SPRECHER, H. (1979) Triene prostaglandins: prostacyclin and thromboxane biosynthesis and unique biological properties. *Proceedings of the National Academy of Sciences of the USA*, **76**, 944–948

NEGUS, P., TANNEN, R. L. and DUNN, M. J. (1976) Indomethacin potentiates the vasoconstriction actions of angiotensin II in normal man. *Prostaglandins*, **12**, 175–180

NISSEN, H. M. and BOJESEN, I. (1979) On lipid droplets in renal interstitial cells. Isolation and identification. *Zeitschrift für Zellforschung und Mikroskopische Anatomie*, **97**, 274–284

NUGTEREN, D. H., VAN EVERT, W. C., SOETING, W. J. and SPUY, J. H. (1980) The effect of different amounts of linoleic acid in the diet on the excretion of urinary prostaglandin metabolite in the rat. *Advances in Prostaglandin and Thromboxane Research*, **8**, 1793–1796

OKAHARA, T., IMANISHI, M. and YAMAMOTO, K. (1983) Zonal heterogeneity of prostaglandin and thromboxane release in the dog kidney. *Prostaglandins*, **25**, 373–381

OLIVER, J. A. and CANNON, P. J. (1978) The effect of altered sodium balance upon renal vascular reactivity to angiotensin II and nonepinephrine in the dog. Mechanism of variation in angiotensin responses. *Journal of Clinical Investigation*, **61**, 610–623

OLIVER, J. A., PINTO, J., SCIACCA, R. R. and CANNON, P. J. (1980) Increased renal secretion of norepinephrine and prostaglandin E_2 during sodium depletion in the dog. *Journal of Clinical Investigation*, **66**, 748–756

OLIW, E., KOVER, G., LARSSON, C. and ANGGARD, E. (1976) Reduction by indomethacin of furosemide effects in the rabbit. *European Journal of Pharmacology*, **38**, 95–100

OLIW, E. H., LAWSON, J. A., BRASH, A. R. and OATES, J. A. (1981) Arachidonic acid metabolism in rabbit renal cortex. Formation of two novel dihydroxyeicosatrienoic acids. *Journal of Biological Chemistry*, **256**, 9924–9931

OSTER, P., ARAB, L., SCHELLENBERG, B., KOHLMEIER, M. and SCHLIERF, G. (1980) Linoleic acid and blood pressure. *Proceedings of Food Nutrition Science*, **4**, 39–40

PACE-ASCIAK, C. R. (1976) Decreased renal prostaglandin catabolism precedes onset of hypertension in the developing spontaneously hypertensive rat. *Nature (London)*, **263**, 510–511

PACE-ASCIAK, C. R., CARRARA, M. C., RANGARAJ, G. and NICOLAOU, K. C. (1978) Enhanced formation of PGI_2. A potent hypotensive substance by aortic rings and homogenates of the spontaneously hypertensive rat. *Prostaglandins*, **15**, 1005–1012

PACE-ASCIAK, C. R., CARRARA, M. C. and NICOLAOU, K. C. (1978) PGI_2 has more potent hypotensive properties than PGE_2 in the normal and spontaneously hypertensive rat. *Prostaglandins*, **15**, 999–1003

PADFIELD, P. L., ALLISON, M. E. M., BROWN, J. J. *et al.* (1975) Effect of intravenous frusemide on plasma renin concentrations. Suppression of response in hypertension. *Clinical Science and Molecular Medicine*, **49**, 353–358

PETRULIS, A. S., AIKAWA, M. and DUNN, M. J. (1981) Prostaglandin and thromboxane synthesis by rat glomerular epithelial cells. *Kidney International*, **20**, 469–474

PIPER, P. J., LETTS, L. G. and GALTON, S. A. (1983) Generation of a leukotriene-like substance from porcine vascular and other tissues. *Prostaglandins*, **25**, 591–599

PIPER, P. J. (1983) Pharmacology of leukotrienes. *British Medical Bulletin*, **39**, 255–259

PUGSLEY, D. J., MULLINS, R. and BEILIN, L. J. (1976) Renal prostaglandin synthesis in hypertension induced by deoxycorticosterone and sodium chloride in the rat. *Clinical Science and Molecular Medicine*, **51** (Suppl. 3), 253S–256S

PUSKA, P., NISSINEN, A., VARTIAINEN, E. *et al.* (1983) Controlled randomised trial of the effect of dietary fat on blood pressure. *Lancet*, **1**, 1–5

RATHAUS, M., BAUMINGER, S. and BERNHEIM, J. (1980) Effect of frusemide on renal prostaglandin E_2 and F_2 in normal subjects and in patients with essential hypertension. *Israel Journal of Medical Science*, **16**, 106–110

RATHAUS, M., KORZETS, Z. and BERNHEIM, J. (1983) The urinary excretion of prostaglandin E_2 and $F_{2\alpha}$ in essential hypertension. *European Journal of Clinical Investigation*, **13**, 13–17

REMUZZI, G., CAVENAGHI, A. E., MECCA, G., DONATI, M. B. and DE GAETANO, G. (1978) Human renal cortex generates prostacyclin-like activity. *Thrombosis Research*, **12**, 363–366

REMUZZI, G., MECCA, G., LIVIO, M. *et al.* (1980) Prostacyclin generation by cultured endothelial cells in haemolytic uraemic syndrome. *Lancet*, **1**, 656–657

RIGHTSEL, W. A., OKAMURA, T., INAGAMI, T. *et al.* (1982) Juxtaglomerular cells grown as monolayer cell culture contain renin, angiotensin I-converting enzyme and angiotensin I and II/III. *Circulation Research*, **50**, 822–829

ROBERTSON, R. M., ROBERTSON, D., ROBERTS, L. J. *et al.* (1981) Thromboxane A_2 in vasotonic angina pectoris: evidence from direct measurements and inhibitor studies. *New England Journal of Medicine*, **304**, 998–1003

ROMERO, J. C. and STRONG, C. G. (1977) The effect of indomethacin blockade of prostaglandin synthesis on blood pressure of normal rabbits, and rabbits with renovascular hypertension. *Circulation Research*, **40**, 35–41

ROSENTHAL, J., SIMONE, P. G. and SILBERGLEIF, A. (1974) Effects of prostaglandin deficiency on natriuresis, diuresis and blood pressure. *Prostaglandins*, **5**, 435–450

SAKR, H. M. and DUNHAM, E. W. (1982) Enhanced renal vasoconstriction in rats fed essential fatty acid-deficient diet. *American Journal of Physiology*, **234**, H61–H67

SAKR, H. M. and DUNHAM, E. W. (1982) Mechanism of arachidonic acid-induced vasoconstriction in the intact rat kidney: possible involvement of thromboxane A_2. *Journal of Pharmacology and Experimental Therapeutics*, **221**, 614–621

SATO, K., ABE, K., SEINO, M. *et al.* (1983) Reduced urinary excretion of prostaglandin E in essential hypertension. *Prostaglandin and Leukotrienes in Medicine*, **11**, 189–197

SCHAEFFER, B. E. and CURTIS, A. S. G. (1977) Effects on cell adhesion and membrane fluidity of changes in plasmalemmal lipids in mouse L929 cells. *Journal of Cell Science*, **26**, 47–55

SCHARSCHMIDT, L. A. and DUNN, M. J. (1983) Prostaglandin synthesis by rat glomerular mesangial cells in culture. Effects of antiotensin II and arginine vasopressin. *Journal of Clinical Investigation*, **71**, 1756–1764

SCHERER, B. and WEBER, P. C. (1979) Urinary prostaglandins in the newborn: relationship to urinary osmolarity, urinary potassium and blood pressure. *Advances in Prostaglandin and Thromboxane Research*, **7**, 1033–1038

SCHNERMANN, J. and BRIGGS, J. P. (1981) Participation of renal cortical prostaglandins in the regulation of glomerular filtration rate. *Kidney International*, **19**, 802–815

SCHOENE, N. W., REEVES, V. B. and FERRETTI, A. (1980) Effects of dietary linoleic acid on the biosynthesis of PGE_2 and $PGF_{2\alpha}$ in kidney medullae in spontaneously hypertensive rats. *Advances in Prostaglandin and Thromboxane Research*, **8**, 1791–1792

SCHWERTSCHLAG, U., STAHL, T. and HACKENTHAL, E. (1982) A comparison of the effects of prostacyclin and 6-keto-prostaglandin E_1 on renin release in the isolated rat and rabbit kidney. *Prostaglandins*, **23**, 129–138

SHEBUSKI, R. J. and AIKEN, J. W. (1980) Angiotensin II stimulation of renal prostaglandin synthesis elevates circulating prostacyclin in the dog. *Journal of Cardiovascular Pharmacology*, **2**, 667–677

SHIBOUTA, Y., INADA, Y., TERASHITA, Z.-I., NISHIKAWA, K., KIKUCHI, S. and SHIMAMOTO, K. (1979) Angiotensin II stimulated release of thromboxane A_2 and prostacyclin (PGI_2) in isolated perfused kidneys of spontaneously hypertensive rats. *Biochemical Pharmacology*, **28**, 3601–3609

SHIBOUTA, Y., TERASHITA, Z.-I., INADA, Y., NISHIKAWA, K. and KIKUCHI, S. (1981) Enhanced thromboxane A_2 biosynthesis in the kidney of spontaneously hypertensive rats during the development of hypertension. *European Journal of Pharmacology*, **70**, 247–256

SHIBOUTA, Y., TERASHITA, Z.-I., INADA, Y., KATO, K. and NISHIKAWA, K. (1982) Renal effects of pinane thromboxane A_2 and indomethacin in saline volume-expanded spontaneously hypertensive rats. *European Journal of Pharmacology*, **85**, 51–59

SIESS, W. and DRAY, F. (1982) Very low levels of 6-keto prostaglandin $F_{1\alpha}$ in human plasma. *Journal of Laboratory and Clinical Medicine*, **99**, 388–398

SIESS, W., ROTH, P., SCHERER, B., KURZMANN, B., BOHLIG, B. and WEBER, P. C. (1980) Platelet-membrane fatty acids, platelet aggregation and thromboxane formation during a mackerel diet. *Lancet*, **1**, 441–444

SIMPSON, L. L. (1974) The effect of prostaglandin E_2 on the arterial blood pressure of normotensive and spontaneously hypertensive rats. *British Journal of Pharmacology*, **51**, 559–564

SIROIS, P. and GAGNON, D. J. (1974) Release of renomedullary prostaglandins in normal and hypertensive rats. *Experientia*, **30**, 1418–1419

SMEDEGARD, G., HEDQVIST, P., DAHLEN, S.-E., REVENAS, B., HAMMARSTROM, S. and SAMUELSSON, B. (1982) Leukotriene C_4 affects pulmonary and cardiovascular dynamics in monkey. *Nature (London)*, **295**, 327–329

SMITH, W. L. and WILKIN, G. G. (1977) Immunochemistry of prostaglandin endoperoxide-forming cyclooxygenases. The detection of cyclooxygenases in rat, rabbit and guinea-pig kidneys by immunofluorescence. *Prostaglandins*, **13**, 873–892

SMITH, W. L. and BELL, T. G. (1978) Immunohistochemical localisation of prostaglandin forming cyclooxygenase in renal cortex. *American Journal of Physiology*, **235**, F451–F457

SPECTOR, A. A., HOAK, J. C., FRY, G. L., DENNING, G. M., STOLL, L. L. and SMITH, J. B. (1980) Effect of fatty acid modification on prostacyclin production by cultured human endothelial cells. *Journal of Clinical Investigation*, **65**, 1003–1012

SRAER, J., STRAER, J. D., CHANSEL, D., RUSSO-MARIE, F., KOUZNETZOVA, B. and ARDAILLOU, R. (1979) Prostaglandin synthesis by isolated rat renal glomeruli. *Molecular Cellular Endocrinology*, **16**, 29–37

STOKES, J. B. and KOKKO, J. P. (1977) Inhibition of sodium transport by prostaglandin E_2 across the isolated perfused rabbit collecting tubule. *Journal of Clinical Investigation*, **59**, 1099–1104

STOKES, J. B. (1979) Effect of PGE_2 on chloride transport across the rabbit thick ascending limb of Henle. *Journal of Clinical Investigation*, **64**, 495–502

STONE, K. J. and HART, M. (1975) Prostaglandin-E_2-9-ketoreductase in rabbit kidney. *Prostaglandins*, **10**, 273–288

STYGLES, V. G., REINKE, D. A., RICKERT, D. E. and HOOK J. B. (1978) Increased blood pressure in the SHR is not related to a deficit in renomedullary PGE_2. *Esperientia*, **34**, 1025–1026

SUSTARSIC, C. L., MC PARTLAND, R. P. and RAPP, J. P. (1981) Development patterns of blood pressure and urinary protein, kallikrein and prostaglandin E_2 in Dahl salt-hypertension-susceptible rats. *Journal of Laboratory and Clinical Medicine*, **98**, 599–606

SWAIN, J. A., HEYNDRICKX, G. R., BOETTCHER, D. H. and VATNER, S. F. (1975) Prostaglandin control of renal circulation in the unanaesthetised dog and baboon. *American Journal of Physiology*, **229**, 826–830

TAI, H. H. and YUAN, B. (1978) On the inhibitory potency of imidazole and its derivatives on thromboxane synthetase. *Biochemical and Biophysical Research Communications*, **80**, 236–242

TAN, S. Y., SWEET, P. and MULROW, P. J. (1978) Impaired renal production of PGE_2: a newly identified lesion in human essential hypertension. *Prostaglandins*, **15**, 139–149

TAYLOR, J. D., WATSON, M. L., THOMSON, D. and UNGAR, A. (1981) Renal interstitial cell granularity in dogs with renal hypertension. *Journal of Laboratory and Clinical Medicine*, **98**, 78–88

TERRAGNO, D. A., CROWSHAW, K., TERRAGNO, N. A. and MC GIFF, J. C. (1975) Prostaglandin synthesis by bovine mesenteric arteries and veins. *Circulation Research*, **36** (Suppl. 1), 76–80

TERRAGNO, N. A., TERRAGNO, D. A. and MC GIFF, J. C. (1977) Contribution of prostaglandins to the renal circulation in conscious, anaesthetised and laparotomized dogs. *Circulation Research*, **40**, 590–595

TERRAGNO, N. A., MC GIFF, J. C. and TERRAGNO, A. (1978) Prostacyclin (PGI_2) production by renal blood vessels: relationship to an endogenous prostaglandin synthesis inhibitor (EPSI). *Clinical Research*, **26**, 545A

TOBIAN, L., ISHII, M. and DUKE, M. (1969) Relationship of cytoplasmic granules in renal papillary interstitial cells to post renal hypertension. *Journal of Laboratory and Clinical Medicine*, **73**, 309–319

TOBIAN, L., GANGULY, M., JOHNSON, M. A. and IWAI, J. (1982) Influence of renal prostaglandins and dietary linoleate on hypertension in Dahl-S rats. *Hypertension*, **4** (*Suppl. 11*), 149–153

UDERMAN, H. D., WORKMAN, R. J. and JACKSON, E. K. (1982) Attenuation of the development of hypertension in spontaneously hypertensive rats by the thromboxane synthetase inhibitor, 4^1-(imidazol-1-YL) acetophenone. *Prostaglandins*, **24**, 237–244

VANE, J. R. (1964) The use of isolated organs for detecting active substances in the circulating blood. *British Journal of Pharmacology and Chemotherapy*, **23**, 360–373

VANE, J. R. (1971) Inhibition of prostaglandin synthesis by aspirin-like drugs. *Nature (London)*, **231**, 232–235

VERGROESEN, A. J., DEDECKERE, E. A. M., TENHOR, F. and HORNSTRA, G. (1980) Cardiovascular effects of linoleic acid. *Progress in Food Nutrition Science*, **4**, 13–25

VIERHAPPER, H., WALDHAUSL, W. and NOWOTNY, P. (1981) Effect of indomethacin upon angiotensin-induced changes in blood pressure and plasma aldosterone in normal man. *European Journal of Clinical Investigation*, **11**, 85–89

WATSON, M. L., LAMBIE, A. T., THOM, A. and UNGAR, A. (1982) Role of prostaglandins in mediating excretion by the kidney of an intravenous infusion of sodium chloride in normal human subjects. *Clinical Science*, **62**, 27–33

WATSON, J. L., HERZER, W. and BRANCH, R. A. (1983) Short-term infusion of angiotensin II does not stimulate systemic prostaglandin I_2 synthesis in conscious dogs. *British Journal of Pharmacology*, **79**, 387

WATSON, M. L., McCORMICK, J. and UNGAR, A. (1984) Angiotensin sensitivity and prostaglandins in dogs with renal hypertension. *Journal of Hypertension* (in press)

WATSON, M. L., GOODMAN, R. P., GILL, J. R. *et al.* (1984) Endogenous prostacyclin synthesis is decreased during activation of the renin–angiotensin system in man. *Journal of Clinical Endocrinology and Metabolism*, **58**, 304–308

WEBER, P. C., LARSSON, C., ANGGARD, E. *et al.* (1976) Stimulation of renin release from rabbit renal cortex by arachidonic acid and prostaglandin endoperoxides. *Circulation Research*, **39**, 868–874

WEBER, P. C., LARSSON, C. and SCHERER, B. (1977) Prostaglandin E_2-9-ketoreductase as a mediator of salt intake-related prostaglandin–renin interaction. *Nature (London)*, **266**, 65–66

WEBER, P. C., SIESS, W. and SCHERER, B. (1980) Possible significance of renal prostaglandins in essential hypertension. *Clinical and Experimental Hypertension*, **2**, 741–760

WHORTON, A. R., MISONO, K., HOLLIFIELD, J., FROLICH, J. C., INAGAMI, T. and OATES, J. A. (1977) Prostaglandins and renin release. *Prostaglandins*, **14**, 1095–1104

WHORTON, A. R., SMIGEL, M., OATES, J. A. and FROLICH, J. C. (1977) Evidence for prostacyclin production in renal cortex. *Prostaglandins*, **13**, 1021 (Abstract)

WHORTON, A. R., SMIGEL, M., OATES, J. A. and FROLICH, J. C. (1978) Regional differences in prostaglandin formation by the kidney. *Biochimica Biophysica Acta*, **529**, 176–180

WHORTON, A. R., YOUNG, S. L., DATA, J. L., BARCHOWSKY, A. and KENT, R. S. (1982) Mechanism of bradykinin-stimulated prostacyclin synthesis in porcine aortic endothelial cells. *Biochimica Biophysica Acta*, **712**, 79–87

WILLIAMS, T. J. (1983) Interactions between prostaglandins, leukotrienes and other mediators of inflammation. *British Medical Bulletin*, **39**, 239–242

WILLIS, A. L., HASSAM, A. G., CRAWFORD, M. A., STEVENS, P. and DENTON, J. P. (1981) Relationships between prostaglandins, prostacyclin and EFA precursors in rabbits maintained on EFA-deficient diets. *Progress in Lipid Research*, **21**, 161–168

WILSON, D. R., HONRATH, U. and SONNENBERG, H. (1982) Prostaglandin synthesis inhibition during volume expansion; collecting duct function. *Kidney International*, **22**, 1–7

WONG, P. Y. K., MALIK, K. U., DESIDERIO, D. M., MC GIFF, J. C. and SUN, F. F. (1980) Hepatic metabolism of prostacyclin (PGI_2) in the rabbit: formation of a potent novel inhibitor of platelet aggregation. *Biochemical and Biophysical Research Communications*, **93**, 486–494

YARGER, W. E., SCHOCKEN, D. D. and HARRIS, R. H. (1980) Obstructive nephropathy in the rat. Possible role for the renin–angiotensin system, prostaglandins, and thromboxanes in post-obstructive renal function. *Journal of Clinical Investigation*, **65**, 400–412

YUN, J., KELLY, G. and BARTTER, F. C. (1979) Effect of indomethacin on renal function and plasma renin activity in dogs with chronic renovascular hypertension. *Nephron*, **24**, 278–282

ZUKOWSKA-GROJEC, Z., BAYORH, M. A., YAAR, I., KOPIN, I. J. and FEUERSTEIN, G. (1983) Leukotriene D_4: divergent cardiovascular and sympathetic effects in spontaneously hypertensive and normotensive Wistar–Kyoto rats. *Advances in Prostaglandin, Thromboxane and Leukotriene Research*, **11**, 407–412

ZOLLNER, N., ADAM, D. and WOLFRAM, G. (1979) The influence of linoleic acid intake on the excretion of urinary prostaglandin metabolites. *Research in Experimental Medicine (Berlin)*, **175**, 149–153

ZUSMAN, R. M. and KEISER, H. R. (1977a) Prostaglandin E biosynthesis by rabbit renomedullary interstitial cells in tissue culture. *Journal of Biological Chemistry*, **252**, 2069–2071

ZUSMAN, R. M. and KEISER, H. R. (1977b) Prostaglandin biosynthesis by rabbit renomedullary interstitial cells in tissue culture. *Journal of Clinical Investigation*, **60**, 215–223

ZUSMAN, R. M., KEISER, H. R. and HANDLER, J. S. (1978) Effect of adrenal steroids on vasopressin-stimulated PGE synthesis and water flow. *American Journal of Physiology*, **234**, F532–F540

10
The renomedullary interstitial cells and their antihypertensive hormone

E. E. Muirhead

INTRODUCTION

Transplants of fragmented renal medulla or renal papilla (Heptinstall, Salyer and Salyer, 1975; Manthorpe, 1973, 1975; Muirhead, Stirman and Jones, 1960; Muirhead *et al.*, 1970, 1972a, 1972b; Susic and Kentera, 1980; Susic, Sparks and Machado, 1976; Tobian and Azar, 1971) and transplants of renomedullary interstitial cells (RIC) grown in monolayer cell culture (Muirhead, 1974, and personal communication; Muirhead *et al.*, 1975, 1977) exert an antihypertensive action. In time, these transplants consist mostly of renomedullary interstitial cells and capillaries, resembling an endocrine-type structure (Muirhead, 1974; Muirhead *et al.*, 1972a, 1975). Some of these transplants exert their antihypertensive action before they are vascularized (Muirhead *et al.*, 1974). It is, therefore, almost impossible to explain their antihypertensive action without invoking the secretion of a substance that circulates, i.e. a hormone (Muirhead, 1974; Muirhead *et al.*, 1970, 1972a, 1974, 1975, 1977).

It is the purpose of this chapter to review more recent observations in support of a renomedullary interstitial cell antihypertensive hormone and to relate evolving data indicating its mechanism of action.

TWO ANTIHYPERTENSIVE LIPIDS DERIVED FROM RENAL PAPILLA, ANRL AND APRL

Two antihypertensive lipids have been derived by the extraction and purification of fresh renal papilla (Blank *et al.*, 1979; Muirhead, 1980a; Muirhead *et al.*, 1976, 1982a, 1983a; Prewitt *et al.*, 1979).

These are the antihypertensive neutral renomedullary lipid (ANRL) and the antihypertensive polar renomedullary lipid (APRL). Flow charts in the appendix to this chapter (pp. 289–291) give the details of the procedures used in deriving ANRL. The procedures used in deriving APRL are described in detail elsewhere (Muirhead *et al.*, 1983a). One of the main structural differences between these two moieties is in their polarity – APRL is quite polar, ANRL is much less polar (being near neutral).

BIOLOGICAL DIFFERENCES BETWEEN APRL AND ANRL

APRL causes a near sudden (within 2 seconds) drop in the arterial pressure (AP) (*Figure 10.1*) when injected intravenously as a bolus dose (Prewitt *et al.*, 1979). The magnitude and duration of this drop is dose-dependent. The effect is much more pronounced in the hypertensive animal (Smith *et al.*, 1981). Given in multiple doses per day or as a lasting infusion APRL causes a prolonged vasodepression, the arterial pressure remaining depressed for 24–48 or more hours (Prewitt *et al.*, 1979; *Figure 10.2*). In some hypertensive animals it is active by mouth (Blank *et al.*, 1979; Muirhead *et al.*, 1981a; *Figure 10.3*).

ANRL injected intravenously as a bolus dose causes a much slower drop in arterial pressure after a lag period, usually lasting about 2 minutes in the

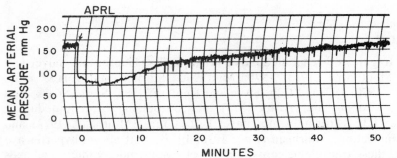

Figure 10.1 The vasodepressor effect of APRL injected as a bolus intravenously into a hypertensive rat is shown. The effect results from a high dose. (From Prewitt *et al.*, 1979)

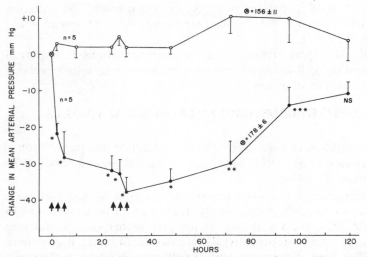

Figure 10.2 The prolonged depressor effect (●——●) due to multiple doses (*at the arrows*) of APRL 25 μg in 20 minutes t.i.d. is depicted. Lecithin vehicle (○——○); $P* < 0.001$; $** < 0.005$; $*** < 0.05$. (From Prewitt *et al.*, 1979)

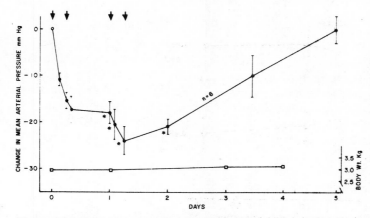

Figure 10.3 This figure relates the prolonged depressor effect following multiple doses of APRL 25µg by mouth to the hypertensive rabbit. $P* < 0.001$. (From Muirhead *et al.*, 1981a)

hypertensive rat (Prewitt *et al.*, 1979; Muirhead *et al.*, 1983; *Figure 10.4*). Depending on the dose, the nadir is reached in 5–15 minutes and recovery requires 15–60 minutes. There is a threshold dose, less potent and more potent responses indicating a type of dose response. The lag period is characteristic and often is associated with a minimal elevation of the AP (~5 mmHg) before the decline occurs. What transpires during the lag remains a major question.

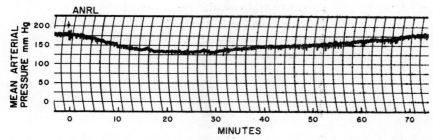

Figure 10.4 The effect of ANRL following a bolus dose intravenously to the hypertensive rat is shown. There was a lag period before the arterial pressure began to drop. In this case the nadir occurred in ~18 minutes and recovery required over 60 min. (From Prewitt *et al.*, 1979)

APRL and ANRL contrast further in their effect on the heart rate (HR) and sympathetic activity (SA). As the arterial pressure drops following a bolus dose or an infusion of APRL, the heart rate and sympathetic activity (measured on the renal nerve efferent pathway) *elevate* (Muirhead *et al.*, 1983a, 1983b; *Figure 10.5*). ANRL behaves entirely differently – as the arterial pressure drops following a bolus dose of ANRL the heart rate and sympathetic activity are *lowered* (Muirhead *et al.*, 1983a; *Figure 10.6*).

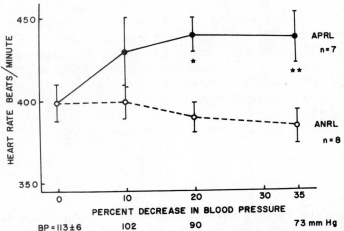

Figure 10.5 The effect of APRL and ANRL on the heart rate is shown after their intravenous injection into normotensive rats. APRL elevates the heart rate, ANRL depresses it. $P* < 0.05$; $** < 0.01$. (From Muirhead *et al.*, 1983b)

APRL is a powerful vasodilator (1000 × more so than papaverine; Muirhead *et al.*, 1983b) (see also Faber *et al.*, 1982; Prewitt *et al.*, 1979). Placed on resistance arterioles it dilates them quickly (Smith *et al.*, 1981; *Figure 10.7*). It also dilates venules – the arterioles of hypertensive animals are more responsive than those of normotensive animals while the venules are equiresponsive (Prewitt *et al.*, 1979). The drop of the arterial pressure due to lower doses of APRL intravenously is due primarily to a reduction of the peripheral vascular resistance (Prewitt *et al.*, 1979; *Figure 10.8*). As the dose is increased the cardiac output is also lowered (Prewitt *et al.*, 1979). These responses suggest a primary effect on resistance vessels and a secondary effect on capacitance vessels.

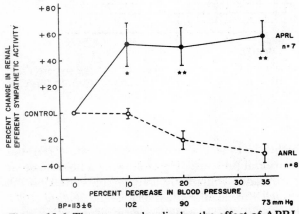

Figure 10.6 These examples display the effect of APRL and ANRL on sympathetic activity of the normal rat. Note that APRL elevates and ANRL depresses sympathetic activity. $P* < 0.01$; $** < 0.001$. (From Muirhead *et al.*, 1983b)

The effect of APRL on resistance vessels is supported by two additional observations. In the isolated hindlimb preparation of the rat, APRL increases flow and overcomes to the same extent the constrictor effect of norepinephrine (NE), vasopressin (VP) and Ba^{2+} (Muirhead *et al.*, 1983b). It also dilates the splanchnic, renal, hindlimb vascular beds (the splanchnic more so) (Faber *et al.*, 1982) and the coronary bed (Crespo *et al.*, 1982). APRL has no effect on the tonic contractures of an isolated portal vein and no negative inotropic effect on the isolated rat heart even at maximum vasodilating doses (Muirhead *et al.*, 1983b). It has no effect on the circulation when injected into the lateral ventricle (Faber *et al.*, 1982).

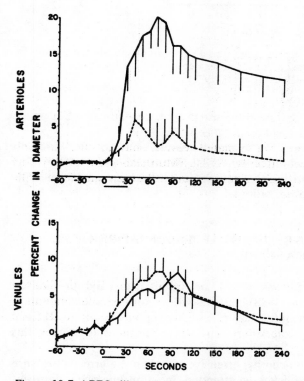

Figure 10.7 APRL dilates tertiary arterioles of the cremaster muscle of the SHR to a greater extent than those of the WKY rat (*upper panel*). Venules of these rats are dilated to the same extent (*lower panel*). (From Smith *et al.*, 1981)

Does APRL interfere with α-adrenergic receptor function? This question is moot. In some isolated systems it appears to interfere (Smith *et al.*, 1981, 1982, 1984). It was suggested that this might be a steric hindrance within the membrane (Smith *et al.*, 1982). The isolated mesenteric artery with its constrictor fiber attached does not support a major α-adrenergic action. The constrictor effect of low frequency stimulation of the nerve is not modified by APRL. This indicates no interference with release of norepinephrine and no interference with its action on

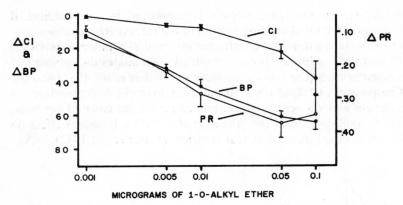

Figure 10.8 Lower doses of APRL depress the arterial pressure of the SHR primarily by decreasing peripheral vascular resistance; higher doses depress the cardiac index as well as peripheral vascular resistance. (From Prewitt *et al.*, 1979)

the vascular smooth muscle. The latter observations appear significant. Yet, more work is needed in this area (Muirhead *et al.*, 1983b).

A few preliminary experiments on isolated vessels and on the hindlimb preparation failed to show a direct effect by ANRL (Muirhead *et al.*, 1983b). This could be due to the absence of the 'lag mechanism' under these circumstances. This is another area requiring more observations.

ANRL IN THE RENAL VENOUS EFFLUENT AFTER UNCLIPPING THE GOLDBLATT HYPERTENSIVE ANIMAL

Unclipping the Goldblatt hypertensive rat or rabbit (the Byrom–Dodson experiment, Byrom and Dodson, 1948) has yielded a considerable amount of information in recent years. This information is highly supportive of ANRL as a hormone of the renomedullary interstitial cells. It is pertinent to review this material.

Unclipping the one-kidney, one-clip hypertensive rat when the arterial pressure is at its sustained hypertensive level is attended by a pronounced diuresis–natriuresis and a fall in arterial pressure to normal in three hours or less (Muirhead and Brooks, 1980; *Figure 10.9*). Anastomosing the ureter to the vena cava slows this process to an average of 20 hours (no loss of sodium and water to the outside) (Muirhead and Brooks, 1980). This is not due to vasodepressor substances in the urine as replacement of the sodium and water of the first experiment above is also attended by a return of arterial pressure in 20 hours (Muirhead and Brooks, 1980). The powerful nature of the renal antihypertensive action under these circumstances is attested by the fact that interposing a saline load equivalent to 1.25–5% of the body weight after the ureteral anastomosis and then unclipping is attended by the arterial pressure still reaching normal but in 45–50 hours. Sham operated controls have no change in arterial pressure.

Degranulation of the renomedullary interstitial cells occurs as the arterial pressure drops following unclipping (Pitcock *et al.*, 1981; *Figure 10.10*). This is fairly complete by five hours post-unclipping. At the same time ANRL and APRL appear in the renal venous effluent. It is to be recalled that ANRL can be derived from the same renomedullary interstitial cells monolayer cell cultures that lower the arterial pressure when transplanted subcutaneously (Muirhead *et al.*, 1977; *Figure 10.11*).

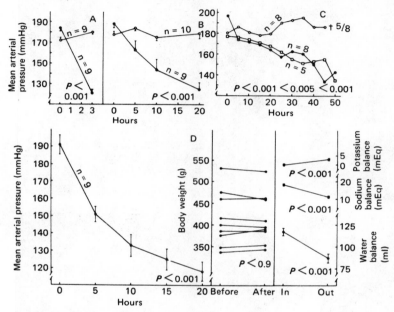

Figure 10.9 The effect of unclipping the one-kidney, one-clip hypertensive rat under different conditions is shown. In A urine was allowed to flow freely and the arterial pressure reached normal levels within three hours. In B the ureter was anastomosed to the vena cava and normal arterial pressure was reached in 20 hours. In C the ureter was anastomosed to the vena cava, a saline load was added intravenously and the clip was removed. The arterial pressure reached normal in 50 hours. Sham controls had no change in arterial pressure. In D urine was allowed to flow freely and the excreted sodium and water were replaced. The arterial pressure reached normal in 20 hours, as in B. (From Muirhead and Brooks, 1980)

Unclipping lowers the arterial pressure primarily by lowering peripheral vascular resistance (Hallback-Norlander, Noresson and Lundgren, 1979). The renal venous effluent of the unclipped isolated kidney lowers the arterial pressure of a normal conscious recipient rat (Göthberg, Lundin and Folkow, 1982; *Figure 10.12*). In other words, unclipping and the blood from the unclipped kidney perform the same function – they lower the arterial pressure. It follows that after unclipping it is the blood from the kidney that is greatly involved in dropping the arterial pressure.

In order for unclipping to be successful in dropping the arterial pressure to normal or near so, the renal papilla of the unclipped kidney must be intact (Bing *et*

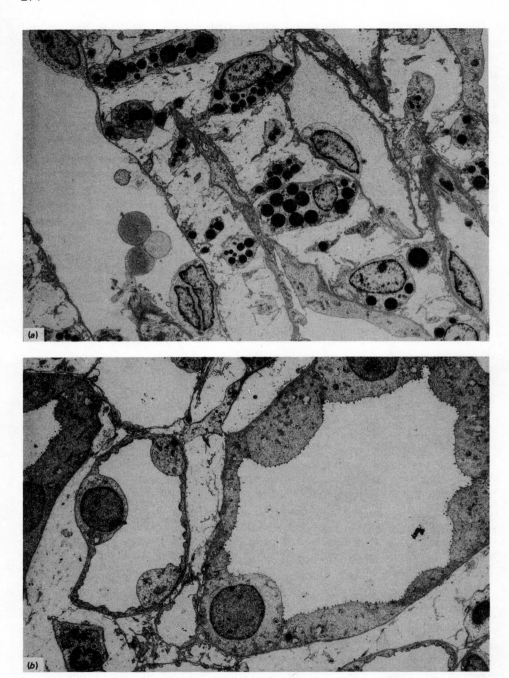

Figure 10.10 (*a*) The renomedullary interstitial cells of the clipped kidney are shown by electron microscopy, note the prominent cytoplasmic granules; (*b*) The renomedullary interstitial cells after unclipping lose most of their granules and the cells lining the collecting duct flatten out. (From Pitcock *et al.*, 1981)

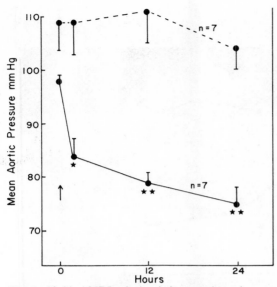

Figure 10.11 ANRL derived from cultured renomedullary interstitial cells lowered the arterial pressure of hypertensive rabbits (●———●). Animals receiving the vehicle (●‒‒‒●) had no change in arterial pressure. $P* < 0.01$; $** < 0.001$. (From Muirhead *et al.*, 1977)

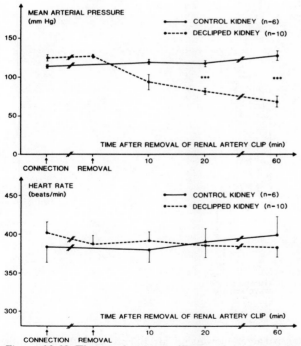

Figure 10.12 The renal venous effluent of the isolated unclipped kidney lowers the arterial pressure of a normal rat without changing the pulse rate. (From Göthberg, Lundin and Folkow, 1982)

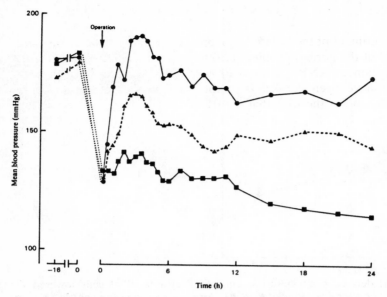

Figure 10.13 Chemical medullectomy interferes with the drop in arterial pressure following unclipping (▲). The upper curve is of the sham group; the lower curve is of the control, unclipped group without medullectomy. (From Bing *et al.*, 1981)

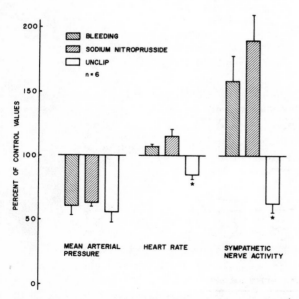

Figure 10.14 Unclipping the hypertensive animal lowers the arterial pressure, the heart rate and sympathetic activity. Lowering the arterial pressure by bleeding or by the use of a vasodilator lowers the arterial pressure while elevating the heart rate and sympathetic activity. $P*<0.01$. (From Göthberg *et al.*, 1982)

al., 1981; *Figure 10.13*). This is the area where the renomedullary interstitial cells are concentrated.

The renal venous effluent of the isolated unclipped kidney lowers heart rate and sympathetic activity of the normal recipient (Göthberg *et al.*, 1982; *Figure 10.14*). This is the same action of ANRL (Muirhead *et al.*, 1983a). Even though both ANRL and APRL have been derived from the renal venous effluent (*Figure 10.15*), these results support the view that ANRL is dominant.

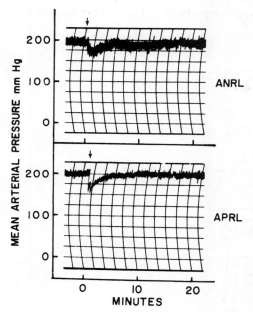

Figure 10.15 The renal venous effluent following unclipping contains both ANRL (*upper panel*) and APRL (*lower panel*). (From Muirhead *et al.*, 1983a)

These major results, singularly complementary, indicate that unclipping is followed by secretion of ANRL by renomedullary interstitial cells into the blood leaving the kidney. So ANRL or a closely related compound appears very likely as the hormone from the kidney that exerts the antihypertensive action.

ANRL VERSUS APRL

It appears that adding APRL to ANRL and giving both intravenously potentiates and prolongs the antihypertensive action (Muirhead, 1983c; *Figure 10.16*). The immediate acute effect remains and is less pronounced but the duration of the ANRL effect is prolonged. Thus, it could be that the relatively smaller amount of APRL in the renal venous effluent after unclipping adds to the antihypertensive action.*

---

* The ultimate effect of these two compounds together seems to depend on the ratio of the mixture. APRL can overwhelm ANRL if it is the dominant compound present.

APRL is *not* likely to be a natural antihypertensive factor. One of its components is identical to the platelet activating factor (PAF) (Benveniste, Henson and Cochrane, 1972; Chesney *et al.*, 1982; Hanahan *et al.*, 1980). PAF causes platelet aggregation (more in rabbit and human than rat) (Benveniste, Henson and Cochrane, 1972; Chesney *et al.*, 1982; Hanahan *et al.*, 1980), liberates leukotrienes (Voelkel *et al.*, 1982), accelerates heart rate and stimulates the sympathetic nervous system (Muirhead *et al.*, 1983a, 1983b). ANRL, conversely, is an ideal antihypertensive substance – it is a natural product that lowers arterial pressure while decreasing heart rate and suppressing sympathetic activity (Muirhead *et al.*, 1983a, 1983b).

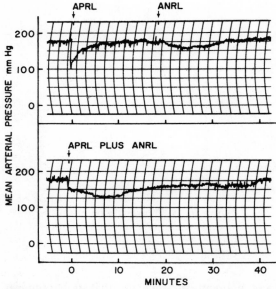

Figure 10.16 (*Upper panel*) APRL and ANRL were injected intravenously as a bolus to a hypertensive rat. (*Lower panel*) the same dose of APRL and ANRL were combined and injected the same way. Note the extension of the effect (from 175–125 mmHg, lasting 40 minutes). (From Muirhead *et al.*, 1983c)

There are indications that APRL and ANRL are related (Muirhead *et al.*, 1983a). For some time it has been apparent that the process deriving ANRL-type activity yields APRL-like activity, in some instances, as refinement progresses. This has been a source of frustration. Recently, however, the data support the proposal that under certain circumstances ANRL may yield APRL. Should this become secure, then APRL may be a precursor of ANRL or somewhat attached to ANRL. This indicates another area for further work, which is being pursued.

ANRL VERSUS ANGIOTENSIN

Our hypothesis considers an opposing effect between ANRL and angiotensin. The greatest support for this possibility comes from the use of the juxtaglomerular cell

(JGC) monolayer cell culture (Rightsel *et al.*, 1982). These cells have the major characteristics of juxtaglomerular cells as observed in the kidney.* Subcutaneous transplants of these cells into syngeneic recipients plus a reduction of renal mass (uninephrectomy or 70% partial nephrectomy) causes hypertension (Muirhead *et al.*, 1983c). The arterial pressure reaches a maximum in an average of 18 days and then levels off. The hypertensive state is of malignant type, being attended by fibrinoid necrosis and musculomucoid hyperplasia of small arteries and arterioles of the viscera. During the developmental phase of the hypertension the plasma angiotensin II/III levels are high but plasma renin concentration (PRC) and plasma renin activity (PRA) are normal (a hyperangiotensinemic–normoreninemic state) and during the maintenance phase, i.e. after 3–4 weeks, the plasma angiotensin II/III level is normal. Saralasin lowers the arterial pressure during the developmental phase but not during the maintenance phase, as would be expected.

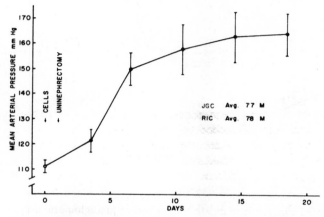

Figure 10.17 These examples received transplants of juxtaglomerular cells (JGC) and renomedullary interstitial cells (RIC) at the same time but at different sites followed by uninephrectomy. The arterial pressure elevated in the usual manner, reaching a plateau at about 15 days. (From Muirhead *et al.*, 1983c)

When cultured juxtaglomerular cells and renomedullary interstitial cells are transplanted into a syngeneic rat at the same time but at different sites and the renal mass is reduced the hypertension develops in the usual manner (*Figure 10.17*). When renomedullary interstitial cells are transplanted after four weeks the arterial pressure is reduced significantly (*Figure 10.18*). Thus, during the developmental phase when plasma angiotensin is high, the renomedullary interstitial cells are ineffective as an antihypertensive structure but during the maintenance phase when plasma angiotensin is low the renomedullary interstitial cells exert their

---

* These include peripheral dense bodies, myofibrils, a prominent Golgi apparatus, rough endoplasmic reticulum containing a precipitate, and granules (lysosomal and secretory types). In addition, they contain renin, angiotensin I and II/III, converting enzyme and by implication renin substrate.

antihypertensive action. In this connection it is of interest that angiotensin II facilitates sympathetic activity (McCubbin, 1974; Trendelenburg, 1966) while ANRL, as already sited, suppresses sympathetic activity.

It is postulated that the clipped kidney generates angiotensin intrarenally (Rightsel *et al.*, 1982) and that in the juxtamedullary area the concentration leading into the papilla can be significant. This local angiotensin generation is considered to constrain the antihypertensive action of the renomedullary interstitial cells. Unclipping, according to this hypothesis, is a major stimulus to the renomedullary interstitial cells to secrete their antihypertensive hormone.

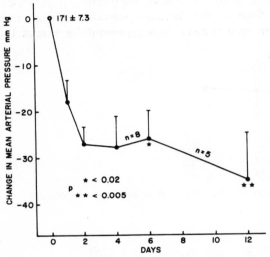

Figure 10.18 Rats having sustained hypertension due to transplants of juxtaglomerular cells (JGC) beyond 30 days post-transplant were transplanted with renomedullary interstitial cells. The arterial pressure dropped as shown. $P*<0.02$; $**<0.005$. (From Muirhead *et al.*, 1983c)

Malignant hypertension of the rabbit has been standardized by use of a narrow rigid clip (Brooks and Muirhead, 1971) and removal of the opposite kidney (Muirhead *et al.*, 1972a). Under these conditions all animals die within three weeks and display encephalopathy, renal failure, fibrinoid necrosis and musculomucoid hyperplasia of visceral small arteries and arterioles. This is a hyper-reninemic state. The converting enzyme inhibitor teprotide prevents the malignant phase when it is started at the time of the application of the clip and removal of the opposite kidney (Muirhead, Brooks and Arora, 1974). Stopping the teprotide intake after 21 days is followed by a sudden rise in arterial pressure and death. Teprotide is not effective in preventing the malignant phase if started eight or more days after the clip is applied and the opposite kidney is removed. After eight days the renomedullary interstitial cells of the clipped kidney are reduced in number and markedly degenerated (Muirhead *et al.*, 1981c). It is of interest that transplantation of the renal papilla at the time of the application of the clip and uninephrectomy prevents

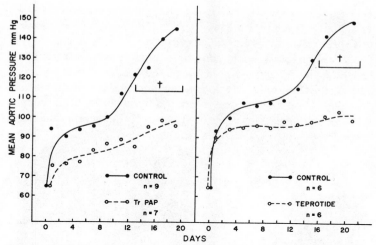

Figure 10.19 The malignant hypertension was induced by a narrow clip plus uninephrectomy. Left alone all animals die in three weeks. Autotransplant of renal papilla (*left panel*) prevents the malignant phase in a manner comparable to teprotide (*right panel*). (From Muirhead *et al.*, 1980b)

the malignant phase in the same manner as teprotide (*Figure 10.19*). Removal of the transplant after 21 days is followed by a sudden rise in arterial pressure and death. Thus, the secretion of a hormone by the transplanted renomedullary interstitial cells, presumably ANRL, blocks the development of malignant hypertension in the same manner as blocking the renin–angiotensin system. It is speculated that teprotide acts partly by allowing the renomedullary interstitial cells to function unimpeded by angiotensin generated intrarenally.

IN SITU DEGENERATION OF RENOMEDULLARY INTERSTITIAL CELLS

Electronmicroscopy and morphometric studies indicate that in some hypertensive states the renomedullary interstitial cells within the kidney are significantly reduced in numbers and degenerated in appearance (Muirhead *et al.*, 1981c). These include partial nephrectomy–salt hypertension of the rat (Pitcock *et al.*, 1980), malignant hypertension of the rabbit (Muirhead *et al.*, 1981c; *Figure 10.20*), angiotensin–salt hypertension plus a high salt intake of the rat (Muirhead *et al.*, 1981b) and malignant hypertension of the human (Muehrcke, Mandal and Voline, 1970). In renoprival hypertension the renomedullary interstitial cells and their hormone, naturally, are absent. The latter makes the organism sensitive to salt and volume in terms of elevation of the arterial pressure (Ledingham, 1971; Merrill, Giordano and Hertderks, 1961).

The *in situ* degeneration and reduction of renomedullary interstitial cells is considered to contribute to the pathogenesis of a hypertensive state by interfering with the secretion of the antihypertensive hormone. Malignant hypertension, for

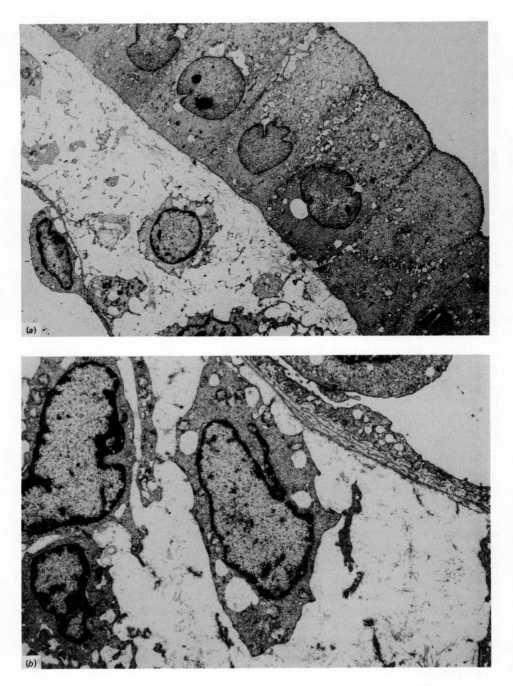

Figure 10.20 The renomedullary interstitial cells of rabbits having malignant hypertension are (*a*) markedly degenerated – rounded and with few granules, (*b*) vacuolated and with few organelles. (From Muirhead *et al.*, 1980c)

instance, may well result from a mixture of elevated angiotensin levels (circulating and within the kidney), renal failure and salt retention and a deficiency of the renomedullary interstitial cells antihypertensive hormone.

DISCUSSION

Modern experimental approaches indicate the near-ubiquitous distribution of positive and negative feedback systems. Thus, if the kidney exerts prohypertensive actions, such as by the secretion of renin and angiotensin and the retention of sodium and water, then antihypertensive systems would be expected. It is proposed that the kidney exerts antihypertensive actions not only by the excretion of sodium and water but by the secretion of an antihypertensive hormone. The generation and secretion of renin–angiotensin is in the renal cortex. The generation and secretion of the antihypertensive hormone is in the renal medulla and its papilla.

The existence of the renopapillary antihypertensive hormone has been established by classic endocrinological techniques, as indicated by the following.

The ablation of the tissue at issue is accompanied by either removal of the kidneys (the renoprival state) or by removal of the renal papilla (papillectomy). Ablation was first proposed by Thomas Addison (1868) in a syndrome later carrying his name (Addison's disease) and ascribed to the *destruction* of the 'suprarenal capsules'. Gull (1874) described myxedema and Horsley (1890) reproduced it in monkeys by the ablation of the thyroid gland. Von Mering and Minkowski (1889) ablated the pancreas of the dog and caused diabetes mellitus. MacCallum and Voegtlin (1909) ablated the parathyroid glands of the rabbit and induced hypocalcemic tetany, etc. The renoprival state by itself does not necessarily cause hypertension (nor hypotension). Rather, it makes the organism susceptible to the action of prohypertensive factors, especially sodium and volume (Ledingham, 1971; Merrill, Giordano and Hertderks, 1961; Muirhead, Stirman and Jones, 1959). The sodium may be derived either endogenously (Floyer, 1957; Muirhead, Stirman and Jones, 1959; Muirhead, Jones and Graham, 1953) or from an exogenous source (Ledingham, 1971; Merrill, Giordano and Hertderks, 1961).

The reintroduction of the tissue prevents the abnormality induced by the ablation. This was first shown by A. A. Berthold of Gottingen (Berthold, 1849; Biedl, 1913). He studied two groups of young roosters. One group had orchiectomies and became capons. The other had orchiectomies followed by introduction of one testicle into the peritoneal cavity. The latter group remained muscular, retained their cock's comb, fought other roosters and chased hens but were sterile. At autopsy, Berthold described a vascularized nodule attached to the peritoneum and seemingly without nerves. He concluded, '*the testicles act upon the blood and the blood acts correspondingly upon the entire organism*'. These observations and conclusions preceded those of Bayliss and Starling (1902) by about 50 years. The autotransplantation route was used to prevent hypothyroidism and Addison's disease by Schulz (1900). It established the existence of sex hormones by Knauer (1896). Autotransplants of fragmented renal papilla prevent renoprival hypertension.

The reintroduction of the tissue reverses the abnormality at issue. Foges (1898), showed that transplantation of segments of a testicle reverses major features of capons. Transplants of fragmented renal papilla reverse the hypertensive state (Manthorpe, 1973, 1975; Muirhead *et al.*, 1970, 1975, 1977; Tobian and Azar, 1971).

Evidence that a substance formed by the tissue is transported by the blood stream Bayliss and Starling (1902), demonstrated that pancreatic juice was secreted when acid chyme was introduced into the duodenum, even though the pancreas was disconnected from the nervous system. An extract of chyme and duodenal mucosa did the same thing when injected into the blood. The substance was termed a 'hormone' and labelled secretin. This placed the endocrine concept on secure grounds. Transplants of cultured renomedullary interstitial cells may lower the arterial pressure before they become vascularized. It is almost certain, then, that a substance formed by the transplanted renomedullary interstitial cells seeps out and is circulated by the blood. In time a close relationship develops between the renomedullary interstitial cells and capillaries (positive tropism), a finding consistent with the endocrine nature of these cells. Moreover, the blood leaving the kidney after unclipping the Goldblatt hypertensive animal has antihypertensive properties.

Extracts of the tissue yield an active principle that replaces the action of the tissue. Murray and Catab (1892), prepared extracts of thyroid gland and demonstrated their curative properties toward myxedema. Takamine (1901) isolated a pressor substance from the adrenal gland (later termed adrenaline and structurally identified as epinephrine). Antidiuretic hormone (ADH) was discovered by Oliver and Schafer (1895). Banting and Best discovered insulin (1922) and Collip (1925) discovered parathormone by the extraction route. Extracts of fresh renal papilla and of cultured renomedullary interstitial cells yield ANRL, a substance found in the renal venous effluent after unclipping the Goldblatt hypertensive animal. The same renal venous effluent has properties identical to those of extracted ANRL. It appears inescapable that ANRL is secreted by the kidney, most likely its renomedullary interstitial cells. As the kidney secretes ANRL the renomedullary interstitial cells degranulate. Degranulation of these cells implies that the lipids stored in their granules are either transposed elsewhere or transformed into other substances.

CONCLUSION

The renomedullary interstitial cells constitute an endocrine organ that secretes an antihypertensive hormone. ANRL appears to be this hormone.

References

ADDISON, T. (1868) On the constitutional and local effects of disease of the supra-renal capsules. In *A Collection of the Published Writings of the Late Thomas Addison, Physician to Guy's Hospital*, edited by Wilks and Daldy. London: The New Sydenham Society

BANTING, F. G. and BEST, C. H. (1922) The internal secretion of the pancreas. *Journal of Laboratory and Clinical Medicine*, **VII** (5), 251–266

BAYLISS, W. M. and STARLING, E. H. (1902) The mechanisms of pancreatic secretion. *Journal of Physiology*, **28**, 325

BENVENISTE, J., HENSON, P. M. and COCHRANE, C. G. (1972) Leukocyte dependent histamine release from rabbit platelets. *Journal of Experimental Medicine*, **136**, 1356–1377

BERTHOLD, A. A. (1849) Transplantation der Hoden. *Archives of Anatomy and Physiology*, 42–46

BIEDL, A. (1913) *The Internal Secretory Organs: Their Physiology and Pathology*, translated by Linda Foster, p. 3. New York: William Wood and Company

BING, R. F., RUSSELL, G. I., SWALES, J. D., THURSTON, H. and FLETCHER, A. (1981) Chemical renal medullectomy: effect upon reversal of two-kidney, one-clip hypertension in the rat. *Clinical Science*, **6**, 335S

BLANK, M. L., SNYDER, F., BYERS, L. W., BROOKS, B. and MUIRHEAD, E. E. (1979) Antihypertensive activity of an alkyl ether analog of phosphatidylcholine. *Biochemical and Biophysical Research Communications*, **90**, 1194–1200

BROOKS, B. and MUIRHEAD, E. E. (1971) Rigid clip for standardized hypertension in the rabbit. *Journal of Applied Physiology*, **31**, 307–308

BYROM, F. B., DODSON, L. F. (1949) The mechanism of the vicious circle in chronic hypertension. *Clinical Science*, **8**, 1

CHESNEY, C. McI., PIFER, D. D., BYERS, L. W. and MUIRHEAD, E. E. (1982) Effect of platelet-activity factor (PAF) on human platelets. *Blood*, **59** (3), 582–585

COLLIP, J. B. (1925) The extraction of a parathyroid hormone on normal animals. *Journal of Biological Chemistry*, **63**, 439–460

CRESPO, M. S., ALONSA, F., ALVAREZ, V., INARREA, P. and EGIDO, J. (1982) Vascular actions of synthetic PAF-acether (a synthetic platelet-activating factor) in the rat. Evidence for a platelet-independent mechanism. *Immunopharmacology*, **4**, 173–185

FABER, J. E., BARRON, K. W., LAPPE, R. W., MUIRHEAD, E. E. and BRODY, M. J. (1982) Regional hemadynamic effects of antihypertensive polar renomedullary lipid (APRL) in conscious rats. *Circulation*, **66**, II-164 (abstract)

FLOYER, M. A. (1957) Role of kidney in experimental hypertension. *British Medical Bulletin*, **13**, 29–32

FOGES, A. (1898) Zur Hoden transplantation ber Hahnen. *Centralblatt fur Physiologie*,

GÖTHBERG, G., LUNDIN, S. and FOLKOW, B. (1982) Acute vasodepressor effect in normotensive rats following extracorporeal perfusion of the declipped kidney of two-kidney, one-clip hypertensive rats. *Hypertension*, **3**, II-101–II-105

GÖTHBERG, G., LUNDIN, S., FOLKOW, B. and THOREN, P. (1982) Suppression of tonic sympathetic nerve activity by depressor agents released from the declipped kidney. *Acta Physiologica Scandinavica*, **116**, 93–95

GULL, W. W. (1874) On a cretinoid state supervening in adult life in women. *Transactions of the Clinical Society of London*, **7**, 180–185

HALLBACK-NORLANDER, M., NORESSON, E. and LUNDGREN, Y. (1979) Haemodynamic alterations after reversal of renal hypertension in rats. *Clinical Science*, **57**, 15S–17S

HANAHAN, D. J., DEMOPOULOS, C. A., LIEHR, J. and PINCKARD, R. N. (1980) Identification of platelet activating factor isolated from rabbit basophils as acetyl glyceryl ether phosphorylcholine. *Journal of Biological Chemistry*, **225** (12), 5514–5516

HEPTINSTALL, R. H., SALYER, D. C. and SALYER, W. R. (1975) Experimental hypertension: the effects of chemical ablation of the renal papilla on the blood pressure of rats with and without silver-clip hypertension. *American Journal of Pathology*, **78**, 297–308

HORSLEY, V. (1890) Note on a possible means of arresting the progress of myxoedema, cachexia strumipriva, and allied diseases. *British Medical Journal*, **1**, 287

KNAUER, E. (1896) Einige versuche von ovarientransplantation am baninchen, *Zentralblaft für Gynäkologie*, **20**, 524–528

LEDINGHAM, J. M. (1971) Blood pressure regulation in renal failure. *Journal of the Royal College of Physicians*, **5**, 103

MacCALLUM, W. G. and VOEGLLIN, C. (1908) On the relation of the parathyroid to calcium metabolism and the nature of tetany. *Bulletin of Johns Hopkins Hospital*, **19**, 91

MANTHORPE, T. (1973) The effect on renal hypertension of subcutaneous isotransplantation of renal medulla from normal or hypertensive rats. *Acta Pathologica et Microbiologica Scandinavica*, **81** (5), 725–733

MANTHORPE, T. (1975) Antihypertensive and hypertensive effects of the kidney. *Acta Pathologica et Microbiologica Scandinavica*, **83**, 395–405

McCUBBIN, J. W. (1974) *Peripheral Effects of Angiotensin on Autonomic Nervous System in Angiotensin*, edited by J. H. Page and F. M. Bumpus, pp. 417–423. New York: Springer-Verlag

MERING, VON and MINKOWSKI, A. (1932) quoted by MacCallum (1932) in *Textbook of Pathology*. Philadelphia: W. B. Saunders

MERRILL, J. P., GIORDANO, C. and HERTDERKS, D. K. (1961) The role of the kidney in human hypertension: failure of hypertension to develop in the renoprival subject. *American Journal of Medicine*, **31**, 931–940

MUEHRCKE, R. C., MANDAL, A. K. and VOLINE, F. I. (1970) Renal interstitial cells: prostaglandins and hypertension. *Circulation Research*, **26** and **27** (*Suppl. I*), 109–119

MUIRHEAD, E. E., JONES, F. and GRAHAMS, P. (1953) Hypertension in bilaterally nephrectomized dogs in absence of exogenous sodium excess: maintenance of fluid balance during peritoneal irrigation. *Archives of Pathology*, **56**, 286–292

MUIRHEAD, E. E., STIRMAN, J. A. and JONES, F. (with the assistance of B. Brooks) (1959) Further observations on the potentiation of post-nephrectomy hypertension of the dog by dietary protein. *Circulation Research*, **7**, 68–78

MUIRHEAD, E. E., STIRMAN, J. A. and JONES, F. (1960) Renal autoexplanation and protection against renoprival hypertensive cardiovascular disease and hemolysis. *Journal of Clinical Investigation*, **39**, 266–281

MUIRHEAD, E. E., BROWN, G. B., GERMAIN, G. S. and LEACH, B. E. (1970) The renal medulla as an antihypertensive organ. *Journal of Laboratory and Clinical Medicine*, **76**, 641–651

MUIRHEAD, E. E., BROOKS, B., PITCOCK, J. A. and STEPHENSON, P. (1972a) Renomedullary antihypertensive function in accelerated (malignant) hypertension: observations on renomedullary interstitial cells. *Journal of Clinical Investigation*, **51**, 181–190

MUIRHEAD, E. E., BROOKS, B., PITCOCK, J. A., STEPHENSON, P. and BROSIUS, W. L. (1972b) Role of the renal medulla in the sodium-sensitive component of renoprival hypertension. *Laboratory Investigation*, **27**, 192–198

MUIRHEAD, E. E. (1974) The role of the renal medulla. In *Advances in Internal Medicine*, edited by G. H. Stollerman, pp. 81–107. Chicago: Year Book Medical Publishers, Inc.

MUIRHEAD, E. E., BROOKS, B. and ARORA, K. K. (1974) Prevention of malignant hypertension by the synthetic peptide SQ 20,881. *Laboratory Investigation*, **30**, 129–135

MUIRHEAD, E. E., GERMAIN, G. S., ARMSTRONG, F. B. *et al.* (1974c) Renomedullary endocrine system. Its antihypertensive action. *Transactions of the Association of American Physicians*, **87**, 288–297

MUIRHEAD, E. E., GERMAN, G. S., ARMSTRONG, F. B. *et al.* (1975) Endocrine-type antihypertensive function of renomedullary interstitial cells. *Kidney International*, **8** (Suppl. V), 271–282

MUIRHEAD, E. E., LEACH, B. E., BYERS, L. W. and BROOKS, B. (1976) Enhanced potency of depressor renomedullary lipid. *Circulation*, **53**, II-175 (abstract)

MUIRHEAD, E. E., RIGHTSEL, W. A., LEACH, B. E., BYERS, L. W., PITCOCK, J. A. and BROOKS, B. (1977) Reversal of hypertension by transplants and lipid extracts of cultured renomedullary interstitial cells. *Laboratory Investigation*, **35**, 162–172

MUIRHEAD, E. E. (1980a) Antihypertensive functions of the kidney. *Hypertension*, **2**, 444–464

MUIRHEAD, E. E. (1980b) In *Captopril and Hypertension*, edited by D. B. Case., E. H. Donnenblick and J. H. Laragh, pp. 25–38. New York: Plenum Medical Book Company

MUIRHEAD, E. E. and BROOKS, B. (1980) Reversal of one-kidney, one-clip hypertension by unclipping: the renal sodium–volume relationship re-examined. *Proceedings of the Society of Experimental Biology and Medicine*, **163**, 540–546

MUIRHEAD, E. E., BYERS, L. W., DESIDERIO, D. M. JR, SMITH, K. A., PREWITT, R. L. and BROOKS, B. (1981a) Alkyl ether analogs of phosphatidylcholine are orally active in hypertensive rabbits. *Hypertension*, **3** (Suppl. 1), 107–111

MUIRHEAD, E. E., PITCOCK, J. A., BROOKS, B. and BROWN, P. (1981b) Captopril in angiotensin–salt hypertension: a possible linkage between angiotensin, salt, vascular disease and renomedullary interstitial cells. In *Frontiers in Hypertension Research*, edited by J. H. Laragh, F. Buhler and D. W. Seldin, pp. 559–566. New York: Springer-Verlag

MUIRHEAD, E. E., PITCOCK, J. A., BROWN, P. S. and BROOKS, B. (1981c) Possible link between converting enzyme inhibition and renomedullary interstitial cells. *Federation Proceedings*, **40** (8), 2262–2267

MUIRHEAD, E. E., BYERS, L. W., DESIDERIO, D. M. JR, BROOKS, B. and BROSIUS, W. L. (1982a) Derivation of antihypertensive neutral renomedullary lipid from renal venous effluent. *Journal of Laboratory and Clinical Medicine*, **99**, 64–75

MUIRHEAD, E. E., RIGHTSEL, W. A., PITCOCK, J. A. *et al.* (1982b) Cultured juxtaglomerular cells cause hypertension by secreting angiotensin. *Transactions of the Association of American Physicians*, **95**, 110–119

MUIRHEAD, E. E., FOLKOW, B., BYERS, L. W. *et al.* (1983a) Cardiovascular effects of antihypertensive polar and neutral renomedullary lipids. *Hypertension*, **5** (Suppl. I), I-112–I-118

MUIRHEAD, E. E., FOLKOW, B., BYERS, L. W. *et al.* (1983b) Cardiovascular effects of antihypertensive renomedullary lipids (APRL and ANRL). *Acta Physiologica Scandinavica*, **117**, 465–467

MUIRHEAD, E. E., BYERS, L. W., FOLKOW, B., GÖTHBERG, G., THORÉN, P. and BROOKS, B. (1983c) Antihypertensive polar and neutral renopapillary lipids: which is a hormone? *Hypertension*, **5**, V-61–V-65

MURRAY, B. R. and CATAB, M. R. (1892) Remarks on the treatment of myxoedema with thyroid juice with notes of four cases. *British Medical Journal*, **2**, 449–454

OLIVER, G. and SCHAFER, E. A. (1895) On the physiological action of extract of pituitary body and certain other glandular organs. *Journal of Physiology*, **18**, 277–279

PITCOCK, J. A., BROWN, P., BROOKS, B., CLAPP, W. L. and MUIRHEAD, E. E. (1980) Renomedullary deficiency in partial nephrectomy–salt hypertension. *Hypertension*, **2**, 281–290

PITCOCK, J. A., BROWN, P., BYERS, J. W.*et al.* (1981) Degranulation of renomedullary interstitial cells during reversal of hypertension. *Hypertension*, **3**, II-75–II-80

PREWITT, R. L., LEACH, B. E., BYERS, L. W., BROOKS, B., LANDS, W. E. and MUIRHEAD, E. E. (1979) Antihypertensive polar renomedullary lipid, a semisynthetic vasodilator. *Hypertension*, **1**, 299–308

RIGHTSEL, W. A., PITCOCK, J. A., INAGAMI, T. *et al.* (1982) Juxtaglomerular cells grown as monolayer cell culture contain renin, angiotensin I converting enzyme angiotensin I and II/III. *Circulation Research*, **50** (6), 822–829

SCHULZ, O. (1900) Uber die lebensuichtigkeit und des Schilddrusenapparates. *Deutsche Medizinische Wochenshrift*

SMITH, K. A., CORNETT, L. E., NORRIS, J. S., BYERS, L. W. and MUIRHEAD, E. E. (1982) Blockade of alpha-adrenergic receptors by analogues of phosphatidylcholine. *Life Sciences*, **31**, 1891–1902

SMITH, K. A., BROOKS, B., DOW, A. W. and MUIRHEAD, E. E. (1984) Decreased vascular response to norepinephrine after 1-alkyl-2-actyl-glycophosphocholine in unclipped hypertensive rats (in preparation)

SMITH, K. A., PREWITT, R. L., BYERS, L. W. and MUIRHEAD, E. E. (1981) Analogues of phosphatidylcholine: α-adrenergic antagonists from the renal medulla. *Hypertension*, **3**, 281–297

SUSIC, D. and KENTERA, D. (1980) Role of the renal medulla in the resistance of rats to salt hypertension. *Pflügers Archives*, **384**, 283–285

SUSIC, D., SPARKS, J. C. and MACHADO, E. A. (1976) Salt-induced hypertension in rats with hereditary hydronephrosis: the effect of renomedullary transplantation. *Journal of Laboratory and Clinical Medicine*, **87**, 232–239

TAKAMINE, J. (1901) The isolation of the active principle of the suprarenal gland. *Journal of Physiology*, **27**, 29–30

TOBIAN, L. and AZAR, S. (1971) Antihypertensive and other functions of the renal papilla. *Transactions of the Association of American Physicians*, **84,** 281–288

TRENDELENBURG, V. (1966) Observations on the ganglion-stimulating action of angiotensin and bradykinin. *Journal of Pharmacology and Experimental Therapy*, **154,** 418–425

VOELKEL, N. F., WORTHEN, S., REEVES, J. T., HINSON, P. M. and MURPHY, R. C. (1982) Nonimmunological production of leukotrienes by platelet-activating factor. *Science*, **218,** 286–289

Appendix: Flow charts

Isolation of ANRL from rabbit renal papilla

Kidneys from 900 rabbits (1800 kidneys)

↓

Fresh renal papilla 240 g

↓ + 240 ml pH 7.5 Sorensen's phosphate buffer.   0.268 M

| Blend in Waring blender
| 15 sec – slow
↓   2 min – fast

↓   Transfer to Erlenmeyer flask with 240 ml saline

Slurry

↓ Incubate for 30 min, with gentle swirling, at 37°C

↓ Pour on to lyophiliser tray and freeze-dry overnight

Dry powder, 40–48 g

Total lipid extraction of renal papilla (Bligh and Dyer)

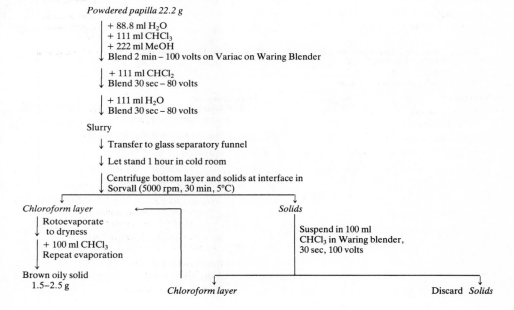

Powdered papilla 22.2 g

| + 88.8 ml H₂O
| + 111 ml CHCl₃
| + 222 ml MeOH
↓ Blend 2 min – 100 volts on Variac on Waring Blender

| + 111 ml CHCl₂
↓ Blend 30 sec – 80 volts

| + 111 ml H₂O
↓ Blend 30 sec – 80 volts

Slurry

↓ Transfer to glass separatory funnel

↓ Let stand 1 hour in cold room

| Centrifuge bottom layer and solids at interface in
↓ Sorvall (5000 rpm, 30 min, 5°C)

Chloroform layer   *Solids*

| Rotoevaporate
↓ to dryness

| + 100 ml CHCl₃   Suspend in 100 ml
| Repeat evaporation   CHCl₃ in Waring blender,
                                     30 sec, 100 volts

Brown oily solid
   1.5–2.5 g
                        Chloroform layer   Discard *Solids*

Unisil column chromatography of papillary lipids

Unisil – Clarkson Chemical Company

↓ Resecreened – 100–200 mesh 140 g

| Suspended in freshly opened CHCl₃
↓ Poured into 2.5 cm Pharmacia column

| Allowed fresh CHCl₃ to drip through at
↓ 1 drop/sec overnight – 700–800 ml

Column (uniform, nearly transparent-bluish color)

| + 1.5–2.5 g papilla lipids
↓ Dissolved in fresh CHCl₃ (50 ml)

↓ 2–15 ml CHCl₃ washes

| Attach CHCl₃ reservoir and collect effluent-flow rate
| rate 2–3 drops/sec
↓ 380 ml collected (1800 drop fractions, 20 of them)

| *NOTE:* Light yellow band comes through
↓ at tubes 12 and 13

↓ Effluent discarded

↓ CHCL₃ elution continued for another 200 ml effluent

| *NOTE:* This fraction contains considerable white
| crystalline material (cholesterol) and some
| antihypertensive activity (sometimes
↓ APRL-like, sometimes ANRL-like).

↓ Effluent saved, but kept separate; 150–224 mg solids

| 10% MeOH in CHCl₃ elution started and continued
| for 500 ml effluent
↓ Effluent rotoevaporated to dryness

  100–250 mg brown oily solid ANRL

Thin layer chromatography of Unisil column fraction of papillary lipids

Dimension 1st   Starting material – Unisil column fraction ANRL – mass 15 mg

                        +600 μl CHCL₃

15 μl   Remainder

| Spotted on | Streaked on
| 5 × 20 cm marker | preparative
| plate | plate

  NOTE: These plates previously up-washed with CHCL₃ and dried. Plates subjected to TLC in solvent system:
          CHCl₃:MeOH:NH₄OH
           60   35   8
  NOTE: Plates air dried for 30 min

Marker plate   *Preparative plate*

| Sprayed with | Plate cut into fractions according
↓ Conc. H₂SO₄   ↓ to burned marker plate

| Heated on hot | Fractions scraped off plate, one at
↓ plate   ↓ a time, and kept separate

                                  | Each eluted:

                                  | + 7 ml H₂O – swirl
                                  | + 14 ml 2% HOAc in MeOH –
                                  | invert 20 times
                                  | + 14 ml CHCl₃ – shake 1 minute
                                  ↓ + 7 ml H₂O – shake 1 minute

                                  | Each centrifuged: 25000 rpm, 5°C,
                                  ↓ 15 min

                                  | Each filtered: sintered glass –
                                  ↓ 5 ml CHCl₃ – rinse

                                  ↓ Each N₂ ⟶ dryness

Thin layer chromatography of Unisil column fraction of papillary lipids

Dimension 2nd   Starting material cut # 4 mass   1st Dimension TLC

+600 μl CHCL$_3$

15 μl

Spotted on
5 × 20 cm marker
plate

Remainder

Streaked on
preparative
plate

NOTE: These plates previously up-washed with CHCL$_3$ and dried. Plates subjected to TLC in solvent system:
Hexane:Ether:HOAc
40   60   1
NOTE: Plates air dried for 30 min

Marker plate

↓ Sprayed with
  Conc. H$_2$SO$_4$

↓ Heated on hot
  plate

Preparative plate

↓ Plate cut into fractions according
  to burned marker plate

↓ Fractions scraped off plate, one at
  a time, and kept separate

Each eluted:

  + 7 ml H$_2$O – swirl
  + 14 ml 2% HOAc in MeOH –
    invert 20 times
  + 14 ml CHCl$_3$ – shake 1 minute
↓ + 7 ml H$_2$O – shake 1 minute

↓ Each centrifuged: 25000 rpm, 5°C,
  15 min

↓ Each filtered: sintered glass –
  5 ml CHCl$_3$ – rinse

↓ Each N$_2$ ⟶ dryness
             2.4 mg

Dimension 3rd   Starting material cut # 2 of 2nd dimension – mass 2.4–3.6 g

+600 μl CHCL$_3$

15 μl

Spotted on
5 × 20 cm marker
plate

Remainder

Streaked on
preparative
plate

NOTE: These plates previously up-washed with CHCL$_3$ and dried. Plates subjected to TLC in solvent system:
Ether:HOAc:H$_2$0
100   0.5   0.5
NOTE: Plates air dried for 30 min

Marker plate

↓ Sprayed with
  Conc. H$_2$SO$_4$

↓ Heated on hot
  plate

Preparative plate

↓ Plate cut into fractions according
  to burned marker plate

↓ Fractions scraped off plate, one at
  a time, and kept separate

Each eluted:

  + 7 ml H$_2$O – swirl
  + 14 ml 2% HOAc in MeOH –
    invert 20 times
  + 14 ml CHCl$_3$ – shake 1 minute
↓ + 7 ml H$_2$O – shake 1 minute

↓ Each centrifuged: 25000 rpm, 5°C,
  15 min

↓ Each filtered: sintered glass –
  5 ml CHCl$_3$ – rinse

↓ Each N$_2$ ⟶ dryness
             700 μg

11
Pregnancy and hypertension

Peter C. Rubin

INTRODUCTION

In posing the question: Is hypertension during pregnancy an endocrine disease? one immediately encounters problems of definition. In the broadest sense hypertension which occurs during pregnancy can be of two general forms. The hypertension might be associated specifically with the pregnancy, developing at some stage during gestation and resolving within a few weeks or months of delivery, or the pregnancy might be superimposed on a pre-existing hypertensive state which is unrelated to the pregnancy itself. In this latter situation the differentiation into essential or secondary hypertension is going to be no different from that which would be applicable to any young woman who is found to have hypertension, and the question concerning endocrine aetiology will be as discussed in the earlier chapters of this text. It is pertinent to mention here, however, that the diagnosis of one rare but important endocrine cause of hypertension is very difficult during pregnancy but that misdiagnosis may have fatal consequences. Phaeochromocytoma is among the least common of the secondary causes of hypertension, but its well-known symptoms of variable blood pressure – anxiety, sweating, palpitations and so on – might well be mistaken for manifestations of pregnancy (Hendee, Martin and Waters, 1969). This has resulted in the regrettable fact that most cases of phaeochromocytoma occurring during pregnancy are actually diagnosed at autopsy. This is perhaps illustrated with no greater clarity than in the confidential report into maternal deaths in England and Wales (Department of Health and Social Services, London, 1978) in which three of the 39 maternal deaths attributed to hypertension were caused by phaeochromocytoma. This is grossly out of proportion to the situation in the non-obstetric population. Although this is a very striking figure, it remains the case that the great majority of women who are found to be hypertensive during pregnancy have neither essential hypertension nor a readily identifiable secondary cause. They have high blood pressure which is associated with that pregnancy and it is with this very particular form of hypertension that the remainder of the chapter will be concerned.

Physicians who are accustomed to dealing with hypertension in the non-obstetric population sometimes find it difficult to appreciate just how different pregnancy-associated hypertension is with regard to presentation, clinical significance and priorities for management. Any attempt to provide an aetiological basis for pregnancy-associated hypertension must explain its unique clinical features and its epidemiological characteristics. The problem of definition is still with us even if we have decided that the hypertension is pregnancy-related. Medical students will have no difficulty in reciting the classical triad which forms the basis of diagnosing pre-eclampsia: any two symptoms of hypertension, proteinuria and oedema. However, oedema occurs with such regularity during pregnancy – around 80% of women develop oedema at some stage – that it is virtually useless as a diagnostic sign (Thomson, Hytten and Billewitz, 1967). Hypertension can be specifically related to pregnancy without being associated with proteinuria, and the presence of proteinuria is important primarily because it places the condition in a more severe category from the standpoint of fetal survival (MacGillivray, 1961). There is always, therefore, the possibility that one woman's pre-eclampsia is another's essential hypertension with oedema, which does nothing to improve the comparability between studies.

The following facts must be explained by any theory concerning the aetiology of hypertension related to pregnancy. The condition is far more common in first than in subsequent pregnancies, developing usually somewhere after 24 weeks and resolving often within a few days of delivery but sometimes taking up to 6 months. The importance of parity is demonstrated by the fact that even a previous abortion greatly reduces the likelihood of developing pre-eclampsia in the first pregnancy to proceed to term (McGillivray, 1958). Interestingly, even if a woman is not in her first pregnancy a change of sexual partner returns her likelihood of developing pre-eclampsia to that of a woman who has had no previous pregnancies (Need, 1975). This taken together with the observation that a prior blood transfusion reduces the likelihood of pre-eclampsia and the finding of deposits of IgM, IgG and complement in renal biopsy specimens (Petrucco *et al.*, 1974) suggests the strong possibility of an immunological basis for the disease.

Pre-eclampsia is also more common in women with large placentae, such as diabetics, those with multiple pregnancies and hydatidiform mole. There is a definite family tendency to the inheritance of pre-eclampsia (Adams and Finlayson, 1961). The disease also shows racial and geographical tendencies, occurring for example more frequently in Jewish people, and also having a tendency to be concentrated in coastal rather than inland areas of large land masses (Davies, 1971).

From all the above it can be seen that we are dealing here with a very different condition from essential hypertension in non-obstetric practice. Indeed, it is almost certainly incorrect to use the term 'condition' in the singular since it is highly likely that pregnancy-related hypertension is in fact comprised of several different conditions with possibly quite diverse pathogenesis. The remainder of this chapter will concern itself with a discussion of such evidence as exists concerning the possible role of various endocrine systems in the aetiology of pregnancy-related hypertension. It will soon become apparent that in all respects the evidence is either negative or inconclusive.

RENIN–ANGIOTENSIN–ALDOSTERONE SYSTEM

There is general agreement that during normal pregnancy all components of this system demonstrate an increase in circulating concentration. This begins within a few weeks of conception and concentrations return rapidly towards normal in the few days following delivery (Becker *et al.*, 1978; Gallery *et al.*, 1980; Gordon *et al.*, 1973; Helmer and Judson, 1967; Jadoul, Broughton-Pipkin and Lamming, 1982; Skinner, Lumbers and Symonds, 1972; Weir *et al.*, 1971). The reason for this stimulation of the renin-angiotensin system in normal pregnancy is not clear although contributing factors might well be the substantial increase in filtered sodium load which occurs during pregnancy (Sims and Krantz, 1958) and the antagonism of aldosterone by progesterone (Landau and Lugibihl, 1958). There is also general agreement that during normal pregnancy there is a diminution of sensitivity to the vasoconstrictor effects of angiotenin II (Chesley *et al.*, 1965) with responsiveness being at a trough by around 14 weeks and being maintained at this level until about 30 weeks (Gant *et al.*, 1973). Sensitivity to angiotensin II is returning to normal by term (Symonds and Broughton-Pipkin, 1978). Interestingly, women who have or who are going to develop pre-eclampsia demonstrate a greater sensitivity to infusions of angiotensin II than do their normotensive counterparts (Chesley *et al.*, 1965; Gant *et al.*, 1973).

It is tempting to infer that, since the relatively increased sensitivity to angiotensin II occurs before the clinical appearance of pre-eclampsia, the renin–angiotensin system must in some way be involved in the pathogenesis of this condition. This interpretation is either complicated or confirmed, depending on your viewpoint, by the knowledge that pregnancy-associated hypertension is a volume-depleted condition (Freis and Kenny, 1948) and by the observation that volume depletion appears, like the changed sensitivity to angiotensin II, before pre-eclampsia becomes clinically evident (Gallery, Hunyor and Gyory, 1979). This reduction in plasma volume could be considered as the trigger for stimulation of the renin–angiotensin system in pre-eclampsia. Alternatively, the reduction in plasma volume associated presumably with a decrease in the diameter of the capacitance vessels, itself might contribute in large part to the apparently increased sensitivity to infused angiotensin II. If the former were the case then it would be expected that circulating concentrations of angiotensin II would be elevated in pre-eclampsia but there is no consistent evidence to support this possibility. While there is agreement that plasma renin concentration in women with pre-eclampsia is either the same (Brown *et al.*, 1966; Gallery *et al.*, 1980), or lower (Helmer and Judson, 1967) than in normotensive pregnancies, there is anything but agreement on what happens to the concentration of angiotensin II in pre-eclampsia. These concentrations have been variously reported as normal (Massani *et al.*, 1967), elevated (Symonds, Broughton-Pipkin and Craven, 1975) or substantially depressed (Weir *et al.*, 1973) in women with pre-eclampsia compared to normotensive controls. The reasons for such disparate findings are not immediately obvious although angiotensin II is not the easiest of substances to analyze and this, together with the probability of differences in diagnosis, could well have made a major contribution.

Current knowledge therefore allows the conclusion that pregnancy itself leads to a stimulation of the renin–angiotensin–aldosterone system, but it is far less clear what role if any this system plays in the aetiology or maintenance of pre-eclampsia.

SYMPATHETIC NERVOUS SYSTEM AND PREGNANCY HYPERTENSION

In common with hypertension occurring in non-obstetric practice, there have been various attempts to investigate the possible role of the sympathetic nervous system in either the pathogenesis or maintenance of pregnancy-associated hypertension. Earlier studies in which urinary catecholamines were measured suggested that there is increased production in women with pregnancy-associated hypertension (Cession, 1966; Zuspan, 1979). In recent years the increasing availability of sensitive and specific analytical methods have permitted the accurate measurement of plasma catecholamine concentrations in plasma. Unfortunately the increase in analytical precision has not led to any clarification of catecholamine behaviour in pregnancy hypertension. One study which involved Cape Coloured women in South Africa produced data suggesting that those women with hypertension during the last trimester of pregnancy had higher plasma adrenaline, noradrenaline and dopamine concentrations than normotensive control subjects (Davey and McNab, 1981). However, a closer inspection of the data reveals that blood samples were taken from women shortly after admission to the hospital, and when the patients were studied subsequently these differences within the two groups had disappeared. Since the control subjects had been admitted to the hospital for obstetric reasons, such as previous caesarean section, it seems possible that the higher catecholamine concentrations seen in the pregnant hypertensives on day 1 of the study could have been a result of anxiety at being admitted with a potentially serious complication. The only other recent study which suggests a possible role for catecholamines in pregnancy hypertension is a finding that catechol-o-methyltransferase (COMT) activity in the erythrocytes of women with pregnancy-induced hypertension is slightly but significantly higher than that found in normotensive control pregnant women (Bates, Whitworth and Jackson, 1982). The remaining studies suggest that the sympathoadrenal system is not involved in pregnancy-associated hypertension. One study measured plasma noradrenaline and adrenaline concentrations in patients with pre-eclampsia, those with essential hypertension during pregnancy, normotensive pregnant control subjects and non-pregnant controls. Measurements were performed both in the second and the third trimesters and at 5 days and 3 months following delivery (Pedersen et al., 1982).

There were no differences in plasma noradrenaline or adrenaline concentration between any of these groups at any time. Another study which investigated 21 patients who developed hypertension during the last trimester found that their plasma noradrenaline concentrations were significantly lower than those found in normotensive gestation matched controls (Tunbridge and Donnai, 1981). In a study of ten women with pregnancy-associated hypertension and eight normotensive pregnant controls we found no difference in plasma noradrenaline concentration in the last trimester (Rubin, Butters and Reid, 1983).

Recently, the plasma concentrations of noradrenaline and adrenaline measured serially during pregnancy have been described. There were 52 normotensive women and nine who developed hypertension. Both noradrenaline and adrenaline concentration fell significantly during normal pregnancy. There was a tendency for both catecholamines to be lower in the women who became hypertensive (Natrajan *et al.*, 1982).

The available evidence would therefore suggest that neither the sympathetic nervous system nor the adrenal gland are involved in pregnancy-associated hypertension.

PROSTAGLANDINS

Not surprisingly, prostaglandins have been implicated in the aetiology of pre-eclampsia. The discovery of prostacyclin and thromboxane A_2 which not only influence vascular reactivity in opposing ways but also influence platelet aggregation, was greeted with enthusiasm as a possible explanation not only for the increased blood pressure but for the well-known observation that pre-eclampsia is accompanied by platelet consumption. It was suggested that perhaps a reduction in prostacyclin or an increase in thromboxane A_2 concentration could be responsible both for the platelet aggregation and hypertension seen in pre-eclampsia. Unfortunately, evidence to support this very interesting and exciting concept is substantially lacking.

The analysis of prostaglandins in general, and prostacyclin and thromboxane A_2 in particular, is very difficult largely because of their instability. Since there is no animal model of pregnancy hypertension, plasma is usually the most accessible tissue and most investigators have studied the more stable metabolites of these compounds. There appears to be agreement that pregnancy itself has no effect on the metabolites of prostacyclin or thromboxane A_2 (Koullapis *et al.*, 1982; Ylikorkala, Kirkiness and Viinikka, 1981). These two studies differed, however, in their findings in women with pre-eclampsia – the former observing no difference from normal pregnancies while the latter obtained statistically significantly elevated concentrations of both prostacyclin and thromboxane A_2 metabolites in women with pre-eclampsia. The standard deviations were, however, very large.

Analyses of the parent prostaglandins have produced equally conflicting results, even from the same laboratory. Thus prostacyclin production has been claimed to be lower in placental vascular tissue from women with pre-eclampsia, although prostacyclin-stimulating factor was found in a separate study to be present in higher concentration in plasma from women with pre-eclampsia (Remuzzi *et al.*, 1980, 1981). Similarly, the concentrations of prostaglandins E and F in placenta from normotensive or hypertensive pregnancies have been shown to be the same or different (Hillier and Smith, 1981).

Until analytical techniques for prostaglandins and their metabolites have improved substantially it is unlikely that much clarification of the above confusion can be expected.

OTHER HORMONES

The major criterion for being considered as a possible agent in pre-eclampsia appears to have been the ability to measure the hormone concerned. The concentrations of various hormones – for example, progesterone and deoxcortico-sterone – have been found to be substantially elevated in pregnancy itself but there is little to suggest that levels are any different in hypertensive pregnancy (Brown, Strott and Liddle, 1972; Parker *et al.*, 1979, 1980). Work on other substances such as kinins has not reached a sufficient level of sophistication even to allow preliminary judgement on what happens in pregnancy let alone pregnancy hypertension.

CONCLUSION

Those of us whose daily work involves the management of patients with pre-eclampsia realize that we are dealing with a very special and unique condition or collection of conditions. Unfortunately, so far no single hypothesis, be it endocrine, haematological or immunological, has satisfactorily explained the diverse features of pre-eclampsia (MacGillivray, 1981). The closest that endocrinology comes to being involved with the hypertensive pregnancy is the observation concerning the enhanced sensitivity to angiotensin II. However, why this should occur in Dar-es-Salaam but not in Riyadh, for example, or why it should occur almost exclusively in primagravidae is far from clear. Despite the intensive research into the subject, pre-eclampsia has not yet divulged its fascinating secrets.

References

ADAMS, E. M. and FINLAYSON, A. (1961) Familial aspects of pre-eclampsia and hypertension in pregnancy. *Lancet*, **2**, 1375–1378

BATES, G. W., WHITWORTH, N. S. and JACKSON, E. (1982) Erythrocyte catechol-o-methyltransferase activity in pregnant women with pregnancy-induced hypertension. *American Journal of Obstetrics and Gynecology*, **142**, 177–178

BECKER, R. A., HAYASHI, R. M., FRANKS, R. C. and SPEROFF, L. (1978) Effect of positional change and sodium balance on the renin–angiotensin–alderosterone system by renin and prostaglandins in normal pregnancy. *Journal of Clinical Endocrinology and Metabolism*, **46**, 467–472

BROWN, J. J., DAVIES, D. L., DOAK, D. B., LEVER, A. F., ROBERTSON, J. I. S. and TRUST, P. (1966) Plasma renin concentration in the hypertensive diseases of pregnancy. *Journal of Obstetrics and Gynaecology of the British Commonwealth*, **73**, 410–417

BROWN, R. D., STROTT, C. A. and LIDDLE, G. W. (1972) Plasma deoxycorticosterone in normal and abnormal human pregnancy. *Journal of Clinical Endocrinology and Metabolism*, **35**, 736–742

CESSION, G. (1966) Sur l'élimination urinaire des catecholamines et de leur metabolite au cours de la dysgravidie due 3me trimestre de la gestation. *Bulletin de la Societé Royale Belge Gynécologie et Obstétrique*, **36**, 196–216

CHESLEY, L. C., TALLEDO, E., BOHLER, C. S. and ZUSPAN F. P. (1965) Vascular reactivity to angiotensin II and norepinephrine in pregnant and non-pregnant women. *American Journal of Obstetrics and Gynecology*, **91**, 837–842

DEPARTMENT OF HEALTH AND SOCIAL SERVICES, LONDON (1978) *Confidential Enquiry into Maternal Deaths in England and Wales, 1973–1975*

DAVEY, D. A. and McNAB, M. F. (1981) Plasma adrenaline, noradrenaline and dopamine in pregnancy hypertension. *British Journal of Obstetrics and Gynaecology*, **88**, 611–618

DAVIES, A. M. (1971) *Geographical Epidemiology of the Toxaemias of Pregnancy*. Springfield, Ill.: Thomas

FREIS, E. D. and KENNY, J. F. (1948) Plasma volume, total circulating protein and available fluid abnormalities in pre-eclampsia and eclampsia. *Journal of Clinical Investigation*, **27**, 283–289

GALLERY, E. D. M., HUNYOR, S. N. and GYORY, A. Z. (1979) Plasma volume contraction: a significant factor in both pregnancy-associated hypertension (pre-eclampsia) and chronic hypertension in pregnancy. *Quarterly Journal of Medicine*, **48**, 593–602

GALLERY, E. D. M., STOKES, G. S., GYORY, A. Z., ROWE, J. and WILLIAMS, J. (1980) Plasma renin activity in normal human pregnancy and in pregnancy associated hypertension, with reference to cryoactivation. *Clinical Science*, **59**, 49–53

GANT, N. F., DALEY, G. L., CHAND, S., WHALLEY, P. J. and MACDONALD, P. C. (1973) A study of antiotensin II pressor response throughout primigravid pregnancy. *Journal of Clinical Investigation*, **52**, 2682–2689

GORDON, R. D., SYMONDS, E. M., WILMSHURST, E. G. and PAWSEY, C. G. K. (1973) Plasma renin activity, plasma angiotensin and plasma and urinary electrolytes in normal and toxaemic pregnancy, including a prospective study. *Clinical Science and Molecular Medicine*, **45**, 115–127

HELMER, O. and JUDSON, W. (1967) Influence of high renin substrate levels on the renin angiotensin system in pregnancy. *American Journal of Obstetrics and Gynecology*, **99**, 9–17

HENDEE, A. E., MARTIN, R. D. and WATERS, W. C. (1969) Hypertension in pregnancy: toxaemia of pheochromocytoma. *American Journal of Obstetrics and Gynecology*, **105**, 64–70

HILLIER, K. and SMITH, M. D. (1981) Prostaglandins E and F concentrations in placentae of normal, hypertensive and pre-eclampsia patients. *British Journal of Obstetrics and Gynaecology*, **88**, 274–277

JADOUL, F. A. C., BROUGHTON-PIPKIN, F. and LAMMING, G. D. (1982) Changes in the renin–angiotensin–aldosterone system in normotensive primigravidae in the four days after normal spontaneous delivery. *British Journal of Obstetrics and Gynaecology*, **89**, 633–639

KOULLAPIS, E. N., NICOLAIDES, K. H., COLLINS, W. P., RODECK, C. H. and CAMPBELL, S. (1982) Plasma prostanoids in pregnancy induced hypertension. *British Journal of Obstetrics and Gynaecology*, **89**, 617–621

LANDAU, R. L. and LUGIBIHL, K. (1958) Inhibition of the sodium-retaining influence of aldosterone by progesterone. *Journal of Clinical Endocrinology and Metabolism*, **18**, 1237–1245

MacGILLIVRAY, I. (1958) Some observations on the incidence of pre-eclampsia. *Journal of Obstetrics and Gynaecology of the British Empire*, **65**, 536–539

MacGILLIVRAY, I. (1961) Hypertension in pregnancy and its consequences. *Journal of Obstetrics and Gynaecology of the British Empire*, **68**, 557–569

MacGILLIVRAY, I. (1981) Aetiology of pre-eclampsia. *British Journal of Hospital Medicine*, **26**, 110–119

MASSANI, Z. M., SANGUINETTI, R., GALLEGOS, R. and RAIMONDI, D. (1967) Angiotensin blood levels in normal and toxemic pregnancies. *American Journal of Obstetrics and Gynecology*, **99**, 313–317

NATRAJAN, P. G., McGARRIGLE, H. H. G., LAWRENCE, D. M. and LACHELIN, G. C. L. (1982) Plasma noradrenaline and adrenaline levels in normal pregnancy and in pregnancy-induced hypertension. *British Journal of Obstetrics and Gynaecology*, **89**, 1041–1045

NEED, J. A. (1975) Pre-eclampsia in pregnancies by different fathers: immunological studies. *British Medical Journal*, **1**, 548–549

PARKER, C. R., EVERETT, R. B., QUIRK, J. G., WHALLEY, P. J. and GRANT, N. F. (1979) Plasma levels of progesterone and 5α-pregnane-3,20-dione throughout pregnancy of normal women and women who developed pregnancy induced hypertension. *American Journal of Obstetrics and Gynecology*, **135**, 778–782

PARKER, C. R., EVERETT, R. B., WHALLEY, P. J., QUIRK, J. G., GANT, N. F. and MacDONALD, P. C. (1980) Plasma levels of deoxycorticosterone throughout pregnancy of normal women and women who developed pregnancy induced hypertension. *American Journal of Obstetrics and Gynecology*, 138, 626–631

PEDERSEN, E. B., RASMUSSESN, A. B., CHRISTENSEN, N. J. *et al.*, (1982) Plasma noradrenaline and adrenaline in pre-eclampsia, essential hypertension in pregnancy and normotensive pregnant control subjects. *Acta Endocrinologica*, **99**, 594–600

PETRUCCO, O. M., THOMSON, N. M., LAWRENCE, J. R. and WELDON, M. W. (1974) Immunofluorescent studies in renal biopsies in pre-eclampsia. *British Medical Journal*, **1**, 473–476

REMUZZI, G., MARCHESI, D., MECCA, G. *et al.* (1980) Reduction of fetal vascular prostacyclins in pre-eclampsia. *Lancet*, **2**, 310

REMUZZI, G. ZOJA, C., MARCHESI, D. *et al.* (1981) Plasmatic regulation of vascular prostacylins in pregnancy. *British Medical Journal*, **282**, 512–514

RUBIN, P. C., BUTTERS, L. and REID, J. L. (1983) Plasma noradrenaline in pregnancy-associated hypertension. *Clinical and Experimental Hypertension*, **B2(3)**, 421–428

SIMS, E. A. H. and KRANTZ, K. E. (1958) Serial studies of renal function during pregnancy and puerperium in normal women. *Journal of Clinical Investigation*, **37**, 1764–1774

SKINNER, S. L., LUMBERS, E. R. and SYMONDS, E. M. (1972) Analysis of changes in the renin–angiotensin system during pregnancy. *Clinical Science*, **42**, 479–488

SYMONDS, E. M., BROUGHTON-PIPKIN, F. and CRAVEN, D. J. (1975) Changes in the renin–angiotension system in primagravidae with hypertensive disease of pregnancy. *British Journal of Obstetrics and Gynaecology*, **82**, 643–646

SYMONDS, E. M. and BROUGHTON-PIPKIN, F. (1978) Pregnancy hypertension, parity and the renin–angiotensin system. *American Journal of Obstetrics and Gynecology*, **132**, 473–479

THOMSON, A. M., HYTTEN, F. E. and BILLEWITZ, Z. (1967) The epidemiology of oedema during pregnancy. *Journal of Obstetrics and Gynaecology of the British Commonwealth*, **74**, 1–10

TUNBRIDGE, R. D. G. and DONNAI, P. (1981) Plasma noradrenaline in normal pregnancy and in hypertension of late pregnancy. *British Journal of Obstetrics and Gynaecology*, **88**, 105–108

WEIR, R. J., PAINTIN, D. B., BROWN, J. J. et al. (1971) A serial study in pregnancy of the plasma concentrations of renin, corticosteroids, electrolytes and proteins and of haematocrit and plasma volume. *Journal of Obstetrics and Gynaecology of the British Commonwealth*, **78**, 590–602

WEIR, R. J., FRASER, R., LEVER, A. F. et al. (1973) Plasma renin, renin substrate, angiotensin II and aldosterone in hypertensive disease of pregnancy. *Lancet*, **1**, 291–294

YLIKORKALA, O., KIRKINESS, P. and VIINIKKA, L. (1981) Maternal plasma prostacyclin concentration in pre-eclampsia and other pregnancy complications. *British Journal of Obstetrics and Gynaecology*, **88**, 968–972

ZUSPAN, F. P. (1979) Catecholamines – their role in pregnancy and the development of pregnancy induced hypertension. *Journal of Reproductive Medicine*, **23**, 143–150

12
Hypertension in diabetes mellitus
Paul L. Drury

INTRODUCTION

There has recently been a marked increase of interest in the pathogenesis of arterial hypertension in patients with diabetes mellitus. The present chapter will concentrate on the possible relevance of endocrine mechanisms to this condition and will necessarily touch upon the issues of epidemiology, other possible pathogenetic mechanisms, the relevance of hypertension to diabetic complications, and treatment of the problem. Several full reviews of the subject with more extensive discussions of the epidemiology and drug treatment are available (Christlieb, 1980, 1982; Drury, 1983; Sowers and Tuck, 1981).

Only recently has there been widespread agreement about the classification of diabetes mellitus (National Diabetes Data Group, 1979; World Health Organization, 1980). As will become apparent, there is evidence that the hypertension seen with Type 1 (insulin-dependent) diabetes and Type 2 (non-insulin-dependent) diabetes may have different clinical accompaniments and, possibly, different pathogenetic mechanisms, though there are obvious metabolic and endocrine parallels between them. As far as possible they will be discussed separately although much of the data comes from reports where subjects with both types of diabetes have been studied.

INTERPRETATION OF PREVIOUS EPIDEMIOLOGICAL STUDIES

Interpretation of, and comparison between, many early studies of hypertension in diabetes is rendered difficult by problems of methodology. The use of non-standardized conditions such as different postures, Korotkoff phases IV or V for diastolic pressure (American Heart Association Committee Report, 1981), and the variable 'definitions' of hypertension and diabetes employed pose major problems. Thus, the use of a fixed level of $\geq 160/95$ mmHg for 'hypertension' (World Health Organization, 1979) will lead to a low prevalence in a young population, even though the blood pressure of the diabetic group may be well above that of a suitable young control group. Confusion between an increased overall prevalence of hypertension and significantly increased blood pressures in specific groups of patients has, until recently, obscured several important areas.

The single most difficult issue, however, is that of body weight. In westernized society, obesity is the greatest risk factor for type 2 (non-insulin-dependent) diabetes and is present in the majority of such patients. Conventional blood pressure recording techniques may, by the use of inappropriate cuff sizes, lead to inaccuracies – recent evidence suggests that correction factors, when applied at all, may previously have underestimated the extent of the adjustment needed (Maxwell *et al.*, 1982). In addition there is a further effect of body weight on true arterial pressure – it has been clearly shown that, both in diabetics and non-diabetics, blood pressure falls with reduction of body weight (Heyden, 1978; Tuck *et al.*, 1981).

SECONDARY HYPERTENSION AND DIABETES

The combination of diabetes (or impaired glucose tolerance) and hypertension as a presentation of other endocrine disorders is well known (*Table 12.1*). Thyrotoxicosis, acromegaly, phaeochromocytoma and Cushing's syndrome are occasionally seen, while the use of synthetic oestrogen/progestogen combinations and primary aldosteronism are less frequent. Apart from the possible relevance of these models to the endocrine mechanisms of hypertension in type 1 and type 2 diabetes, they will not be discussed in detail.

Diabetes and other causes of hypertension may presumably coexist by chance. In the absence of any unequivocal marker for essential hypertension it is not possible

Table 12.1 Secondary causes of hypertension and diabetes and proposed mechanisms

Condition	Postulated mechanism of hypertension	Postulated mechanism of diabetes
Thyrotoxicosis	? increased receptor sensitivity to catecholamines (Sowers and Tuck, 1981; Dratman, 1976)	? increased glycogenolysis and insulin degradation (Young and Landsberg, 1977)
Acromegaly	increased exchangeable sodium; ? direct effect of growth hormone; also ? sympathetic component (Taylor and Bartter, 1977; Sowers and Tuck, 1981)	? direct effect of growth hormone or via hyperinsulinism or insulin resistance (Wass *et al.*, 1980)
Phaeochromocytoma	direct catecholamine effects; vasoconstriction, decreased blood volume (Cryer, 1981)	? suppression of insulin release; other effects on glucose metabolism (Cryer, 1981; Isles and Johnson, 1983)
Cushing's syndrome	glucocorticoid plus mineralocorticoid actions of sodium retention; ? others (Taylor and Bartter, 1977; Krakoff and Elijovich, 1981)	gluconeogenesis and insulin resistance
Primary aldosteronism	mineralocorticoid effects of sodium retention; ? others (Schalekamp, Wenting and Man In 't Veld, 1981)	hypokalaemia leading to decreased insulin secretion (Conn, Knopf and Nesbit, 1964)

to differentiate this from 'diabetic hypertension'. Weidmann (1980) has recently compared pathogenetic mechanisms in essential hypertension with those in 'diabetic hypertension' but there are obvious differences in some areas, especially with the hypertension of diabetic nephropathy. Apart from the secondary conditions listed above, there is no evidence of any significant increase in the prevalence of other causes of hypertension; an early suggestion of an increased frequency of renal artery stenosis has not been substantiated (Shapiro, Perez-Stable and Monsos, 1965; Munichoodappa *et al.*, 1979).

TYPE I (INSULIN-DEPENDENT) DIABETES

Epidemiology

It is now clear that hypertension accompanying insulin-dependent diabetes is often very closely associated with the presence of diabetic renal disease. Progressive diabetic nephropathy affects 20–45% of insulin-dependent diabetic subjects and is

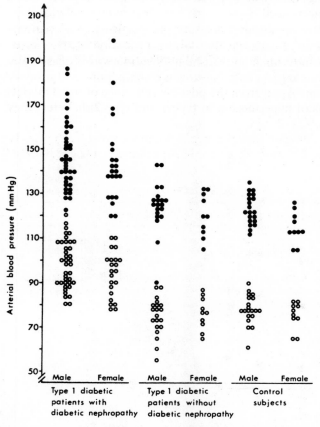

Figure 12.1 Systolic (●) and diastolic (○) blood pressures in Type 1 diabetic patients with (*n* = 61), and without (*n* = 30) diabetic nephropathy, and in healthy subjects (*n* = 30). (From Parving *et al.*, 1983, courtesy of the Publishers, *Diabetologia*)

one of the major causes of death (Anderson *et al.*, 1983; Deckert, Poulsen and Larsen, 1978; Tunbridge, 1981).

The stage of diabetic renal disease at which increased blood pressure becomes apparent has been a matter of considerable debate, which has been greatly clarified by recent Danish data. Many authorities have regarded it as a late accompaniment, only being present when the serum creatinine was clearly elevated (Ireland, Viberti and Watkins, 1982) but Parving *et al.* (1983a) have shown significantly higher blood pressures at a much earlier stage. In 61 Type 1 diabetic patients with persistent proteinuria blood pressure was higher (146/96 mmHg) compared with 30 Type 1 diabetic patients without persistent proteinuria (123/75 mmHg) and 30 normal subjects (120/77 mmHg) (*Figure 12.1*). The groups were well matched for age, sex and body weight, and for disease duration in the two diabetic groups; all had a normal serum creatinine at the time of blood pressure measurement. Though the mean difference between diabetics with and without proteinuria was 23/21 mmHg, only 51% of the former had a diastolic pressure ≥95 mmHg and would thus be considered truly 'hypertensive'. It may well be that use of this arbitrary level, which is most inappropriate for subjects aged 20–40 years, has obscured this relationship.

The same workers have measured blood pressure prospectively in 14 patients with persistent proteinuria (>0.5 g/day) and showed, over a period of 26 months, an increase in blood pressure from 132/88 to 153/101 mmHg, phases I/V; *P* < 0.01).

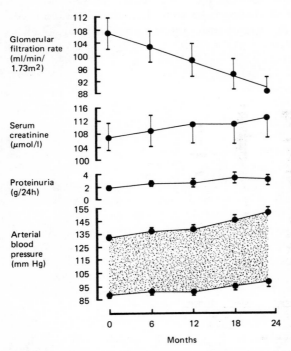

Figure 12.2 The course of blood pressure, proteinuria and renal function in 14 Type 1 diabetic subjects with persistent proteinuria (> 0.5 g/day) over a period of 2 years. Data are mean ± SEM. (From Christiansen *et al.*, 1981; courtesy of the Publishers, *Diabetologia*)

Of the 14 patients 13 showed a linear decline in glomerular filtration rate over this time, the mean declining from 107 to 87 ml/min/1.73 m^2) (Christiansen *et al.*, 1981) (*Figure 12.2*).

It does, however, appear that major increases in blood pressure do not long antedate the development of nephropathy, if the latter is defined as persistent proteinuria. Deckert and Poulsen (1981) compared multiple factors present before the onset of nephropathy in 21 type 1 diabetic patients who subsequently developed clinical nephropathy with 21 carefully matched subjects who had remained free of renal disease; initial blood pressure was marginally but not significantly lower in the group who later developed nephropathy. Examination of the two studies described above (Christiansen *et al.*, 1981; Parving *et al.*, 1983a) does however suggest some elevation in blood pressure: thus the initial pressures in the prospective study (132/88 mmHg) is apparently higher than in those patients free of proteinuria (123/75 mmHg), although the two groups are not strictly comparable; this may relate to the arbitrary definition of persistent proteinuria >0.5 g/day as the selection criteria. Substantive data on blood pressure in those subjects with microalbuminuria (albumin excretion rate >30 μg/min), who are believed to be at high risk of subsequent development of clinical nephropathy (Viberti *et al.*, 1982), are not yet available (see Addendum).

These findings are in general agreement with earlier studies which showed a close temporal relationship between the prevalence of diabetic nephropathy and significant hypertension, however the two entities were defined (Christlieb *et al.*, 1981; Moss, 1962 White, 1956). Several of these reports are, however, open to criticism on the grounds of inadequate definition of hypertension and/or nephropathy or the lack of suitable control populations.

Systolic pressures

Moss (1962) suggested that children with diabetes may have slightly elevated systolic pressures from the time of adolescence onwards; the numbers in each age group in this study were, however, small and no more recent report with adequate numbers and controls has addressed this question. The data from Parving *et al.* (1983a), using age, sex and weight-matched controls, would appear to exclude any increase of more than 2–3 mmHg in patients free of nephropathy.

An interesting observation is the increased systolic pressure shown after heavy exercise by some insulin-dependent diabetic subjects. Though this phenomenon has been mainly described in subjects with some degree of renal impairment, its relationship to complications is not yet clear (Mogensen, 1982b; Mogensen, Vittinghus and Solling, 1979); it has been proposed as a screening method for 'subclinical' renal involvement.

No adequately controlled data on systolic pressure are available for a large cohort of older type 1 diabetic patients. Though there appears to be a high prevalence of hypertension, this is partially because the use of any fixed criteria, such as ≥160 mmHg systolic and/or ≥95 mmHg diastolic (World Health Organization, 1979) will necessarily give an increasing prevalence of hypertension with age in any westernized population. The question of an increased prevalence of systolic or diastolic hypertension in this group is made yet more difficult because of the inevitable fatal progression of diabetic nephropathy and thus selective loss of the most obvious hypertensive group; additionally many of the surviving subjects have extensive vascular disease which may itself be involved in the pathogenesis of systolic hypertension (Janka, Standl and Meinhert, 1980). The true prevalence of raised blood pressure in this group thus remains an open question; such data as there is would be compatible with the hypothesis that systolic hypertension in particular is more frequent in patients with type 1 diabetes over 45–50 years of age (Christlieb *et al.*, 1981).

Nature of the renal lesion leading to hypertension

Diabetic glomerulosclerosis is a frequent occurrence in long-standing Type 1 diabetes irrespective of the presence of clinical renal disease. Similarly, increased renal plasma flow and hypertrophy are seen in the early years of diabetes (Mogensen, 1976), but blood pressure appears to be normal at this stage. The nature of the renal lesion which develops later and is characterized by proteinuria and accompanied by hypertension, remains unknown. The characteristic pattern of excretion of albumin but not β_2-microglobulin strongly suggests a glomerular origin. Hostetter, Rennke and Brenner (1982) have recently proposed mechanisms, based on studies in the streptozotocin-diabetic rat, whereby the haemodynamic changes observed in early diabetes might lead to mesangial changes and progressive deterioration in renal function. The relationship of such changes to the renin–angiotensin system and other local renal hormones such as kallikrein and prostaglandins is not clear although a report of multiple intrarenal haemodynamic and endocrine abnormalities in Type 2 diabetes has recently been published (Olshan *et al.*, 1982).

TYPE 2 (NON-INSULIN-DEPENDENT) DIABETES

Two main categories of Type 2 diabetes are recognized, that associated with significant obesity being much the commoner in western societies (National Diabetes Data Group, 1979). This high prevalence of obesity has led to great difficulty in the design and interpretation of epidemiological data on the prevalence of hypertension among these patients; it is further confounded by apparent differences between newly diagnosed and established diabetics (Jarrett *et al.*, 1978; Keen, Track and Sowry, 1975). Blood pressure in these studies appears to be higher in undiagnosed than in established diabetics.

   Whether there is an increased prevalence of hypertension in Type 2 diabetes remains arguable; detailed references to the many studies performed over the last 70 years may be found in several recent publications (Barrett-Connor *et al.*, 1981; Drury, 1983; Jarrett *et al.*, 1978; Pell and D'Alonzo, 1967). Much hinges on the weight comparability of the control population or the correction factor for obesity employed.

Whether or not the prevalence of hypertension is increased, the condition poses a common problem in diabetic and hypertension clinics. It has also been suggested that the triad of obesity, diabetes and hypertension may all be manifestations of a single central nervous system defect.

POSSIBLE MECHANISMS OF HYPERTENSION IN DIABETES

Not surprisingly, while the cause(s) of essential hypertension remains an enigma, similar ignorance exists about the pathogenesis of hypertension in diabetes. It will become apparent that, at least in certain respects, the endocrine abnormalities in the latter are not identical with those of essential hypertension. However, while no marker for essential hypertension is available, coincidental occurrence of these two common conditions cannot be excluded in the individual patient. Some postulated mechanisms are listed in *Table 12.2*.

Table 12.2 Some postulated mechanisms for hypertension in diabetes mellitus

Theory	Explanation
Increased total sodium	clear evidence of increased exchangeable sodium in diabetic subjects; perhaps leading to hypertension only in susceptible subjects
Renal lesion (type 1 diabetes)	unknown mechanism, but closely linked temporally to development of proteinuira
Renin–angiotensin system	elevated or inappropriate renin/angiotensin II concentrations increased pressor sensitivity to angiotensin II
Aldosterone	? mild inappropriate hyperaldosteronism
Catecholamine sensitivity	increased pressor sensitivity to noradrenaline ? inappropriate noradrenaline concentrations for blood pressure
Growth hormone	possibly via direct effect on sodium retention
Endogenous opiates (type 2 diabetes)	involvement in altered glucose homeostasis, dietary intake and blood pressure regulation
Primary neurogenic origin	
Physical factors	decreased compliance of diabetic vessels from microvascular disease or atheroma raised blood viscosity

The relationship between renal dysfunction and hypertension is much less clear in Type 2 diabetes than in Type 1 disease. In an investigation of 510 patients with type 2 diabetes Fabre *et al.* (1982) found only a weak correlation between protein excretion and hypertension, even though over 40% of his subjects had diastolic pressures greater than 110 mmHg. Among these 510 patients there was only one death from renal failure and few patients showed progressive changes in glomerular filtration rate.

Table 12.3 Exchangeable sodium in diabetic subjects

Author	Number and description of subjects		Exchangeable sodium (%) (control subjects = 100)
de Châtel et al. (1977)	60; Types I and II;	age 25–39 years	109.0 ± 7.4*
		age 40–59 years	106.9 ± 9.1*
		age 60–70 years	111.5 ± 12.2**
Weidmann et al. (1979)	17; Types I and II;	hypertensive	109 ± 9**
	-	no treatment	100 ± 11
	-	chlorthalidone	
Beretta-Piccoli et al. (1979)	100; Types I and II;	normal blood pressure (DBP < 90 mmHg)	110.6 ± 11.9**
		140/90 < blood pressure < 160/95 mmHg	103.8 ± 10.5
		blood pressure > 160/105 mmHg	114.6 ± 11.3**
O'Hare et al. (1982a)	12; Types I and II;	poor control	102.6 ± 4.2
		improved control	106.0 ± 4.5**
O'Hare et al. (1982b)	66; Types I and II;	uncomplicated	107 ± 2**
		nephropathic, hypertensive	119 ± 5***
		hypertensive, no nephropathy	105 ± 3
Beretta-Piccoli and Weidmann (1982a)	126; Types I and II;	all	110 ± 10***
		normal blood pressure	108 ± 12***
		hypertensive	111 ± 9***

Results are mean + SD *P < 0.05; **P < 0.01; ***P < 0.001 versus normal subjects

Exchangeable sodium

Virtually all studies are agreed that exchangeable sodium is increased in diabetic patients when compared with normal subjects; this applies to normotensive as well as hypertensive diabetics and throughout all age groups (*Table 12.3*). Most of these studies have been performed with mixed groups of Type 1 and Type 2 diabetes (Beretta-Piccoli *et al.*, 1979; Beretta-Piccoli and Weidmann, 1982a; de Châtel *et al.*, 1977; Weidmann *et al.*, 1979), but the excess of sodium is usually of the order of 10%, though there are some difficulties in standardization of exchangeable sodium measurements. As can be seen from *Table 12.3*, the abnormality is more obvious with improved rather than poor control.

O'Hare *et al.* (1982b) have recently shown a positive correlation between exchangeable sodium (mean 119% of control values, $P < 0.002$) and mean arterial pressure in 21 patients with diabetic nephropathy, thus presumably mainly of type 1 disease. There was also a less significant correlation in patients without complications of hypertension. Beretta-Piccoli and Weidmann (1982a) have also shown a similar relationship among 126 diabetic patients with the correlation between systolic blood pressure and exchangeable sodium being closest in patients with high blood pressure (> 90 mmHg diastolic).

With the exception of the report from Cork, the majority of patients in these studies have had type 2 diabetes. This was also so in the report by Weidmann *et al.* (1979), who studied 17 patients with borderline hypertension ($>140/90$ mmHg). Mean supine blood pressure was 165/93 mmHg and associated with an exchangeable sodium of 109% of that shown by 90 normal subjects (defined as 100%); treatment with chlorthalidone for 6 weeks reduced blood pressure to 145/82 mmHg while reducing exchangeable sodium to exactly control values.

While there is an undoubted excess of exchangeable sodium in diabetes, its distribution is less certain. There are differing results on blood volume in diabetes (O'Hare *et al.*, 1982a; Weidmann *et al.*, 1979).

Sodium metabolism and insulin

An area worthy of further study is the effect of insulin on renal sodium metabolism, reviewed by DeFronzo (1981). Miller and Bogdonoff (1954) showed a reduction in urinary excretion of sodium when healthy subjects with a solute or a water diuresis were given insulin. In several series of experiments in the dog, using glucose and insulin clamp techniques DeFronzo and colleagues have shown that hyperinsulinaemia and not hyperglycaemia is responsible for the retention of sodium (*Figure 12.3*); later studies suggest that this effect occurs in a distal part of the nephron (DeFronzo *et al.*, 1975; DeFronzo, Goldberg and Agus, 1976). Further studies using somatostatin to suppress insulin release in normal subjects have suggested that insulin concentrations within the normal range may influence sodium balance (DeFronzo *et al.*, 1978).

This work is of potential importance for both type 1 and type 2 diabetes. In the former it is conceivable that excessive exogenous insulin, administered peripherally

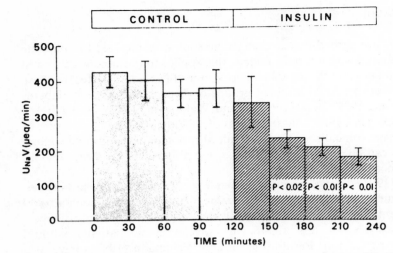

Figure 12.3 The time-course of decrease in sodium excretion ($U_{Na}V$) in men following insulin infusion while maintaining euglycaemia. Data represent mean values + SEM of six subjects. (From DeFronzo *et al.*, 1975; courtesy of the Publishers, *Journal of Clinical Investigation*)

rather than into the portal circulation, could be responsible for sodium retention. The fact that all diabetic subjects, whether hypertensive or not, appear to have increased exchangeable sodium together with the absence of any correlation between insulin dose and blood pressure would suggest that other factors must also be involved. However the recent reports by O'Hare *et al.* (1982b) and Beretta-Piccoli and Weidmann (1982) showing the direct correlation between mean blood pressure and exchangeable sodium is of particular interest; the close relationship between hypertension and diabetic renal disease does suggest involvement of a renal mechanism in the pathogenesis of the raised blood pressure, perhaps early involvement of sodium handling mechanisms. Detailed investigation of the relationships between blood pressure, exchangeable sodium and renal sodium handling in Type 1 diabetic patients is clearly indicated.

The relationship between insulin and sodium retention may be of even greater relevance in Type 2 diabetes associated with obesity. Obesity *per se* is a state of insulin resistance and is characterized by increased fasting insulin levels with excessive responses to glucose stimulation (DeFronzo *et al.*, 1978). The majority of patients with Type 2 diabetes, especially the obese, show insulin levels which correlate more closely with adiposity than with basal glucose. There is an absence of first-phase insulin release after intravenous glucose administration.

Dietary sodium

The relationship of dietary sodium to blood pressure among diabetic subjects has not been studied. In the non-diabetic with essential hypertension there remains conflicting evidence of the efficacy of mild sodium restriction (approximately 80 mmol/day) in reducing arterial pressure (MacGregor *et al.*, 1982; Watt *et al.*, 1983).

Calorie restriction, sodium and blood pressure

A detailed review of the effects of obesity on blood pressure and endocrine factors will be found in Chapter 13. Much hinges upon the secondary changes of sodium in calorie restriction, the natriuresis of fasting. There is conflicting evidence as to whether caloric restriction but maintenance of sodium balance will result in a fall in blood pressure (Dahl, Silver and Christie, 1958; Reisin *et al.*, 1978). A more recent study suggested that calorie restriction produced the same fall in blood pressure whether the patients were receiving a 40 mmol/day or 120 mmol/day sodium intake (Tuck *et al.*, 1981); this does not however exclude a negative sodium balance during the study. As well as effects of calorie restriction on weight and sodium balance, there are profound effects on other endocrine and vasoactive factors.

Endocrine responses to weight loss

In normal non-diabetic subjects there is evidence of significant falls in urinary catecholamines within days of the introduction of a low energy diet, even when sodium balance is positive (Jung *et al.*, 1979); this is accompanied by an acute hypotensive response. Tuck and colleagues (1981) demonstrated significant falls in plasma renin activity, plasma aldosterone, mean blood pressure and body weight in obese patients on a reducing diet with either medium (120 mmol) or low (40 mmol) sodium intake; among the subjects were three patients with Type 2 diabetes. The changes in renin and aldosterone took some weeks to appear while falls in mean arterial pressure correlated with weight loss throughout the study. It thus appears that blood pressure falls with calorie restriction, at least in non-diabetic subjects; weight loss is accompanied by reduction in urinary catecholamines, plasma renin activity and plasma aldosterone. It is possible that the three changes are all interrelated.

A further possible factor is the reduction in fasting insulin concentration with weight loss (Stanik and Marcus, 1980).

Growth hormone

Serum growth hormone concentrations are increased in poorly controlled diabetic subjects (Zadik *et al.*, 1980). While the mechanism of hypertension in acromegaly is not well understood (Sowers and Tuck, 1981), there is clear evidence of increased exchangeable sodium with suppression of the renin–angiotensin aldosterone system. Growth hormone has been shown to promote sodium retention (Biglieri, Waltington and Forsham, 1961) and is, of course, a counter-regulatory hormone to insulin. Acromegaly is also associated with fasting hyperinsulinism, but it is difficult to see how this could be relevant to the pathogenesis of sodium retention in type 1 diabetes when endogenous insulin secretion is deficient; it could, however, be relevant to the situation in type 2 disease.

The renin–angiotensin–aldosterone system

Plasma renin activity

Reports of basal plasma renin activity (PRA) in uncomplicated diabetes are conflicting, high, normal or low values having been reported (Beretta-Piccoli, Weidmann and Keusch, 1981; Burden and Thurston, 1979; De Châtel *et al.*, 1977; Gossain *et al.*, 1975). In diabetic subjects with hypertension, the picture is even more confused.

Christlieb, Kaldany and D'Elia (1976) reported low plasma renin activity in diabetics with hypertension and nephropathy, but normal levels in those with hypertension but no nephropathy. Almost all were receiving insulin, but it is not clear if they were insulin-dependent. Control subjects were younger than the diabetics and weights were not given. Beretta-Piccoli *et al.* (1979), studying 100 diabetic patients (both Type 1 and Type 2) showed reduced plasma renin activity in diabetics with mild hypertension (mean 160/92) but 'normal plasma renin activity' in those with moderate hypertension (mean 192/109 mmHg); all diabetic groups were, however, 20 years older than the control groups, the plasma renin activity falling with age. In the study by Burden and Thurston (1979), plasma renin activity was higher in diabetic patients with hypertension than in normotensive or control subjects and similar to that of normotensive diabetic subjects.

Unfortunately, interpretation of many of these studies is complicated by the heterogeneity of the patients with respect to Type 1 or Type 2 diabetes, the presence or absence of significant complications, and inadequate age/weight matching. In one recent study exclusively of patients with type 1 diabetes, higher plasma renin activity and higher blood pressures were observed in 31 subjects with proliferative retinopathy than in 17 age-matched, sex-matched and weight-matched subjects free of all complications (Drury *et al.*, 1982); the raised plasma renin activity in the setting of higher blood pressures might be considered especially inappropriate, and suggests a failure of autoregulation of renin secretion. Compared with a control group, the diabetics with retinopathy showed no evidence of inverse relationships of renin activity with increasing blood pressure or with increasing sodium output (Drury *et al.*, 1984).

Inactive renin

Several workers have shown abnormalities of inactive renin secretion among diabetic patients, especially in those with nephropathy, but their significance in terms of blood pressure control is unknown (Bryer-Ash, Ammon and Luetscher, 1983).

Angiotensin II

The only report of direct angiotensin II measurements showed lower levels of angiotensin in hypertensive diabetics than in uncomplicated patients, though the former were 14 years older on average. Angiotensin II levels were not significantly different between other diabetic groups and control subjects (Ferriss *et al.*, 1982).

Aldosterone

In contrast to the renin–angiotensin system there are few studies of plasma or urinary aldosterone in patients with diabetes, and fewer still that relate to any possible role of aldosterone in the sodium retention and hypertension of diabetes.

Ferriss *et al.* (1982) showed similar plasma aldosterone levels in diabetic and normal subjects, confirming the observations of others (Beretta-Piccoli *et al.*, 1979; Christlieb *et al.*, 1978), but in conflict with the findings of Weidmann *et al.* (1979), who found lower plasma aldosterone levels in hypertensive diabetics than in healthy controls. It may, however, again be argued that even normal levels of aldosterone are inappropriate for a state of sodium retention. The recent description of reduced plasma aldosterone levels after improved control of non-ketotic diabetes suggest that this may be a significant mechanism for sodium retention (O'Hare *et al.*, 1982a; Quigley *et al.*, 1982) especially as plasma aldosterone levels were still above those of non-diabetic controls. Indirect support for an excess of mineralocorticoid activity comes from the description of reduced total body potassium in poorly controlled but non-ketoacidotic diabetics (Walsh *et al.*, 1974).

Vasopressor sensitivity to angiotensin II

Vascular sensitivity, as measured by the diastolic blood pressure response to infused angiotensin II, has been shown to be increased in both diabetic patients and animals. The human studies have again included groups of both type 1 and type 2 patients with retinopathy, hypertension and a heterogeneous group with and without complications (Beretta-Piccoli and Weidmann, 1981; Christlieb, 1976; Weidmann *et al.*, 1979). The pressor doses for a given increase in pressure in the diabetic subjects were only about 40% of those needed for non-diabetic controls. It is however unclear whether the abnormality relates to diabetes *per se* or to the presence of complications or hypertension.

We have recently infused six Type 1 diabetic patients free of all complications with angiotensin II and compared the pressor response with that seen in six age-matched, sex-matched and weight-matched normal controls; the diabetic patients showed significantly greater pressor responses both of diastolic and systolic pressure (*Figure 12.4*; Drury and Smith, unpublished observations). This would suggest that the increased sensitivity may relate more to the diabetic state than to the presence of complications.

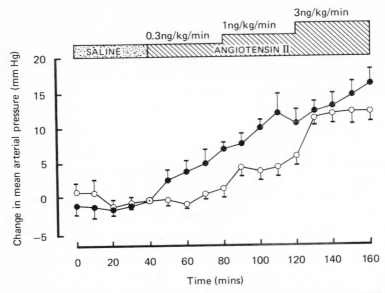

Figure 12.4 Changes in mean arterial pressure during angiotensin II infusion in six Type 1 diabetic subjects without complications (●) and six age-matched, sex-matched and weight-matched normal controls (○). Results are mean ± SEM; basal blood pressure defined as that at end of saline infusion.

The presence of increased vasopressor sensitivity to angiotensin II is especially interesting in view of the apparently normal basal levels; it provides a possible explanation of the increased blood pressure response to exercise (Mogensen, 1982b; Mogensen, Vittinghus and Solling, 1979). The increased sensitivity reported by Weidmann *et al.* (1979) was reversed to 'normal' after treatment with chlorthalidone, as would be expected, though even normal sensitivity might be considered surprising for this situation of increased basal renin activity and volume contraction.

In contrast Rhie *et al.* (1982) have shown vascular insensitivity, as measured by vasoconstriction, to angiotensin II and to noradrenaline in the retina of diabetic subjects. It may thus be that different vascular beds react differently to such stimuli.

Catecholamines

With the exception of autonomic neuropathy, there is a wealth of evidence that plasma catecholamines are close to normal levels in well-controlled diabetic patients (Beretta-Piccoli *et al.*, 1979; Christensen, 1979; Christlieb, 1976; de Châtel *et al.*, 1977). In one study of hypertensive diabetic patients (predominantly type 2) Beretta-Piccoli and colleagues (1979) reported 40% increased plasma levels of noradrenaline among those with mild hypertension but normal levels in the normotensive and moderately hypertensive. 'Normal', let alone increased, levels might again be considered inappropriate in the setting of raised blood pressure. There is also some evidence for an increased integrated concentration of both noradrenaline and adrenaline in patients with poorly controlled type 1 diabetes (Zadik *et al.*, 1980), but levels have not been demonstrated to fall with improved control.

Pressor sensitivity to noradrenaline

Several investigators have shown that the pressor sensitivity to noradrenaline is markedly increased in diabetic patients (*Figure 12.5*); this is not due to increased plasma clearance (Beretta-Piccoli and Weidmann, 1982b). Once again most of

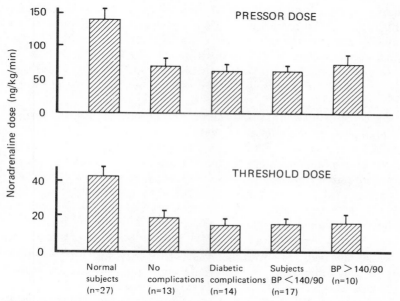

Figure 12.5 Threshold and pressor doses of noradrenaline in normal and diabetic subjects. Data shown as mean ± SEM. (Drawn from the data of Beretta-Piccoli and Weidmann, 1981)

these patients had complications of their diabetes and it remains to be established whether the increased sensitivity is a feature of diabetes alone or related to hypertension or complications (Beretta-Piccoli *et al.*, 1979; Beretta-Piccoli and Weidmann, 1981; Christlieb, 1976; Weidmann *et al.*, 1979). Whether the sensitivity falls with improved control of diabetes is unknown.

Sodium transport mechanisms, calcium and endothelial mechanisms

There have been no studies among diabetic patients of the several sodium transport abnormalities reported in essential hypertension, nor of any possible role of calcium. Endothelial mediation of blood pressure control similarly awaits elucidation.

Opiates

There has been considerable interest in a possible role of endogenous opiates in impaired glucose tolerance and also in blood pressure control. Most of these studies have used the opiate antagonist, naloxone, as a blocker of presumed endogenous opiate activity. Thus high-dose naloxone has been shown to increase both the acute insulin response to glucose and second phase release, as well as enhancing glucose disappearance rate in subjects with non-insulin dependent diabetes (Giugliano *et al.*, 1982); these effects were not seen in normal subjects. Observations that the intriguing phenomenon of chlorpropramide–alcohol flushing may be blocked by naloxone administration provides further evidence that endogenous opiates, or enkephalins, may play some part in this form of diabetes (Leslie, Pyke and Stubbs, 1979). There is also some evidence that high-dose naloxone reduced food intake in massively obese humans, though not in lean controls (Atkinson, 1982). It did not, however, appear that these latter changes were mediated by alterations in insulin secretion.

Naloxone has also been shown to inhibit the normal blood pressure fall during sleep (Rubin, Blaschke and Guilleminault, 1981) and to modulate baroreceptor function (Rubin, McLean and Reid, 1982). It is thus tempting to postulate that an abnormality in control of endogenous opiates might lead simultaneously to obesity, glucose intolerance and abnormal blood pressure regulation.

Intrarenal hormonal and haemodynamic factors

The kidney possesses a wealth of intrarenal vasoactive enzymes. Olshan *et al.* (1982) studied renal haemodynamics and the renin and kallikrein systems in ten type 2 diabetic patients who had subsequently developed hypertension. They found reduced urinary kallikrein activity and reduced erect renin activity compared with normotensive controls but similar to patients with essential hypertension. Aldosterone was however reduced in the diabetics compared with either control group. They postulated an intrarenal abnormality of renal haemodynamics possibly involving kallikrein.

Physical factors

Arterial stiffness and decreased distensibility of the vascular bed in diabetic subjects have been described in diabetic subjects (Faris *et al.*, 1982; McMillan, 1981). The arterial stiffness might be particularly important in relation to the late development of systolic hypertension in diabetic subjects; it would appear likely that atherosclerosis and related vascular damage late in the course of the disease may be largely responsible for the apparent excess of systolic hypertension (Janka, Standl and Meinhert, 1980). In the latter study 623 unselected diabetic outpatients were screened for peripheral vascular disease; multivariate analysis revealed a highly significant association with systolic hypertension. However, it is not clear whether this is cause or effect.

Autoregulation of blood flow in skeletal muscle and subcutaneous tissue has also been shown to be impaired in type 1 diabetic patients with microangiopathy (Faris *et al.*, 1983). Such impairment may clearly affect blood pressure regulatory mechanisms.

CONTROL OF DIABETES

Until the past few years and the work of Ferriss and colleagues, the possible influence of glycaemic control upon blood pressure and relevant hormonal factors has received little attention. O'Hare *et al.* (1982a), investigating nine Type 2 and three Type 1 diabetic subjets, showed small but significant falls in both systolic and diastolic pressures after 3 weeks of improved diabetic control (*Table 12.4*).

Table 12.4 Changes in blood pressure and body fluids with improved diabetic control. (From O'Hare *et al.*, 1982a, courtesy of the Editor and Publishers, *Clinical Science*)

Variable	Diabetic patients (n = 12)			Normal subjects (n = 33)
	Poor control	*Improved control*	*P<*	
Fasting glucose (mmol/l)	13.9 ± 1.1	7.2 ± 0.7	0.001	–
Mean glucose (mmol/l)	16.5 ± 0.9	8.0 ± 0.5	0.001	–
HbA$_1$	12.4 ± 0.5	9.3 ± 0.3	0.001	–
Blood pressure (mmHg)				
systolic	124.8 ± 5.4	121.8 ± 4.7	0.02	120.3 ± 1.7
diastolic	76.2 ± 2.3	71.8 ± 2.3	0.05	72.4 ± 1.4
Plasma angiotensin II (pmol/l)	36.3 ± 9.0	15.7 ± 3.2	0.02	14.9 ± 5.0
Plasma aldosterone (pmol/l)	812 ± 57	525 ± 72	0.02	422 ± 30
Exchangeable sodium (% predicted)	102.6 ± 1.2	106.0 ± 1.3	0.01	100 ± 1.8
Plasma volume (1/1.73 m^2)	2.86 ± 0.12	3.10 ± 0.15	0.05	2.89 ± 0.14
Body weight (kg)	70.5 ± 3.1	71.0 ± 3.1	n.s.	69.4 ± 2.6

Results are mean + SEM. *P* values are for differences between diabetics with poor and improved control. n.s. = not significant

Pressures fell from 124.8/76.2 mmHg to 121.8/71.8 mmHg with a fall in mean glucose from 16.5 mmol/l to 8.0 mmol/l. Simultaneously there were significant falls in plasma angiotensin II (from 36.4 pmol/l to 15.7 pmol/l) and in supine plasma aldosterone (from 812 pmol/l to 525 pmol/l). Total exchangeable sodium rose significantly as did plasma volume. As the patients were on unrestricted sodium intake, this study cannot exclude influences on blood pressure other than those produced by changes in diabetic control. They do, however, extend and confirm previous evidence from the same group of significant falls in plasma angiotensin II and aldosterone following improved control in a larger group of patients (Quigley *et al.*, 1982; Sullivan *et al.*, 1980). It is noteworthy in these studies that values of angiotensin II and aldosterone are high in the uncontrolled diabetic subjects and fall to near-normal rather than subnormal levels with improved control, even though plasma volume and exchangeable sodium are then frankly elevated. This again suggests that the levels of angiotensin II and aldosterone are inappropriate to the sodium/volume situation.

Many of the previous studies on blood pressure in diabetic subjects have failed to provide data on the glycaemic control of the patients. This factor might therefore explain some of the conflicting epidemiological data, especially where blood pressure has been found to be higher in newly diagnosed (markedly hyperglycaemic) patients but not so in established (well or moderately controlled) diabetics. Though the magnitude of the fall in blood pressure might be small for the individual patient (3.0/4.4 mmHg in the study quoted) such a drop could have a significant bearing on overall morbidity in a population, perhaps comparable to that postulated by some for moderate sodium restriction in the population with essential hypertension (MacGregor *et al.*, 1982)!

HYPERTENSION AND DIABETIC COMPLICATIONS

Full discussion of the possible role of hypertension in the pathogenesis of diabetic complications is beyond the scope of this chapter and may be found elsewhere (Drury, 1983; Jarrett, Keen and Chakrabarti, 1982; Mogensen, 1982b).

Diabetic nephropathy

As detailed above, it appears that hypertension arises at approximately the same time as development of persistent proteinuria (Parving *et al.*, 1983a). Present evidence suggests that higher blood pressure is not a risk factor for the development of nephropathy, though once established, blood pressure shows a clear rise with time (Christiansen *et al.*, 1981). A single study has suggested that the rate of progression of established renal failure was proportional to blood pressure (Mogensen, 1976, 1982a), but several other workers have been unable to substantiate these observations prospectively. Substantive data on the blood pressure changes during the phase of 'micro-albuminuria' (albumin excretion rate of 15–300 μg/min, Viberti *et al.*, 1982) are not yet available, although at this stage there may be abnormal increases in systolic pressure with heavy exercise (Mogensen, 1982b); these have been proposed as a possible screening method for early renal/hypertensive disease.

Perhaps most important is the suggestion that effective antihypertensive therapy may reduce the rate of deterioration in renal function. Mogensen (1981, 1982a) has shown this effect in six patients whose otherwise inexorable rate of decline of glomerular filtration rate has been ameliorated, albeit to a highly variable extent. The statistical analysis of this data (*Figure 12.6*) is open to some question, being based on relatively few observations before the initiation of treatment and with no placebo-treated group; further studies are urgently required to confirm the observation. Despite the use of triple therapy (beta-blocker, diuretic and vasodilator) blood pressure control was less than optimal (mean pressures on treatment 144/95 mmHg). In view of the mixed therapy used it is not possible to speculate whether the improvement relates to blood pressure control *per se* or to a more specific mechanism of particular drugs.

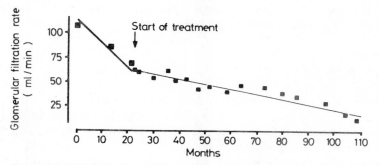

Figure 12.6 Course of glomerular filtration rate before and after start of antihypertensive medication in one patient. Regression lines are shown from before (———) and after (————) treatment. (From Mogensen, 1982, courtesy of the Publishers, *British Medical Journal*)

At an earlier stage of nephropathy Parving *et al.* (1983b) have produced evidence that antihypertensive treatment started during the phase of persistent proteinuria will slow the rate of deterioration of renal function. The study was again not placebo-controlled and the degree of benefit varied greatly between patients, but it does appear likely that such treatment may modify the rate of decline in renal function. If confirmed, these two studies are of immense importance in the prevention (or at least delay) of end-stage renal failure.

Present evidence does not suggest that even excellent control of diabetes will decrease the rate of deterioration in renal function once clinical nephropathy is established (Viberti *et al.*, 1983), though this may be possible at an earlier stage (Holman *et al.*, 1983).

Diabetic retinopathy

The association of diabetic retinopathy with hypertension has long been known. In the best study yet performed Knowler, Bennett and Ballintine (1980) investigated Pima Indians who have a high incidence of type 2 diabetes. When all known risk factors for the development of retinopathy were taken into account there was a two-fold excess of exudates developing over a period of 6 years in those with systolic pressures greater than 145 mmHg compared with those less than 125 mmHg. The association was not present for haemorrhages and the report has since been criticized on several grounds. There are a number of reports from cross-sectional studies of excess hypertension among patients with type 1 diabetes and retinopathy (Bodansky *et al.*, 1982; Dornan, Mann and Turner, 1982) but it is far from clear that hypertension *per se* is a risk factor for the development of retinopathy (*see* Dornan, Mann and Turner, 1982), especially as there is a marked association between retinopathy and nephropathy. It is therefore possible that any excess of hypertension represents subclinical renal disease among these patients rather than being an independent risk factor. Studies to investigate this relationship and to demonstrate whether antihypertensive treatment may inhibit the development or worsening of retinopathy are needed.

Macrovascular disease

While diabetic nephropathy is the cause of premature death of 20–35% of patients with Type 1 diabetes, the major killer later in life in Type 1 diabetes and in all patients with Type 2 diabetes is macrovascular disease (Jarrett, Keen and Chakrabati, 1982). There is a greatly increased incidence of coronary artery disease, cerebrovascular disease and peripheral vascular disease in these patients, whether hypertensive or not, and the relative risk and contribution of hypertension to the mortality and morbidity in diabetes remains controversial (Dawber, 1980; Kannel and McGee, 1979).

ISSUES OF TREATMENT IN HYPERTENSION ASSOCIATED WITH DIABETES

General measures such as reduction of excessive sodium intake (perhaps if greater than 150 mmol/day) are generally advised, though evidence to support such advice is based on non-diabetic subjects. While the efficacy of mild reduction of dietary sodium intake (to about 80 mmol/day) is still disputed in the treatment of essential hypertension (MacGregor *et al.*, 1982; Watt *et al.*, 1983), it cannot be confidently advocated in diabetes; again data are not available. The value of weight loss in Type 2 diabetes is better established; studies of the effect of calorie restriction on blood pressure have included some diabetic subjects (Heyden, 1978; Tuck *et al.*, 1981); sufficient weight loss (if achieved!) may avoid the need for any drug therapy in many patients and reduce the need in many others. There is a conspicuous lack of controlled data on the relative hypotensive efficacy of antihypertensive agents in diabetes mellitus, and still less about the long-term benefits of treatment. The evidence is reviewed by Passa (1980), Sowers and Tuck (1981) and Christlieb (1982). All the commonly used agents pose particular problems, practical and/or theoretical, when used in diabetic subjects (*Table 12.5*).

Table 12.5 Endocrine and other effects of commonly used antihypertensive drugs in patients with diabetes

Drug	Pros (in addition to reduction of blood pressure)	Cons
Diuretics	reduce excess exchangeable sodium reduce vascular sensitivity to angiotensin II and catecholamines	diabetogenic activity (type 2 diabetes) may precipitate hyperosmolar states deleterious effect on lipid profile
Beta-blockers	? reduce vascular sensitivity to catecholamines ? 'cardioprotective' action	may impair recovery from hypoglycaemia may impair awareness of hypoglycaemia ? deleterious effect on lipid profile
Vasodilators (hydralazine, prazosin)	? preservation of renal blood flow	orthostatic hypotension
Potassium-retaining diuretics		deaths and cases of severe hyperkalaemia reported, especially if renal function impaired
Methyldopa		orthostatic hypotension impotence deleterious effect on lipid profile

Drug therapy

Thiazide and loop diuretics

Given the increased exchangeable sodium observed in diabetic patients (*see above*), the use of thiazide or loop diuretics to reduce the excess appears obvious. Weidmann *et al.* (1979), using chlorthalidone for 6 weeks, showed a fall in mean blood pressure from 165/93 to 145/82 mmHg in a group of mild to moderately hypertensive diabetic subjects. At the same time, exchangeable sodium fell from 109% of that of control subjects to normal levels. Also reduced were the increased vasopressor response to angiotensin II and to noradrenaline. Equivalent data from a significant group of patients with Type 1 diabetes are not available.

These agents do, however, cause several problems. Thiazides have been shown to worsen glucose tolerance in normal subjects and those with Type 2 diabetes (Bengston, 1979) and have also been implicated in the precipitation of ketoacidosis and hyperosmolar coma (Alberti and Hockaday, 1973), although this may possibly be prevented if no potassium depletion is allowed (Helderman *et al.*, 1983). They may also worsen lipid profiles. Recent data (Medical Research Council Working Party, 1981) suggest that they are associated with more side-effects than previously realized, including impotence.

Beta-blockers

The immediate case for the use of β-blockade in diabetic subjects is more tenuous, given that increased exchangeable sodium is likely to form some part of the mechanism of the hypertension. Actual evidence of their effect on blood pressure in patients with diabetes is highly variable (Barnett, Leslie and Watkins, 1980; Wright *et al.*, 1979), but they might have the additional advantage of the postulated reduction in sudden deaths and myocardial infarction in what is a high-risk group for these conditions.

Most attention has been focused on the effect of beta-blockers on diabetic control and the occurrence, awareness of, and recovery from hypoglycaemia. The problem has been reviewed by Waal-Manning (1979) and Passa (1980). In general, it appears that cardioselective (β₂) blockers do not significantly affect recovery from hypoglycaemia or, apart from reducing the tachycardia, affect symptoms. In a study of 50 insulin-treated diabetics taking β-blockers compared with 100 matched diabetic controls not taking them, the incidence of loss of consciousness from hypoglycaemia was the same and did not thus appear to be increased by β-blockers (Barnett, Leslie and Watkins, 1980). The recent availability of home blood glucose monitoring should prove an additional benefit where this problem is feared.

Where one agent, diuretic or β-blocker, proves insufficient to control blood pressure most physicians would use a combination of the two. No data are available on what proportion of diabetic subjects are satisfactorily controlled by this combination.

Vasodilators

The usual addition to β-blockers and diuretic therapy, when the two together are inadequate, is a 'vasodilator', hydralazine or prazosin. This is widespread practice but has the potential disadvantage in diabetic subjects of increasing the chance of orthostatic hypertension if there is sympathetic autonomic neuropathy. Both drugs may additionally cause impotence.

Potassium-retaining diuretics

There are a number of reports of death or severe hyperkalaemia occurring in diabetic patients on these agents, especially if initial renal function is impaired. It is not clear if these were cases with the postulated syndrome of 'hyporeninaemic hypoaldosteronism' and thus a particular tendency to hyperkalaemia, but it is obvious that these agents must be used with especial care, and perhaps at reduced dosage, in the diabetic; regular checks of plasma potassium are essential.

Other drugs

Methyldopa, in addition to its effect in causing orthostatic hypotension, also affects lipid profiles adversely and is associated with a relatively high incidence of impotence.

There is relatively little experience, and even less published information, on the controlled use of clonidine, labetolol, minoxidil or such recently introduced agents as captopril, indapamide and nifedipine. Informed advocacy of their use must await publication of adequate data showing their effect on diabetic control, blood pressure responses to orthostasis and sodium and potassium balance.

In any diabetic patient whose hypertension proves resistant to two or three first-line drugs, the possibility of a secondary cause of the hypertension warrants careful re-examination. While it is commonly stated that the hormonal causes of hypertension are rare and do not occur with any greater frequency in the diabetic population than in the normal, this was not found to be so in the only systematically investigated hospital series yet described (Freedman *et al.*, 1958).

The choice of therapy

It will be clear from the foregoing that there are far too few published studies on drug treatment to permit well-founded advice about the initial or subsequent choice of therapy, either in insulin-dependent or non-insulin-dependent diabetic subjects. Passa (1980) provides a full review.

PRACTICAL MANAGEMENT OF HYPERTENSION IN DIABETES

Many patients with Type 1 diabetes found to be hypertensive will have underlying renal disease, shown by reduced creatinine clearance or raised serum creatinine values. If these are absent, proteinuria will often be present in significant quantities. With the known relentless progression of diabetic nephropathy and the available evidence (Mogensen, 1981, 1982a) effective control of blood pressure should be achieved with whichever agents are chosen. Serial measurement of glomerular filtration rate or creatinine clearance will allow an estimate to be made of the benefit achieved; at present it would seem worthwhile to aim for pressures approximating to the 50th centile for control subjects of the appropriate age before concluding that no further benefit can be gained.

If evidence of nephropathy (including elevated microalbumin excretion) is lacking and there is no evidence of any other underlying cause, the hypertension should probably be treated along similar lines as a non-diabetic with essential hypertension; a family history of hypertension is often present in such subjects (Tarn and Drury, unpublished data).

With Type 2 diabetes, the situation is less clear. Although weight loss will produce considerable falls in blood pressure, and parallel improvements in glucose tolerance, this is infrequently achieved. Again, if evidence of renal disease is lacking, these patients should, in the absence of further information, be treated similarly to other overweight patients with essential hypertension.

A particular problem is that of systolic hypertension, often clinically associated with large vessel disease. Yet again information is sparse, but in the face of recent evidence that cerebrovascular and overall morbidity and mortality are more closely linked to systolic than diastolic pressure (Kannel *et al.*, 1981), my own personal (and unsubstantiated) policy is to treat systolic hypertension in the diabetic as in the non-diabetic, at least before old age. Others would differ (Christlieb, 1979).

Other measures

Improved diabetic control, by whatever means, is advised on the basis of a reduced likelihood of other diabetic complications (Tschobroutsky, 1978). An additional likely benefit from improved control is that of a small fall in blood pressure (O'Hare *et al.*, 1982a). Other risk factors for macrovascular disease such as smoking, which also may affect blood pressure, also require attention.

IS HYPERTENSION IN DIABETES AN ENDOCRINE CONDITION?

No clear answer can yet be given to this question. The majority of cases of hypertension in Type 1 diabetes are associated with underlying diabetic nephropathy, the detailed mechanism of which remains obscure. There are, however, profound indications of the involvement of several endocrine mechanisms in the condition: increased exchangeable sodium, inappropriate angiotensin II, catecholamine and aldosterone levels and increased vascular sensitivity to both these pressor agents. It appears that blood pressure may be influenced by changes in glycaemic control, poor control causing a small increase in pressure, and it is likely that at least part of this effect is mediated by endocrine changes.

Whether there is indeed an increased prevalance of hypertension in Type 2 diabetic subjects remains uncertain. Much of the apparent excess is related directly, or indirectly, to obesity. There are clear suggestions that the mediation of the hypertension of obesity, and its accompanying impairment of glucose tolerance, may have direct endocrine mechanisms (*see* also Chapter 13).

FUTURE DEVELOPMENTS

The importance of these relationships is considerable. They may provide insight into the underlying pathogenetic mechanisms of diabetic complications and might, in a number of cases, allow treatment to be directed at mediators of blood pressure control where the underlying condition remains unknown or as yet inaccessible to cure. Thus, if increased or inappropriate catecholamine or angiotensin II levels are relevant, use of β-blockers or converting enzyme inhibitors could be of especial value. As can be seen there is a pressing need for further information on many of these points; hopefully future studies will delineate the type of patients involved more carefully, and use control subjects appropriate for the variables such as obesity that have made interpretation of much previous work so difficult. If adequate treatment of hypertension is effective in preventing or delaying complications, in particular nephropathy, then the potential benefit to many diabetics is enormous.

Acknowledgements

I would like to thank my wife, Dr Susan Rudge, for invaluable assistance in the preparation of this chapter and Miss Fennella Moore and Mrs Celia Burrage for their excellent and patient secretarial help.

References

ALBERTI, K. G. M. M. and HOCKADAY, T. D. R. (1973) Thiazides and hypokalaemia in diabetic ketoacidosis. *Postgraduate Medical Journal*, **49**, 29–31

AMERICAN HEART ASSOCIATION COMMITTEE REPORT (1981) Recommendations for human blood pressure determination by sphygmomanometers. *Hypertension*, **3**, 510A–519A

ANDERSON, A. R., CHRISTIANSEN, J. S., ANDERSEN, J. K., KREINER, S. and DECKERT, T. (1983) Diabetic nephropathy in type 1 (insulin-dependent) diabetes: an epidemiological study. *Diabetologia*, **25**, 496–501

ATKINSON, R. L. (1982) Naloxone decreases food intake in obese humans. *Journal of Clinical Endocrinology and Metabolism*, **55**, 196–198

BARNETT, A. H., LESLIE, D. and WATKINS, P. J. (1980) Can insulin-treated diabetics be given beta-adrenergic blocking agents? *British Medical Journal*, **280**, 976–978

BARRETT-CONNOR, E., CRIGNI, M. H., KLAUBER, M. R. and HOLDBROOK, M. (1981) Diabetes and hypertension in a community of older adults. *American Journal of Epidemiology*, **113**, 276–284

BENGSTON, C. (1979) Impairment of glucose metabolism during treatment with antihypertensive drugs. *Acta Medica Scandinavica (Copenhagen) (Suppl.)*, **628**, 63–67

BERETTA-PICCOLI, C., WEIDMANN, P. and KEUSCH, G. (1981) Responsiveness of plasma renin and aldosterone in diabetes mellitus. *Kidney International*, **20**, 259–266

BERETTA-PICCOLI, C. and WEIDMANN, P. (1981) Exaggerated pressor responsiveness to norepinephrine in non-azotemic diabetes mellitus. *American Journal of Medicine*, **71**, 829–835

BERETTA-PICCOLI, C. and WEIDMANN, P. (1982a) Body sodium-blood volume state in nonazotemic diabetes mellitus. *Mineral Electrolyte Metabolism*, **7**, 36–47

BERETTA-PICCOLI, C. and WEIDMANN, P. (1982b) Total plasma clearance of infused norepinephrine in non-azotaemic diabetes mellitus. *Klinische Wochenschrift*, **60**, 555–560

BERETTA-PICCOLI, C., WEIDMANN, P., ZIEGLER, W., GLUCK, Z. and KEUSCH, G. (1979) Plasma catecholamines and renin in diabetes mellitus. *Klinische Wochenschrift*, **57**, 681–691

BIGLIERI, E. G., WALTINGTON, C. O. and FORSHAM, P. H. (1961) Sodium retention with human growth hormone and its subfractions. *Journal of Clinical Endocrinology and Metabolism*, **21**, 361–366

BODANSKY, H. J., CUDWORTH, A. G., DRURY, P. L. and KOHNER, E. M. (1982) Risk factors associated with severe proliferative retinopathy in type 1 (insulin-dependent) diabetics. *Diabetes Care*, **5**, 97–100

BRYER-ASH, M., AMMON, R. A., LUETSCHER, J. A. (1983) Increased inactive renin in diabetes mellitus without evidence of nephropathy. *Journal of Clinical Endocrinology and Metabolism*, **56**, 557–561

BURDEN, A. C. and THURSTON, H. (1979) Plasma renin activity in diabetes mellitus. *Clinical Science*, **56**, 255–259

CHRISTENSEN, N. J. (1979) Catecholamines and diabetes mellitus. *Diabetologia*, **16**, 211–224

CHRISTIANSEN, J. S., GAMMELGAARD, J., FRANDSEN, M. and PARVING, H. H. (1981) A prospective study of glomerular filtration rate and arterial blood pressure in insulin-dependent diabetics with diabetic nephropathy. *Diabetologia*, **20**, 457–461

CHRISTLIEB, A. R. (1976) Vascular reactivity to angiotensin II and to norepinephrine in diabetic subjects. *Diabetes*, **25**, 268–274

CHRISTLIEB, A. R. (1979) Should you treat systolic hypertension in the diabetic? *Geriatrics*, **34 (11)**, 53–59

CHRISTLIEB, A. R. (1980) Diabetes and hypertension. *Cardiovascular Reviews*, **1**, 609–616

CHRISTLIEB, A. R. (1982) The hypertensions of diabetes. *Diabetes Care*, **5**, 50–58

CHRISTLIEB, A. R., KALDANY, A. and D'ELIA, J. A. (1976) Plasma renin activity and hypertension in diabetes mellitus. *Diabetes*, **25**, 969–974

CHRISTLIEB, A. R., KALDANY, A., D'ELIA, J. A. and WILLIAMS, G. H. (1978) Aldosterone responsiveness in patients with diabetes mellitus. *Diabetes*, **27**, 732–737

CHRISTLIEB, A. R., WARRAM, J. H., KROLEWSKI, A. S. *et al.* (1981) Hypertension: the major risk factor in juvenile-onset insulin-dependent diabetics. *Diabetes*, **30**, (*Suppl. 2*), 90–96

CONN, J. W., KNOPF, R. F. and NESBIT, R. M. (1964) Clinical characteristics of primary aldosteronism from an analysis of 145 cases. *American Journal of Surgery*, **107**, 159–172

CRYER, P. E. (1981) Physiology and pathophysiology of the human sympatho-adrenal neuroendocrine system. *New England Journal of Medicine*, **303**, 436–444

DAHL, L. K., SILVER, L. and CHRISTIE, R. W. (1958) The role of salt in the fall of blood pressure accompanying reduction in obesity. *New England Journal of Medicine*, **258**, 1186–1192

DAWBER, T. R. (1980) Diabetes and cardiovascular disease. In: *The Framingham Study*, pp. 190–201, Cambridge, Mass.: Harvard University Press

DE CHÂTEL, R., WEIDMANN, P., FLAMMER, J. *et al.* (1977) Sodium, renin, aldosterone, catecholamines and blood pressure in diabetes mellitus. *Kidney International*, **12**, 412–421

DECKERT, T. and POULSEN, J. E. (1981) Diabetic nephropathy: fault or destiny? *Diabetologia*, **21**, 178–183

DECKERT, T., POULSEN, J. E. and LARSEN, M. (1978) Prognosis of diabetics with diabetes onset before the age of thirty-one. *Diabetologia*, **14**, 363–377

DeFRONZO, R. A. (1981) The effect of insulin on renal sodium metabolism. A review with clinical implications. *Diabetologia*, **21**, 165–171

DeFRONZO, R. A., COOKE, C. R., ANDRES, R., FALOONA, G. R. and DAVIS, P. J. (1975) The effect of insulin on renal handling of sodium, potassium, calcium and phosphate in man. *Journal of Clinical Investigation*, **55**, 845–855

DeFRONZO, R. A., GOLDBERG, M. and AGUS, Z. (1976) The effects of glucose and insulin on renal electrolyte transport. *Journal of Clinical Investigation*, **58**, 83–90

DeFRONZO, R. A., SHERWIN, R. S., DILLINGHAM, M., HENDLER, R., TAMBORLANE, W. T. and FELIG, P. (1978) Influence of basal insulin and glucagon secretion on potassium and sodium metabolism. *Journal of Clinical Investigation*, **61**, 472–479

DORNAN, T. L., MANN, J. I. and TURNER, R. C. (1982) Factors protective against retinopathy in insulin-dependent diabetics free of retinopathy for 30 years. *British Medical Journal*, **285**, 1073–1077

DRATMAN, M. B. (1976) Thyroid function and high blood pressure. *Cardiovascular Medicine*, **1**, 319–331

DRURY, P. L. (1983) Diabetes and arterial hypertension. *Diabetologia*, **24**, 1–9

DRURY, P. L., BODANSKY, H. J., ODDIE, C. J., CUDWORTH, A. G. and EDWARDS, C. R. W. (1982) Increased plasma renin activity in Type 1 diabetes with microvascular disease. *Clinical Endocrinology*, **16**, 453–461

DRURY, P. L., BODANSKY, H. J., ODDIE, C. J. and EDWARDS, C. R. W. (1984) Factors in the regulation of plasma renin activity and concentration in Type 1 diabetes. *Clinical Endocrinology*, **20**, 607–618

FABRE, J., BALANT, L. P., DAYER, P. G., FOX, H. M. and VERNET, A. T. (1982) The kidney in maturity onset diabetes mellitus: a clinical study of 510 patients. *Kidney International*, **21**, 730–738

FARIS, I., AGERSKOV, K., HENRIKSEN, O., LASSEN, N. A. and PARVING, H. H. (1982) Decreased distensibility of a passive vascular bed in diabetes mellitus: an indicator of microangiopathy. *Diabetologia*, **23**, 411–414

FARIS, I., VAGN NIELSEN, H., HENRIKSEN, O., PARVING, H. H. and LASSEN, N. A. (1983) Impaired autoregulation of blood flow in skeletal muscle and subcutaneous tissue in long-term type 1 diabetic patients with microangiopathy. *Diabetologia*, **25**, 486–488

FERRISS, J. B., SULLIVAN, P. A., GONGGRIJP, H., COLE, M. and O'SULLIVAN, D. J. (1982) Plasma angiotensin II and aldosterone in unselected diabetic patients. *Clinical Endocrinology*, **17**, 261–269

FREEDMAN, P., MOULTON, R., ROSENHEIM, M. L., SPENCER, A. G. and WILLOUGHBY, D. A. (1958) Phaeochromocytoma, diabetes and glycosuria. *Quarterly Journal of Medicine*, **27**, 301–321

GIUGLIANO, D., CERIELLO, A., DI PINTO, P., SACCOMANNO, F., GENTILE, S. and CAPPIAPUOTI, F. (1982) Impaired insulin secretion in human diabetes mellitus. The effect of naloxone-induced opiate receptor blockade. *Diabetes*, **31**, 367–370

GOSSAIN, V. V., WERLE, E. E., SHOLITON, L. J., SRIVASTAVA, L. and KNOWLES, H. C. (1975) Plasma renin activity in juvenile diabetes mellitus and effect of diazoxide. *Diabetes*, **24**, 833–835

HELDERMAN, J. H., ELAHI, D., ANDERSEN, D. K. *et al.* (1983) Prevention of the glucose intolerance of thiazide diuretics by maintenance of body potassium. *Diabetes*, **32**, 106–111

HEYDEN, S. (1978) The workingman's diet II: effect of weight reduction in obese patients with hypertension, diabetes, hyperuricaemia and hyperlipidaemia. *Nutrition and Metabolism*, **22**, 141–159

HOLMAN, R. R., DORNAN, T. L., MAYON-WHITE, V. *et al*. (1983) Prevention of deterioration of renal and sensory-nerve function by more intensive management of insulin-dependent diabetic patients. *Lancet*, **1**, 208–210

HOSTETTER, T. H., RENNKE, H. G. and BRENNER, B. M. (1982) The case for intrarenal hypertension in the initiation of diabetic and other glomerulopathies. *American Journal of Medicine*, **72**, 375–380

IRELAND, J. T., VIBERTI, G. C. and WATKINS, P. J. (1982) The kidney and renal tract. In: *Complications of Diabetes* (2nd Edition), edited by H. Keen and J. Jarrett, pp. 166–172. London: Edward Arnold

ISLES, C. G. and JOHNSON, J. K. (1983) Phaeochromocytoma and diabetes mellitus: further evidence that alpha-2-receptors inhibit insulin release in man. *Clinical Endocrinology*, **18**, 37–41

JANKA, H. U., STANDL, E. and MEINHERT, H. (1980) Peripheral vascular disease in diabetes mellitus and its relation to cardiovascular risk factors: screening with the Doppler ultrasonic technique. *Diabetes Care*, **3**, 207–213

JARRETT, R. J., KEEN, H., McCARTNEY, M. *et al*. (1978) Glucose tolerance and blood pressure in two population samples, their relation to diabetes mellitus and hypertension. *International Journal of Epidemiology*, **7**, 15–24

JARRETT, R. J., KEEN, H. and CHAKRABARTI, R. (1982) Diabetes, hyperglycaemia and arterial disease. In: *Complications of Diabetes*, (2nd Edition), edited by H. Keen and J. Jarrett, pp. 187–190. London: Edward Arnold

JUNG, R. T., SHETTY, P. S., BARRAND, M., CALLINGHAM, B. A. and JAMES, W. P. T. (1979) Role of catecholamines in hypotensive response to dieting. *British Medical Journal*, **1**, 12–13

KANNEL, W. B. and McGEE, D. L. (1979) Diabetes and cardiovascular risk factors: the Framingham study. *Circulation*, **59**, 8–13

KANNEL, W. B., WOLF, P. A., McGEE, D. L., DAWBER, T. R., McNAMARA, P. and CASTELLI, W. P. (1981) Systolic blood pressure, arterial rigidity, and risk of stroke. The Framingham study. *Journal of the American Medical Association*, **245**, 1225–1229

KEEN, H., TRACK, N. S. and SOWRY, G. C. (1975) Arterial pressure in clinically apparent diabetics. *Diabète et Metabolisme*, **1**, 159–164

KNOWLER, W. C., BENNETT, P. H. and BALLINTINE, E. J. (1980) Increased incidence of retinopathy in diabetics with elevated blood pressure. *New England Journal of Medicine*, **302**, 645–650

KRAKOFF, L. R. and ELIJOVICH, F. (1981) Cushing's syndrome and exogenous glucocorticoid hypertension. *Clinics in Endocrinology and Metabolism*, **10**, 479–488

LESLIE, R. D. G., PYKE, D. and STUBBS, W. A. (1979) Sensitivity to enkephalin as a cause of non-insulin dependent diabetes. *Lancet*, **1**, 341–343

MacGREGOR, G. A., MARKANDU, N., BEST, F. *et al*. (1982) Double-blind randomised crossover trial of moderate sodium restriction in essential hypertension. *Lancet*, **1**, 351–354

MAXWELL, M. H., WAKS, A. V., SCHROTH, P. C., KARAM, M. and DORNFELD, L. P. (1982) Error in blood pressure measurement due to incorrect cuff size in obese patients. *Lancet*, **2**, 33–35

McMILLAN, D. E. (1981) Physical factors important in the development of atherosclerosis in diabetes. *Diabetes*, **30**, *(Suppl. 2)*, 97–104

MEDICAL RESEARCH COUNCIL WORKING PARTY (1981) Adverse reactions to bendrofluazide and propranolol for the treatment of mild hypertension. *Lancet*, **2**, 539–543

MILLER, J. H. and BOGDONOFF, F. (1954) Antidiuresis associated with administration of insulin. *Journal of Applied Physiology*, **6**, 509–512

MOGENSEN, C. E. (1976) Renal function changes in diabetes. *Diabetes*, **25**, 872–879

MOGENSEN, C. E. (1981) Long-term anti-hypertensive treatment inhibiting the progression of diabetic nephropathy. *Acta Endocrinologica (Copenhagen)* *(Suppl.)*, **242**, 31–32

MOGENSEN, C. E. (1982a) Long-term antihypertensive treatment inhibiting the progression of diabetic nephropathy. *British Medical Journal*, **285**, 685–688

MOGENSEN, C. E. (1982b) Hypertension in diabetes and the stages of diabetic nephropathy. *Diabetic Nephropathy*, **1**, 2–7

MOGENSEN, C. E., VITTINGHUS, E. and SOLLING, K. (1979) Abnormal albumin excretion after two provocative renal tests in diabetes: physical exercise and lysine injection. *Kidney International*, **16**, 385–393

MOSS, A. J. (1962) Blood pressure in children with diabetes mellitus. *Pediatrics*, **30**, 932–936

MUNICHOODAPPA, C., D'ELIA, J. A., LIBERTINO, J. A., GLEASON, R. E. and CHRISTLIEB, A. R. (1979) Renal artery stenosis in hypertensive diabetics. *Journal of Urology*, **121**, 555–558

NATIONAL DIABETES DATA GROUP (1979) Classification and diagnosis of diabetes mellitus and other categories of glucose intolerance. *Diabetes*, **28**, 1039–1057

O'HARE, J. A., FERRISS, J. B., TWOMEY, B. M., GONGGRIJP, H. and O'SULLIVAN, D. J. (1982a) Changes in blood pressure, body fluids, circulating angiotensin II and aldosterone, with improved diabetic control. *Clinical Science*, **63**, 415s–418s

O'HARE, J. A., BRADY, D., FERRISS, J. B., TWOMEY, B. M. and O'SULLIVAN, D. J. (1982b) Total exchangeable sodium and blood pressure in diabetes. *Diabetologia*, **23**, 472 (Abstract)

OLSHAN, A. R., O'CONNOR, D. T., COHEN, I. M. and STONE, R. A. (1982) Hypertension in adult-onset diabetes mellitus; abnormal renal hemodynamics and endogenous vasoregulatory factors. *American Journal of Kidney Diseases*, **2**, 271–280

PARVING, H. H., ANDERSEN, A. R., SMIDT, V. M., OXENBOLL, B., EDSBERG, B. and SANDAHL CHRISTIANSEN, J. (1983a) Diabetic nephropathy and arterial hypertension. *Diabetologia*, **24**, 10–12

PARVING, H. H., ANDERSEN, A. R., SMIDT, V. and SVENDSEN, P. A. (1983b) Early aggressive antihypertensive treatment reduces rate of decline in kidney function in diabetic nephropathy. *Lancet*, **1**, 1175–1179

PASSA, P. (1980) Le traitement de l'hypertension artérielle chez les diabétiques. *Diabète et Metabolisme*, **6**, 287–298

PELL, S. and D'ALONZO, C. A. (1967) Some aspects of hypertension in diabetes mellitus. *Journal of the American Medical Association*, **202**, 104–110

QUIGLEY, C., SULLIVAN, P. A., GONGGRIJP, H., CROWLEY, M. J., FERRISS, J. B. and SULLIVAN, D. J. (1982) Hyperaldosteronism in ketoacidosis and in poorly controlled non-ketotic diabetes. *Irish Journal of Medical Science*, **151**, 135–139

REISIN, E., ABEL, R., MODAN, M., SILVERBERG, D. S., ELIAHOU, H. E. and MODAN, B. (1978) Effect of weight loss without salt restriction on the reduction of blood pressure in overweight hypertensive patients. *New England Journal of Medicine*, **298**, 1–6

RHIE, F. H., CHRISTLIEB, A. R., SANDOR, T. *et al.* (1982) Retinal vascular reactivity to norepinephrine and angiotensin II in normals and diabetics. *Diabetes*, **31**, 1056–1060

RUBIN, P., BLASCHKE, T. F. and GUILLEMINAULT, C. (1981) Effect of naloxone, a specific opioid inhibitor, on blood pressure fall during sleep. *Circulation*, **63**, 117–121

RUBIN, P. C., McLEAN, K. and REID, J. L. (1982) Endogenous opiates modulate central nervous system blood pressure control in man. *Clinical Science*, **63**, 331s–333s

SCHALEKAMP, M. A. D. H., WENTING, G. J. and MAN IN 'T VELD, A. J. (1981) Pathogenesis of mineralocorticoid hypertension. *Clinics in Endocrinology and Metabolism*, **10**, 397–418

SHAPIRO, A. P., PEREZ-STABLE, E. and MONSOS, S. E. (1965) Co-existence of renal arterial hypertension and diabetes mellitus. *Journal of the American Medical Association*, **192**, 813–816

SOWERS, J. R. and TUCK, M. L. (1981) Hypertension associated with diabetes mellitus, hypercalcaemic disorders, acromegaly and thyroid disease. *Clinics in Endocrinology and Metabolism*, **10**, 631–650

STANIK, S. and MARCUS, R. (1980) Insulin secretion improves following dietary control of plasma glucose in hyperglycaemic obese patients. *Metabolism*, **29**, 346–350

SULLIVAN, P. A., GONGGRIJP, H., CROWLEY, M. J., FERRISS, J. B. and O'SULLIVAN, D. J. (1980) Plasma angiotensin II and the control of diabetes mellitus. *Clinical Endocrinology*, **13**, 387–392

TAYLOR, A. A. and BARTTER, F. C. (1977) Hypertension in licorice intoxication, acromegaly and Cushing's syndrome. In *Hypertension*, edited by J. Genest, E. Koiw, E. Kuchel and E. pp. 755–767. New York: McGraw-Hill

TSCHOBROUTSKY, G. (1978) Relation of diabetic control to development of microvascular complications. *Diabetologia*, **15**, 143–152

TUCK, M. L., SOWERS, J., DORNFELD, L., KLEDZIK, G. and MAXWELL, M. (1981) The effect of weight reduction on blood pressure, plasma renin activity and plasma aldosterone levels in obese patients. *New England Journal of Medicine*, **304**, 930–933

TUNBRIDGE, W. M. G. (1981) Factors contributing to deaths of diabetics under fifty years of age. *Lancet*, **2**, 569–572

VIBERTI, G. C., HILL, R. D., JARRETT, R. J., ARGYROPOULAS, A., MAHMUD, V. and KEEN, H. (1982) Microalbuminuria as a predictor of clinical nephropathy in insulin-dependent diabetes mellitus. *Lancet*, **1**, 1430–1432

VIBERTI, G. C., BILOUS, R. W., MACKINTOSH, D., BENDING, J. J. and KEEN, H. (1983) Long-term correction of hyperglycaemia and progression of renal failure in insulin-dependent diabetes. *British Medical Journal*, **286**, 598–601

WAAL-MANNING, H. J. (1979) Can β-blockers be used in diabetic patients? *Drugs*, **17**, 157–160

WALSH, C. H., SOLER, N. G., JAMES, H., FITZGERALD, M. G. and MALINS, J. M. (1974) Studies on whole-body potassium in non-ketoacidotic diabetics before and after treatment. *British Medical Journal*, **4**, 738–740

WASS, J. A. H., CUDWORTH, A. G., BOTTAZZO, G. F., WOODROW, J. C. and BESSER, G. M. (1980) An assessment of glucose intolerance in acromegaly and its response to medical treatment. *Clinical Endocrinology*, **12**, 53–59

WATT, G. C. M., EDWARDS, C., HART, J. F., HART, M., WALTON, P. and FOY, C. J. W. (1983) Dietary sodium restriction for mild hypertension in general practice. *British Medical Journal*, **286**, 432–436

WEIDMANN, P. (1980) Recent pathogenic aspects in essential hypertension and hypertension associated with diabetes mellitus. *Klinische Wochenschrift*, **58**, 1070–1089

WEIDMANN, P., BERETTA-PICCOLI, C., KEUSCH, G. (1979) Sodium-volume factor, cardiovascular reactivity and hypotensive mechanism of diuretic therapy in mild hypertension associated with diabetes mellitus. *American Journal of Medicine*, **67**, 779–784

WHITE, P. (1956) Natural course and prognosis of juvenile diabetes. *Diabetes*, **5**, 445–450

WORLD HEALTH ORGANIZATION (1979) Report of a WHO Expert Committee on Hypertension. *Who Technical Report Series*. Geneva: WHO

WORLD HEALTH ORGANIZATION (1980) Report of a WHO Expert Committee on Diabetes Mellitus. *Technical Report Series*, No 646, Geneva

WRIGHT, A. D., BARBER, S. G., KENDALL, M. J. and POOLE, P. H. (1979) Beta-adrenoceptor-blocking drugs and blood sugar control in diabetes mellitus. *British Medical Journal*, **1**, 159–161

YOUNG, J. B. and LANDSBERG, L. (1977) Catecholamines and the regulation of hormone secretion. *Clinics in Endocrinology and Metabolism*, **6**, 657–695

ZADIK, Z., KAYNE, R., KAPPY, M., PLOTNICK, L. P. and KOWARSKI, A. A. (1980) Increased integrated concentration of norepinephrine, epinephrine, aldosterone and growth hormone in patients with uncontrolled juvenile diabetes mellitus. *Diabetes*, **29**, 655–658

Addendum

Since completion of this chapter (January, 1984), several significant studies have been published.

Tarn, Lister and Drury (1984) reported very similar systolic and diastolic blood pressures in a large group of children, adolescents and young adults with Type 1 diabetes and in their age-matched non-diabetic siblings. The study was community-based and all pressures were recorded by a single observer using a random zero sphygmomanometer. This suggests that there is no systematic difference in blood pressure in the young diabetic population as a whole.

Three simultaneously published studies have shown that blood pressure is slightly, but significantly, elevated in Type 1 diabetic patients with microalbuminuria (albumin excretion rate $>15–30\,\mu g$/min but without persistent proteinuria)

when compared with their normo-albuminuric age-matched controls (Wiseman *et al.*, 1984; Mathiesen *et al.*, 1984; Mogensen and Christensen, 1984). Interestingly the arterial pressures in the microalbuminuric groups were similar in these three studies (136/87, 131/85 and 138/89 mmHg respectively), though the definition of microalbuminuria varied slightly. The latter study (Mogensen and Christensen, 1984) also confirmed the earlier report of Viberti *et al.* (1982) that microalbuminuria, in this instance >15 μg/min, does accurately predict those subjects who will develop clinical nephropathy. It thus appears that blood pressure is raised from an earlier stage of diabetic renal disease than has hitherto been recognized, though the pressures are clearly not 'hypertensive' by conventional criteria.

Finally a major symposium on hypertension associated with diabetes was held in June, 1984; the proceedings are shortly to be published (Weidmann and Mogensen, 1985).

References

MATHIESON, E. R., OXENBOLL, B., JOHANSEN, K., SVENDSEN P. Aa. and DECKERT, T. (1984) Incipient nephropathy in Type 1 (insulin-dependent) diabetes. *Diabetologia*, **26**, 406–410

MOGENSEN, C. E. and CHRISTENSEN, C. K. (1984) Predicting diabetic nephropathy in insulin-dependent patients. *New England Journal of Medicine*, **311**, 89–93

TARN, A. C., LISTER, J. and DRURY, P. L. (1984) Correlates of high blood pressure among children, adolescents and young adults with Type 1 (insulin-dependent) diabetes. *Diabetic Medicine*, **1**, (In press)

WEIDMANN, P. and MOGENSEN, C. E. (eds) (1985) Proceedings of the First International Symposium on Hypertension associated with Diabetes Mellitus. *Hypertension* (In press)

WISEMAN, M., VIBERTI, G., MACKINTOSH, D., JARRETT, R. J. and KEEN, H. (1984) Glycaemia, arterial pressure and micro-albuminuria in Type 1 (insulin-dependent) diabetes mellitus. *Diabetologia*, **26**, 401–405

13
Endocrine factors in obesity hypertension
Michael L. Tuck

INTRODUCTION

A relationship between obesity and elevated blood pressure has been noted for decades but beyond the observation of this association very few scientific advances were made in delineating the pathogenesis. In the last few years renewed interest in this subject has focused on a number of underlying metabolic and cardiovascular aberrations in obesity that could contribute to elevating blood pressure. One has to take special care in defining obesity hypertension because of the high incidence of essential hypertension in the population. The question of whether there is a unique form of 'obesity hypertension' or whether elevated blood pressure in obese subjects is merely coexisting essential hypertension is currently not resolved. As essential hypertension lacks any specific clinical marker, this differentiation is difficult. Based on a number of aberrations in sympathetic nervous system activity, sodium metabolism and cardiovascular hemodynamics in obesity, it is entirely possible that there is a 'hormonal' cause of hypertension in obesity. It is equally feasible that these metabolic changes could aggravate underlying essential hypertension. Care must also be taken in separating subjects with obesity, defined here as 25% above ideal body weight, from those subjects who are overweight but weigh less than this body weight criterion. Hypertension existing in these two categories of excess body weight may be quite different in its etiology and its response to weight reduction.

This chapter defines the many potential underlying metabolic abnormalities and changes in pressor hormone levels that occur in obesity. One or all of these hormonal changes could contribute to blood pressure elevation in these subjects. The temporal association with reductions in body weight, lowering of blood pressure and normalization of many of the hormonal disturbances offers strong support for a relationship between these events.

EPIDEMIOLOGY

Substantial clinical and epidemiological information supports a strong association between blood pressure levels and body size or fatness (Berchtold, Sims and Brandau, 1981; Berchtold et al., 1981; Chiang, Perlman and Epstein, 1969; Kannel *et al.*, 1967; Lew, 1973; Stamler *et al.*, 1978; Tyrolar, Heyden and Hames, 1975). These findings in obese adults have also been extended to children and adolescents (Ellison *et al.*, 1980). In the Bogalusa Heart study, height was an important determinant of blood pressure, but also within height groups body mass also was an important determinant (Voors *et al.*, 1977). A relationship between body weight and blood pressure is also seen in black children (Lynds, Seyler and Morgan, 1980) and in a mixed-school population of adolescents (McCue, Miller and Mauck, 1979). In obese children whether male or female there is approximately a 2 to 3-fold increase in the incidence of high blood pressure compared to age-matched non-obese children. These findings imply that hypertension in obesity may have its inception early in life. There is, however, in westernized, acculturated societies a generalized increase in body fat to lean body mass with advancing age. The well-established age-dependent increase in blood pressure was also correlated to the change in body fat, as documented in the National Health and Nutrition Examination Survey (NHANES) (Roberts and Maurer, 1976). Conversely, in primitive, unacculturated tribal societies an age-dependent increase in these parameters is not seen (Mann *et al.*, 1964; Page, 1976; Severs *et al.*, 1980). Thus, retrospective epidemiological data would support a strong relationship between body weight and hypertension. Prospectively, normotensive obese subjects have a greater chance of developing hypertension than lean normal subjects. In both the Framingham Study (Kannel and Gordon, 1979) and the Evans County Study (Tyrolar, Heyden and Hames, 1975) subjects who were overweight but normotensive at entry into the study had a higher probability of developing hypertension at some point in the study period compared to lean individuals. A follow-up examination of former college students revealed that excess body weight at that time predicted onset of hypertension later in life (Paffenberger, Thorne and Wing, 1968). This has been extended in a 20–32 year follow-up study of young college men showing that increased body weight over time increased blood pressure but the impact was more on systolic than diastolic pressure (Gillum *et al.*, 1982). There is also some relationship between the type of obesity and the probable development of hypertension. Body cell mass and fat cell number were unrelated to blood pressure level but fat cell size (hypertrophic obesity) was positively correlated (Berglund *et al.*, 1982). Obese men with relative abdominal obesity have greater fat cell size, more hyperinsulinemia and a higher incidence of hypertension compared to obese women, who more often have a greater distribution of fat in the lower segment around the hips and buttocks areas. Circumference measurements of the abdominal region can be important predictors of cardiovascular risk and complications including hypertension. This concept has been examined in an unselected essential hypertensive population where a significant segment of the study group had hyperinsulinemia and glucose intolerance (Berglund and Anderson, 1981). As many subjects in this group (although having increased abdominal girth) were considered to be in a near-normal weight range, the term 'metabolically obese' was given to these subjects (Ruderman, Schneider and Berchtold, 1981). Thus, distribution of body fat may have a very important bearing on recognition and prevention of high risk individuals, giving rise to the concept of hypertensive-prone obesity subtypes. These observations also bring up the consideration that hypertrophic obesity and essential hypertension may be related by common pathogenetic pathways. Again in the few prospective studies dealing with this issue, Tyrolar, Hayden and Hames (1975) in the Evans County Study noted that subjects who had high blood pressure at the outset gained significantly more weight during the 6-year study period than subjects who were normotensive at that time.

Although the cardiovascular risks of being overweight *per se* have been debated, it is clear that obesity either directly or indirectly confers a major risk for cardiovascular disease. The Framingham study showed that overweight subjects have a 4-fold increase in coronary artery disease as manifest by angina pectoris and sudden death and a 7-fold greater incidence of stroke compared to normal weight subjects (Kannel *et al.*, 1967). Hypertension in obese subjects appears to be the leading cause for these cardiovascular complications (Noppa *et al.*, 1980). Obese subjects with normal blood pressure may not be at greater risk for cardiovascular disease and stroke (Andres, 1980; Gunby, 1980; Patel, Eggen, Strong, 1980). Thus, obesity itself may not be an atherogenic factor, and as suggested by Gunby (1980): 'a little body fat may not hasten death'. However, evidence indicates that obesity itself independent of blood pressure increases cardiac work and is associated with a much higher incidence of congestive heart failure and its complications (Messerli, 1982). The compounding effects of other risk factors such as hypertriglyceridemia, hypercholesterolemia, hyperinsulinemia, low serum HDL-cholesterol, and hyperuricemia, although probably less important than hypertension, certainly do contribute to cardiovascular risk in obesity. Less than 10% of obese subjects are entirely free of one or more of these risk factors and those that are tend to be younger, less obese subjects (Berchtold *et al.*, 1981). In this study from Düsseldorf the most frequent risk factor in obesity was diastolic hypertension (68%) followed by systolic hypertension (56%); the incidences of other risk factors such as glucose intolerance, hypertriglyceridemia, hyperuricemia and hypercholesterolemia were lower. There was a stronger influence of age than body weight on blood pressure and certain other risk factors. HDL-cholesterol was lower in obese subjects, serum insulin levels were higher and both these factors correlated with body weight alone and not with age (Clarke, Schlenker and Merrow, 1981).

INSULIN AND CARBOHYDRATES

There is considerable evidence that insulin can effect electrolyte transport in the kidney and several other tissues. This was first demonstrated by André and Crabbé (1966) and Herrera, Whittemburgy and Planchart (1963) who reported that insulin increases sodium transport in frog skin and by Herrera (1965) in toad urinary bladder. A direct effect of insulin on sodium and potassium transport in renal tissue was reported by Nizet, Lefebvre and Crabbé (1971) from the isolated dog kidney. These observations were extended to human studies by Miller and Bogdonoff (1954) and by DeFronzo *et al.* (1975) who reported that insulin can directly increase sodium reabsorption in man. In order to delineate the possible separate effects of glucose versus insulin on renal sodium transport, the glucose clamp technique has been employed (DeFronzo, Tobin and Andres, 1979). In this study in dogs, conditions were altered to create a hyperglycemic, hyperinsulinemic state and a euglycemic, hyperinsulinemic state and renal sodium handling was studied both pre- and post-sodium chloride loading. Under both conditions absolute sodium excretion, sodium clearance and fractional excretion of sodium was decreased after salt loading compared to the control responses. This suggested that hyperinsulinemia *per se* and not hyperglycemia was the proximate cause of renal sodium retention. Further studies by this group (DeFronzo, Goldberg and Agus, 1978; DeFronzo, 1981) have suggested that the site of insulin action for sodium reabsorption is in the distal convoluted tubule and the thick ascending limb of Henle as originally reported by Schloeder and Stinebaugh (1970).

Whether the effect of insulin on renal sodium transport is directly on cellular transport proteins or represents a secondary response to changes in renal metabolism remains uncertain. Based on the early studies on amphibian tissue and several recent studies using *in vitro* systems, a direct effect of insulin on the $Na^+ - K^+$-ATPase pump may be implied. Insulin has been noted to increase intracellular potential in muscle cells (Moore and Rabovsky, 1979) and in adipocytes (Zierler and Rogus, 1981). A direct effect of insulin in stimulating sodium transport has also been described in cultured toad kidney cells (Fidelman *et al.*, 1982). Insulin along with other biologically important compounds has been proposed as a regulator of the sodium–potassium (Na–K) ATPase enzyme for active cation transport. Recently, insulin at physiological concentrations has been shown not only to stimulate purified sodium–potassium ATPase from dog kidney outer medulla but also to bind specifically to the purified enzyme (McGeoch, 1982). This suggests specific insulin receptor sites on this major cellular transport enzyme.

The effects of insulin on sodium reabsorption may explain certain observations on sodium excretion seen in patients with uncontrolled diabetes mellitus, and during the early period of dietary fasting. Some of the earliest observations on the action of insulin on renal sodium handling were made in patients with diabetes mellitus. Rapid withdrawal of insulin in diabetics was accompanied by a natriuresis that resolved with reinstitution of insulin therapy (Atchley *et al.*, 1933). Such additional factors as glycosuria, osmotic diuresis and ketonuria could also contribute to the observed natriuresis in poorly controlled diabetics. Saudek *et al.* (1974) studied six poorly controlled diabetics who had very high levels of urinary sodium showing that it was insulin deficiency and not glucosuria or ketonuria that produced the sodium wasting in these subjects.

During the early phase of fasting consisting of the first 7–10 days, there is a marked increase in sodium excretion that is promptly corrected with refeeding of carbohydrate or protein. Mechanisms put forth to explain this observation have included insulin deficiency, ketonuria, glucagon excess, aldosterone resistance and reduced sympathetic nervous system activity (Kolanowski, 1981). Of these factors, the role of insulin in the natriuresis of fasting seems very crucial. Although glucagon has a natriuretic effect in high doses and blood levels do rise with onset of fasting, several lines of evidence indicate that it has only a minor role in the natriuresis of fasting (Kolanowski *et al.*, 1977). These workers have also noted a correlation between sodium output and ketone excretion in the early part of fasting but concluded that this was not a major factor influencing sodium excretion in fasting (Kolanowski *et al.*, 1978). A prompt reduction in serum insulin levels along with a less consistent rise in glucagon concentration is a major feature of the metabolic adaptation to starvation. Administration of somatostatin to block both insulin and glucagon release in fasting subjects is accompanied by increased renal sodium excretion suggesting that insulin predominates in sodium regulation in fasting (Kolanowski, Ketelslegers and Crabbe, 1980). The temporal association of fasting and natriuresis with the prompt decline in insulin levels and the opposite effect with carbohydrate refeeding suggest a major role for insulin in this adaptation to fasting. Likewise, the change in insulin concentration under these conditions should be capable of altering sodium excretion.

From the above considerations of the effect of insulin on sodium transport it should be theoretically possible that hyperinsulinemia associated with obesity could contribute through sodium retention to the onset or maintenance of hypertension. This proposition has not been adequately investigated to make definitive conclusions. Although insulin resistance, glucose intolerance and elevated serum insulin levels are part of the metabolic consequences of the obese state, very few studies have examined these abnormalities as related to hypertension or sodium balance. The opposite, that is the reversibility of these abnormalities with weight loss, might imply an association between reductions in serum insulin concentration and the decline in blood pressure.

Evidence for a relationship between insulin and hypertension has been noted in studies of the effect of exercise on blood pressure. Krotkiewski *et al.* (1979) have shown that obese subjects after a period of physical training had significant reductions in serum insulin concentration that occurred without major changes in body weight. There were also reductions in blood pressure in those patients after the exercise program and a better correlation was found between insulin and blood pressure changes than with changes in body weight. Björntorp (1982) has suggested that the decrease in serum insulin with exercise leads to less sodium retention and a fall in blood pressure. Berglund *et al.* (1981) have detected hyperinsulinemia in essential hypertensive subjects who were not obese by the usual measurement standards. Along this line, essential hypertensive subjects have been found to have increased body fat relative to lean body mass. The type of obesity and distribution of body fat may also be important in this regard. Male subjects with predominantly abdominal obesity are more prone to complications such as hyperinsulinism and hypertension. In these subjects who do not display major deviations in body weight the term 'metabolic obesity' was proposed suggesting that the metabolic disorder including hyperinsulinism may be a more significant determinant of blood pressure level than obesity (Ruderman, Schneider and Berchtold, 1981).

SYMPATHETIC NERVOUS SYSTEM

An established relationship exists between nutrient intake and activity of the sympathetic nervous system. This adaptive response of the sympathetic nervous system to changes in nutrient availability has a certain survival value especially in times of famine. Contrary to the belief that caloric excess would diminish sympathetic nervous system activity, excess caloric intake appears to stimulate the sympathetic nervous system. A more precise definition of this relationship is hampered by limitations in quantitation of sympathetic nervous system activity in man. Measurement of urinary or circulating levels of catecholamines offers the only practical means of assessing the sympathetic nervous system in man and is only a partial measurement because of the complex disposal of these compounds. Tissue catecholamine levels and turnover rates in animals offer some improvement in estimating the activity of this system. Determination of radiolabelled catecholamine production and metabolic turnover in humans, when feasible, could offer additional information on sympathetic nervous system activity.

The effect of fasting and sucrose feeding on cardiac norepinephrine turnover in rats was first reported by Young and Landsberg (1977, 1979). In this technique rats are injected with ^{3}H-norepinephrine and at specific times hearts were removed for determination of specific activity. Calculated norepinephrine turnover rate was decreased by 39% in fasted rats and increased by 129% in sucrose-overfed rats compared to controls (*Figure 13.1*). Thus, fasting suppressed and overfeeding stimulated sympathetic nervous system outflow. These adaptations appear to occur rapidly within 1 or 2 days of initiation of the diet and persist as long as the diet is maintained. These investigations also demonstrated that not just fasting but reductions of 30–40% in energy intake can suppress sympathetic nervous system activity and that this effect can persist throughout the life of an animal maintained on reduced calories.

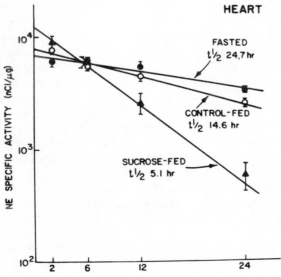

Figure 13.1 Effect of fasting and sucrose overfeeding on cardiac norepinephrine turnover in the rat. Fasting suppressed and overfeeding sucrose stimulated cardiac norepinephrine turnover. (From Landsberg and Young, 1978, courtesy of the Publisher, *International Journal of Obesity*)

The nature of the caloric signal to sympathetic nervous system regulation also has been elucidated. Although carbohydrate and protein overfeeding stimulate sympathetic activity, the response to the latter is much delayed suggesting conversion of protein to glucose as a necessary step. The importance of carbohydrate in this response also suggests that the insulin response to glucose could participate in altering sympathetic activity. Increased plasma norepinephrine levels have been observed after glucose ingestion in man (Robertson *et al.*, 1979; Welle, Lilavivanthana and Campbell, 1980). The independent roles of glucose and insulin on sympathetic activity were examined utilizing insulin and glucose clamp techniques in human subjects (Rowe *et al.*, 1981). During maintenance of euglycemia and an infusion of insulin at 2 and 5 mU/kg/hour there were significant, dose-dependent increments in plasma norepinephrine and blood pressure (*Figure 13.2*). These changes were not seen during the hyperglycemic clamp study

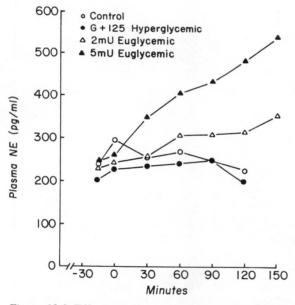

Figure 13.2 Effect of hyperglycemia and euglycemic hyperinsulinism of plasma norepinephrine level in normal human subjects. (From Rowe *et al.*, 1981, courtesy of the Publisher, *Diabetes*)

suggesting that insulin is a major signal in the sympathetic activation process. The physiological implication of these findings are uncertain, as high doses of insulin were infused. These investigators have also examined the central control of nutrient-induced sympathetic stimulation in gold-thioglucose-induced obesity in mice (Young and Landsberg, 1980). This compound destroys portions of the hypothalamus and in these mice there were no differences in cardiac norepinephrine turnover between fasted and sucrose-fed animals. They have proposed that the ventral medial region of the hypothalamus has an inhibitory action on sympathetic outflow. In this model sucrose overfeeding would induce a suppression of the inhibitory effect on sympathetic outflow. The signal for these centrally mediated events could be insulin-induced changes in neuronal glucose metabolism.

Excess energy intake through induction of increased sympathetic nervous system outflow could result in an increase in blood pressure. A major function of the sympathoadrenal system is regulation of blood pressure and it would seem reasonable to expect an effect of energy excess through stimulation of this system on blood pressure. Although blood pressure regulation is under the influence of several other hormonal systems, sympathetic nervous system activity and ambient norepinephrine levels are important determinants of blood pressure especially with changes in posture, intravascular volume and with stress (Cryer, 1980). The 24-hour circadian fluctuations in blood pressure also correlate highly with fluctuations in plasma norepinephrine suggesting a very important role for

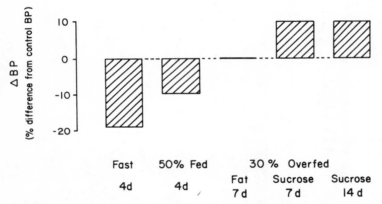

Figure 13.3 Diet-induced changes in blood pressure in the spontaneously hypertensive rat. (From Landsberg and Young, 1981, courtesy of the Publisher, *International Journal of Obesity*)

sympathetic activity in minute-to-minute changes in arterial pressure (Stene *et al.*, 1980). Overactivity of the sympathetic nervous system has been implicated by some investigators in the pathogenesis of blood pressure elevation in subjects with essential hypertension (Franco-Morselli *et al.*, 1977; Sever *et al.*, 1977; Goldstein, 1983) as well as its established role in the hypertension of pheochromocytoma. In the spontaneously hypertensive rat (SHR), considered a genetic model that closely resembles several aspects of human essential hypertension, caloric restriction lowers blood pressure (Young, Mullen and Landsberg, 1978) and sucrose feeding increases blood pressure (Young and Landsberg, 1981). The hypocaloric diet reduced blood pressure by 14% in the spontaneously hypertensive rats compared to control, fed hypertensive animals. Overfeeding with sucrose produced a significant increment in blood pressure from 8 to 10% higher than the control, normal intake spontaneously hypertensive rats (*Figure 13.3*). These studies imply a pronounced influence of diet on development and maintenance of blood pressure in this animal model of hypertension. Although the exact cause of hypertension in this animal model is still uncertain, several studies have noted evidence for increased sympathetic nervous system activity (Hallbäck and Weiss, 1977; Judy *et al.*, 1976). Whether a similar situation applies to certain forms of human hypertension is not certain. In the acute studies in normotensive man using the euglycemic pump, infusion of insulin in relatively high doses produced significant increases in plasma norepinephrine levels accompanied by an increase in blood pressure (Rowe *et al.*, 1981) (see *Figure 13.1*). This would indicate a sequence whereby carbohydrate assimilation, perhaps mediated through the increases in circulating insulin levels, would stimulate sympathetic activity and increase arterial pressure.

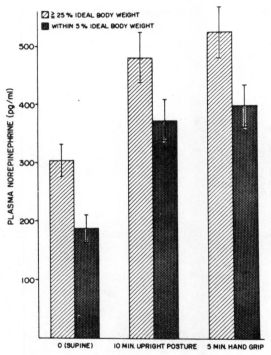

Figure 13.4 Mean (± SEM) plasma norepinephrine responses to upright posture and isometric handgrip exercise in obese subjects and nonobese controls. (From Sowers *et al.*, 1982, courtesy of the Publisher. *Journal of Clinical Endocrinology and Metabolism*)

Several recent observations support the concept that sympathetic nervous system activity may be increased in obese subjects (DeHaven *et al.*, 1980; James *et al.*, 1981; Jung *et al.*, 1979; Sowers *et al.*, 1982a; Tuck *et al.*, 1983). In obese patients, who were greater than 25% over ideal body weight, both supine and upright plasma norepinephrine levels were approximately 30% greater than values in matched non-obese subjects (*Figure 13.4*). Mean ambulatory levels of plasma norepinephrine ranged from 420 to 1440 pg/ml in obese subjects; values in a range that could produce adrenergically mediated changes in cardiovascular function. Plasma norepinephrine responses to the stimuli of upright posture and isometric handgrip in obese subjects also displayed greater absolute increases, but the increments over baseline did not differ from those in non-obese subjects (*Figure 13.4*). Thus, the release of norepinephrine in response to acute stimuli was not enhanced in obese individuals despite the higher ambient circulating levels. Obese subjects were placed on a supplemented fasting program at two different sodium intakes and blood pressure, body weight and plasma norepinephrine levels monitored at 1 to 2 weekly intervals for 8 weeks. Weight reduction by supplemented fasting was accompanied by significant reductions in blood pressure. Both of these events directly correlated with significant, stepwise declines in ambient plasma norepinephrine levels (*Figure 13.5*). These changes were first observed approximately 2 weeks after the subjects started the low caloric diet and plasma

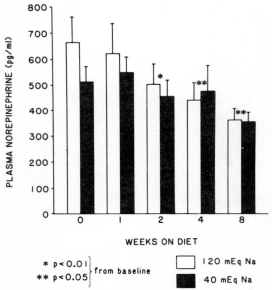

Figure 13.5 Mean ± SEM changes in plasma norepinephrine responses to 10 min upright posture during 8 weeks of supplemented fasting on two sodium intakes. (From Tuck *et al.*, 1983, courtesy of the Publishers, *Acta Endocrinologica*)

norepinephrine concentration fell to levels of non-obese controls by 8 weeks. The decline in blood pressure and norepinephrine often occurred before obese subjects reached ideal body weight. From these observations it would appear that the decrease in blood pressure that occurs during weight reduction is secondary to reduction of circulating norepinephrine as a function of reduced sympathetic nervous system activity. These changes also took place independently of dietary sodium intake as plasma norepinephrine and blood pressure decrements were similar on 120 and 40 mEq sodium intakes (Tuck *et al.*, 1983) (*Figure 13.5*). The lack of an effect of salt balance on plasma norepinephrine levels in obese individuals is at variance with reports in normal weight subjects where salt restriction elevates basal and posture stimulated norepinephrine levels (Stene *et al.*, 1980). Thus, another aspect of the changes in sympathetic nervous system activity with obesity may be loss of normal sodium and volume influences on catecholamine release. It is known, however, that epinephrine and norepinephrine can cause renal sodium reabsorption independently of changes in renal hemodynamics (Besarab, Silva and Landsberg, 1977; DiBona, 1978). Thus, a catecholamine-mediated increase in sodium reabsorption could also contribute to blood pressure increases through sodium retention in obese subjects.

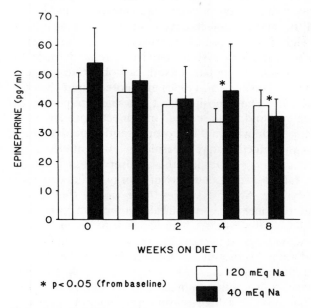

Figure 13.6 Mean ± SEM changes in plasma epinephrine responses to 10 min upright posture during 8 weeks of supplemented fasting in obese patients on two sodium intakes. (From Tuck *et al.*, 1983, courtesy of the Publishers, *Acta Endocrinologica*)

Plasma epinephrine levels also were higher in obese subjects and showed significant reductions on the low calorie diet (*Figure 13.6*). These changes were not as dramatic as those of plasma norepinephrine and reached significance only at the end of the 8-week dietary period. Likewise, the correlation between decrements in body weight and blood pressure to changes in plasma epinephrine were not as strong as with norepinephrine. The third major catecholamine, dopamine, has been reported to increase while circulating levels of norepinephrine and epinephrine are decreasing during early caloric deprivation in obese subjects (Sowers *et al.*, 1982c). Dopamine has a renal natriuretic effect that could account in part for the early natriuresis of fasting and contribute to blood pressure reductions during this phase of weight loss.

Whether stimulation of sympathetic nervous system activity in obese subjects relates to increased nutrient intake alone or also is a function of increased body fat is unresolved. The acute sucrose overfeeding studies in animals would suggest a direct effect of nutrient intake on sympathetic activity (Landsberg and Young, 1978, 1981). Jung *et al.* (1979) noted that a significant reduction in the excretion of the catecholamine urinary metabolite 4-hydroxy-3-methoxymandelic acid and in plasma norepinephrine levels occurred within 24–48 hours after energy restriction in obese adult subjects suggesting a strong role for acute food deprivation in this process. These acute changes in sympathetic activity were accompanied by decrements in pulse rate and blood pressure and were rapidly reversed by refeeding (Jung, Shetty and James, 1980). Our results in obese subjects during weight loss by supplemented fasting demonstrated that blood pressure and catecholamine levels had returned towards normal in many subjects even when they were still significantly above ideal body weight (Tuck *et al.*, 1983; Sowers *et al.*, 1982a). This would imply that basal sympathetic nervous system activity is related more to caloric intake than to obesity. Using a similar mixed carbohydrate–protein low-calorie diet in obese subjects, DeHaven *et al.* (1980) also noted rapid changes in sympathetic nervous system activity. The opposite effect also seems to pertain as catecholamine metabolism has been found to be reduced in subjects with anorexia nervosa (Gross *et al.*, 1979) but this finding has not been consistently noted in other malnourished states where stress and infection may override the nutrient effects on sympathetic activity (Ramirez *et al.*, 1978). Despite these observations it is still conceivable that obesity or body fat mass independently of energy intake can alter catecholamine release or metabolism. Several studies have noted that obese subjects have a reduced thermic response to energy intake compared to normal weight subjects (Kaplan, Leveille, 1976; Pittet, Chappuis and Acheson, 1976). Sympathetic nervous system activity as reflected by plasma norepinephrine responses may play a role in mediating this thermic response to food intake (Welle, Lilavivanthana and Campbell, 1981). Jung *et al.* (1979) noted that obese subjects demonstrate less increase in oxygen consumption than do lean subjects in response to a norepinephrine infusion that produced high plasma norepinephrine levels, implying a possible relative resistance to the effect of catecholamines in obesity. Similar findings were noted after acute meal ingestion in obese subjects who had higher preprandial and postprandial plasma norepinephrine levels but diminished thermic responses to feeding (Schwartz, Halter and Bierman, 1983). This could suggest an insensitivity to catecholamines in mediating the thermic response to feeding. These workers did note, however, enhanced plasma norepinephrine responses to acute administration of a test formula meal in obese subjects substantiating the rapid effect of food intake on this system in obesity. It is also possible that increases in body weight somehow impair norepinephrine removal from the plasma. Detailed studies of norepinephrine metabolism and clearance rates in obese individuals would answer this question. A recent report of norepinephrine infusion in overweight normotensive and essential hypertensive subjects did observe normal pressor sensitivity to norepinephrine infusion and normal norepinephrine clearance in these patients (Boehringer *et al.*, 1982). Another study has compared changes in vascular volume and systemic and regional hemodynamics with changes in plasma norepinephrine before and after weight reduction (Reisin *et al.*, 1983). Total circulating and cardiopulmonary blood volumes were reduced after weight reduction resulting in decreased cardiac output and arterial blood pressure accompanied by a significant decline in resting mean plasma norepinephrine from 591 ± 22 pg/ml to 261 ± 51 pg/ml. These data suggested that reduced adrenergic activity could contribute to the redistribution of intravascular volume away from the cardiopulmonary area reducing venous return, cardiac output and arterial pressure.

An additional link between nutritional status and sympathetic nervous system activity is the regulation of thyroid hormone metabolism by energy intake. The integration of catecholamine and thyroid hormone metabolism by nutritional factors appears to be a major mechanism for regulating energy expenditure during changes in energy availability. The interaction of these two systems under these conditions has been reviewed by Jung, Shetty and James (1980). These workers have proposed that during overfeeding there may be undesirable cardiovascular effects of sympathetic nervous system and thyroid hormone increases in addition to their beneficial effects on regulation of thermogenesis and oxygen consumption. A direct effect of overfeeding might involve an interaction between catecholamines and thyroid hormone at a cellular level to increase cardiovascular function and blood pressure. Similar to the nutrient effects on catecholamines, it has now been shown that overfeeding also produces an increase in the rate of deiodination of thyroxine to triiodothyronine (Danforth *et al.*, 1979). As with fasting, net availability of carbohydrate probably is the major nutrient that determines the deiodination rate in overfeeding. One report has found moderate but significantly higher levels of triiodothyronine in both adolescent and late-onset obese subjects (Schwartz, Halter and Bierman, 1980). Whether these relatively small changes in triiodothyronine blood levels could influence blood pressure in obesity was not addressed in this study. Since thyroid hormone can modulate adrenergic receptor activity at the cellular level (Williams *et al.*, 1977), it is possible that this effect of thyroid hormone in vascular tissue could alter vascular reactivity to catecholamines. Certainly the consideration of a synergistic effect of thyroid hormone and catecholamine overactivity in the pathogenesis of obesity hypertension deserves further attention.

SODIUM INTAKE AND HOMEOSTASIS

There is ample evidence that abnormal sodium intake and balance contribute to the etiology of certain forms of hypertension (Tobian, 1979). A relationship between sodium intake and high blood pressure has been debated for decades with varying degrees of acceptance and rejection. Currently there are important areas of information offering new insights into this relationship that may extend into the pathogenesis of obesity hypertension. These new areas, examined mainly in essential hypertension, include the concept of individual variations in sensitivity of blood pressure to salt intake that may be genetically determined either by recently defined abnormalities in cellular sodium transport pathways or by renal capacity to excrete sodium. A wealth of epidemiological information supports the relationship between salt intake and hypertension. In unacculturated societies where salt intake is low, the incidence of hypertension is low compared to the more acculturated, industrialized nations, where the opposite pertains (Freis, 1976). Examination of the effect of salt intake on the incidence of hypertension within groups in the industrialized nations where salt intake is uniformly high fails to substantiate this relationship. Recently, a more careful examination of individuals in these groups has revealed a wide variation in blood pressure responses to salt loading. These heterogeneous responses have given rise to the concept that some individuals are 'salt-sensitive' in their blood pressure responses whereas others show very little effect on blood pressure to a wide range of sodium intake (Kawasaki, Delea, Bartter, 1978; Luft *et al.*, 1979). Certain demographic factors such as race, age and family history of hypertension may also be important determinants,of the degree of blood pressure response to salt loading (Luft, Weinberger and Grim, 1982). Interestingly, a genetic animal model for salt-sensitivity and resistance of blood pressure has been well established and extensively studied for years (Dahl, 1962).

Support for a possible genetically determined differential blood pressure response to salt in humans emerges from studies of cellular sodium transport in essential hypertension. Because of ease of accessibility, most studies have employed erythrocytes or other circulating blood elements to examine cation transport in human subjects. Much of the interest in cellular sodium transport arises from observations that erythrocyte or lymphocyte intracellular sodium levels are higher in essential hypertensive subjects (Ambrosioni *et al.*, 1979; Fadeke-Aderounmu and Salako, 1979; Losse, Wehmeyer and Wessels, 1960). This observation, however, has not been confirmed by others (Canessa *et al.*, 1980; Wambach *et al.*, 1979). The human erythrocyte has several transport pathways that move sodium across its membrane, including the ouabain-sensitive Na–K-ATPase pump and several ouabain-insensitive pathways (the Na–K cotransport system and the Na^+,Na^+ or Na^+,Li^+ countertransport systems). It is in the ouabain-insensitive pathways that genetically transmitted abnormalities in sodium transport have been found in erythrocytes from essential hypertensive subjects. Garay *et al.* (1980a and b) have noted reduced Na–K cotransport in a significant number of essential hypertensive patients and in normotensive offspring from families with a strong history of hypertension. Canessa *et al.* (1980) have described elevated erythrocyte Na^+,Li^+ countertransport in essential hypertensive subjects and have also noted high countertransport in normotensive offspring from hypertensive first-degree relatives. In other studies abnormalities in the major cellular cation transport system, the ouabain-sensitive Na–K pump have been noted in experimental hypertensive animals (Haddy, Pamnani and Clough, 1978) and in human essential hypertension (DeWardener and MacGregor, 1980). Recent interest has focused on a circulating inhibitor of the Na,K pump that may be elevated in experimental and human hypertension (DeWardener and MacGregor, 1980; Hamlyn *et al.*, 1982). Purification of plasma of volume-expanded animals and from experimental hypertensive animals reveals that certain chromatographic fractions that inhibit pump activity also crossreact with antidigoxin antibodies suggesting that the pump inhibitor may be an endogenous cardiac glycoside-like material (Gruber, Whitaker and Buckalew, 1980; Gruber, Rudel and Bullock, 1982). Thus, several lines of evidence point toward new avenues of investigation that may clarify the relationship between salt intake and the development of arterial hypertension.

One of the earliest proposed etiologies for the development of hypertension in obese subjects was that they had a higher sodium intake than non-obese individuals (Dahl, 1958, 1972). Since obese subjects presumably ingest more calories they therefore should be taking in more salt. Very little data exist on dietary histories of salt intake or urinary sodium excretion rates in obese hypertensive subjects. We did note in a small group of obese subjects with variable ranges of blood pressure that urinary sodium excretion (mean 193 mEq/24 hours) on a free dietary intake was moderately increased over average levels reported for the United States (Tuck *et al.*, 1981) (*Figure 13.7*). However, these individuals when placed on constant 120 or 40 mEq sodium intake did display normal ability to reach and maintain sodium balance for a given sodium intake, suggesting that there was no major defect in renal sodium regulation.

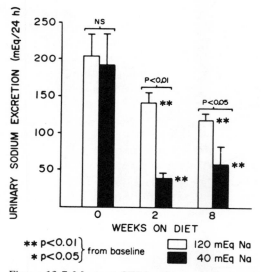

Figure 13.7 Mean ± SEM urinary sodium excretion before (0) and during 8 weeks of supplemented fasting in obese patients on a constant 120 and 40 mmol sodium intake (From Tuck *et al.*, 1983, courtesy of the Publishers, *Acta Endocrinologica*)

Dahl, Silver and Christie (1958) were the first to propose a relationship between salt intake and development of hypertension in obesity. They noted that when the intake of sodium is markedly restricted in obese hypertensives but caloric intake is held constant, blood pressure levels decrease. This observation was left unchallenged for years, but recent studies suggest that excess salt intake may not be as important as previously believed in obesity hypertension. In a report of 81 obese hypertensive subjects in Israel, Reisien *et al.* (1978) placed individuals on a low calorie diet but specifically instructed them to eat generous servings of salty, low-caloric foods. Blood pressure reductions were quite striking (mean of 26 mmHg systolic; 20 mmHg diastolic) and were highly correlated with loss of body weight, occurring independently of salt intake during the 2-month weight loss period. In a second group of obese hypertensives studied while still on antihypertensive medication, the reductions in blood pressure during the high-salt, low-calorie diet were also striking. In an extension of this original report, Eliahou *et al.* (1981) noted that two-thirds of 212 obese, hypertensive subjects on a balanced hypocaloric diet but advised to eat salt freely achieved normal blood pressure levels with loss of only one-half of their weight excess. Urinary sodium measurements documented that salt intake remained high despite the drop in blood pressure that accompanied their weight loss. It was concluded that whatever the role of high sodium intake in the maintenance of hypertension in obesity, this effect could be overridden by the effects of weight loss. These studies also brought out the important observation that overweight, hypertensive subjects can attain normal blood pressure levels by weight reduction long before achieving ideal body weight.

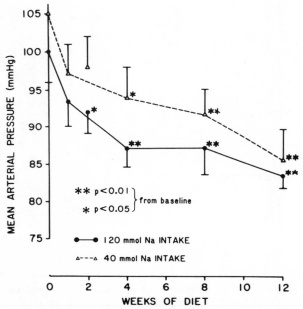

Figure 13.8 Decrements in mean arterial pressure (mean ± SEM) during supplemented fasting in obese patients on a constant sodium intake. (From Tuck *et al.*, 1981, courtesy of the Publishers, *New England Journal of Medicine*)

We have also examined the influence of sodium intake on the hypotensive response to weight reduction by maintaining obese subjects on constant sodium intake and carefully monitering urinary sodium excretion (Tuck *et al.*, 1981). During weight loss by supplemental fasting the fall in blood pressure was similar in subjects on 120 or 40 mEq sodium diets (*Figure 13.8*). Compliance to the dietary sodium intake during the 12 weeks was documented by showing that urinary sodium excretion matched sodium intake. This study provided further proof that the potent hypotensive effect of weight reduction in the obese occurs independently of sodium balance. Our findings also confirmed that only a 10–30% reduction towards ideal body weight was often sufficient to normalize blood pressure in most obese subjects. None of the above studies, however, was so designed to adequately separate the effects of sodium and adiposity in the regulation of blood pressure during caloric maintenance in obese subjects. As is the case in lean hypertensives, one is left with the possibility that abnormal sodium balance or cellular transport could contribute to their hypertension. Several hormones that regulate sodium metabolism are abnormal in obese subjects. High serum insulin levels in obesity could contribute to sodium retention as could elevated circulating catecholamines which can enhance renal sodium reabsorption. Whether the circulating concentration of these hormones in obese subjects could have an effect on renal sodium reabsorption can only be delineated by careful sodium balance studies. Compatible with a role for sodium retention in obesity is the finding of increased fluid volume in obese subjects. However, proper frames of reference to express fluid volumes is difficult to attain in obese individuals, rendering these measurements open to criticism.

Certain of the abnormalities described in sodium cellular transport in essential hypertension have also been noted in obese animals and humans. The obese (ob/ob) mouse which serves as a model for defective thermogenesis and retains a greater proportion of energy than lean animals, also has reduced levels of $Na+-K^+$-ATPase in muscle and liver (Lin *et al.*, 1978; York, Bray and Yukimura, 1978). Obese human subjects also demonstrate reductions in the number of erythrocyte Na^+-K^+ pump units as quantitated by radiolabelled ouabain binding and cation transport activity measured by [86]rubidium uptake (DeLuise, Blackburn and Flier, 1980). Intracellular erythrocyte sodium concentration is also higher in obese subjects. Weight reduction in these subjects did not change erythrocyte Na–K pump activity. Klimes *et al.* (1982) confirmed these findings, noting an inverse correlation between erythrocyte membrane Na^+-K^+-ATPase activity and erythrocyte [86]rubidium uptake with body mass index in Pima Indians. Using erythrocyte vesicles, Mir *et al.* (1981) was unable to confirm these findings in obese subjects in whom he actually noted higher erythrocyte Na^+-K^+-ATPase levels. A relationship between these cellular sodium transport abnormalities, sodium balance, and development of hypertension in obesity were not addressed in these studies. Our group has further examined the relationship between erythrocyte sodium transport, blood pressure levels and sympathetic nervous system activity in obese subjects during a weight loss period (Sowers *et al.*, 1982b). Confirming other studies, obese subjects had reduced erythrocyte membrane Na–K-ATPase activity, erythrocyte [86]rubidium uptake and higher intracellular sodium levels. During the 12-week weight reduction period by supplemented fasting there were no significant changes in these red cell sodium transport parameters despite very significant reductions in arterial pressure and plasma norepinephrine levels. These results would imply a lack of relationship between erythrocyte pump activity and blood pressure levels in obese subjects before or during weight reduction.

RENIN–ANGIOTENSIN–ALDOSTERONE SYSTEM

The renin–angiotensin system is an important hormonal regulatory system for the maintenance of blood pressure and detailed examples of abnormalities of this system in the genesis of hypertension are provided elsewhere in this volume. Correlations between levels of plasma renin activity and body weight have not been reported. Some studies have found normal ambient levels of plasma renin activity in obese subjects using variable standardization for salt intake, age and other factors that effect this measurement (Boehringer *et al.*, 1982; Messerli *et al.*, 1981; Mujais *et al.*, 1982). One investigation found relatively low levels of renin but normal aldosterone values in obese hypertensive subjects (Hiramatsu *et al.*, 1981). The aldosterone:plasma renin activity ratio was found to increase progressively with increases in relative body weight. These investigators proposed a role for the inappropriately higher aldosterone levels compared to renin activity in the genesis of hypertension in obese subjects. These observations have not been confirmed as very limited information exists on either mineralocorticoid or glucocorticoid levels in obesity. This is quite surprising since very early work in steroid hormones described altered glucocorticoid metabolism in obese subjects (Dunkelman *et al.*, 1964). The hallmark of Cushing's syndrome includes obesity and hypertension, yet careful examination of glucocorticoid regulatory dynamics and metabolism have not been extended to an obese, hypertensive population who do not have classic findings of hypercortisolism. One early proposal noted that patients who were obese and hypertensive had scattered findings of Cushingoid-like features but not the full-blown picture of Cushing's syndrome (Esanu *et al.*, 1968). Whether a true intermediate form of this disorder exists in obesity has never been substantiated but seems doubtful. Certain obese animal models of hypertension do have evidence for increased adrenal enzymatic activity of 18-hydroxylation and 11-β-hydroxylation and have higher circulating levels of the mineralocorticoid hormone 11-deoxycorticosterone (Angelin and Kalmar, 1979). In the genetically obese, spontaneously hypertensive rat, adrenalectomy has an ameliorative effect on the hypertension and metabolic derangements suggesting mediation of these effects by the hypothalamic–pituitary–adrenal axis similar to Cushing's disease in man (Wexler and McMurtry, 1981). Circulating levels of several aldosterone biosynthetic precursors including 11-deoxycorticosterone, 18-hydroxycorti-costerone, 18-hydroxy-11-deoxycorticosterone and 19-nor-deoxycorticosterone have been reported to be elevated in certain types of experimental and human hypertension, but these steroids have not been related to obesity and hypertension.

We examined the effect of weight reduction by supplemented fasting on plasma renin activity and aldosterone concentrations in obese subjects on constant 120 mEq and 40 mEq sodium intakes (Tuck *et al.*, 1981). After 2 weeks on the diet plasma renin levels started to decline and at 8 and 12 weeks were 40–50% below baseline levels (*Figure 13.9*). The magnitude of reduction in renin activity was similar on the normal and sodium restricted diets implying an overriding effect of weight loss in counteracting the usual stimulatory effect of sodium restriction on renin release. There was a positive correlation between reductions in plasma renin activity and blood pressure from weeks 4 through 12. Baseline sitting levels of plasma renin activity (mean 3.56 ± 0.42 ng/ml/hour) were high when related to the mean urinary sodium level (197 ± 30 mEq/24 hours) but the study group was too small to make firm conclusions on this relationship. The changes in aldosterone during the weight loss period were quantitatively less but did fall significantly from baseline by week 12 of the diet. These results demonstrate that relatively short-term weight loss is accompanied by reductions in plasma renin activity that may contribute to the decline in blood pressure. Since levels of plasma norepinephrine and epinephrine also fell during this period it is possible that the decline in sympathetic nervous system modulation of renin release contributed to the reduction in plasma renin activity. Whether similar changes in renin and aldosterone occur with more-prolonged, less-calorie restricted diets is uncertain. Reisin *et al.* (1983) reported in 12 obese, hypertensive subjects that during an average of 9 months of weight loss with a balanced hypocaloric diet, that plasma

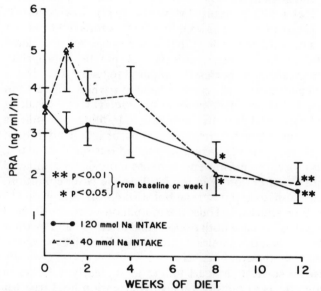

Figure 13.9 Changes in plasma renin activity (mean ± SEM) during weight loss by supplemented fasting in obese patients. (From Tuck *et al.*, 1981, courtesy of the Publishers, *New England Journal of Medicine*)

norepinephrine levels fell significantly but not plasma renin activity. It also appears that the pressor response to infusion of angiotensin II in mild to moderately obese hypertensives is similar to that in normal weight hypertensive subjects (Boehringer *et al.*, 1982). These investigators concluded that there was no unique aberration in the renin–angiotensin system and in the cardiovascular responses to angiotensin II in overweight compared to lean hypertensive subjects.

HEMODYNAMICS

Several careful studies have helped to clarify the changes in cardiovascular hemodynamics that accompany obesity and how these changes might relate to the hormonal aberrations found in this disorder. A better definition of the relationship between the cardiovascular and humoral changes associated with increased body weight becomes important in further dissecting out the mechanisms of hypertension in obesity. Much of the difficulty in interpreting hemodynamic and blood volume measurements in obesity has been selecting the proper frame of reference related to body weight to express these parameters. This problem is compounded by the onset of hypertension which produces its own set of hemodynamic and volume aberrations. Cardiac output is an important determinant of blood pressure and if elevated can produce hypertension. Increased metabolic demands and total body oxygen consumption in obesity lead to expanded intravascular volume, increased cardiac output due to increases in stroke volume but not heart rate (Messerli *et al.*, 1981; Woodward, Quinones and Alexander, 1978). Cardiac output is high in obese subjects irrespective of level of blood pressure (Messerli, 1982). Correction of cardiac output for body surface area (cardiac index), however, results in normal or subnormal values in obese subjects. Messerli (1982) has emphasized that such frames of reference as body weight in obese subjects may not be appropriate especially since fat tissue is relatively underperfused compared to lean tissue. These correction factors may artificially normalize cardiac function when, in fact, in obesity the heart pumps more blood per given amount of time. The end result of this high preload with increased end-diastolic volume and filling pressure is ventricular dilatation and congestive heart failure that can occur independently of blood pressure levels. Messerli *et al.* (1982) have also pointed out the contrasting cardiovascular adaptations that occur in normotensive obese individuals compared to normal weight subjects with hypertension (*Figure 13.10*). In the latter condition, vascular volume is constricted, cardiac output normal but stroke work is high due to increased peripheral resistance or afterload. Thus, the mutual onset of obesity and hypertension would be expected to increase both preload and afterload and by their opposing effects on volume and hemodynamics could 'normalize' the measured hemodynamic values. Nonetheless, the combined changes would act synergistically to increase markedly the risk of congestive heart failure as is clearly the case in obesity. The same contrasting effects of obesity versus hypertension hold true for vascular volume which is usually expanded in obesity and contracted in non-obese, essential hypertensives. Current evidence suggests that intracellular body water is increased compared to interstitial fluid volume in obese hypertensives and that weight reduction shifts this ratio of volume distribution along with reductions in blood pressure (Raison *et al.*, 1983). Total peripheral resistance is often low in obesity because of high cardiac output, so theoretically in obese subjects developing hypertension this measurement should still be lower compared to peripheral resistance in lean hypertensives. It has been proposed that the vascular resistance-lowering effect of obesity could result in less impact on target organ disease compared to lean subjects with the same degree of hypertension. Severity of obesity may also have some bearing on the hemodynamic picture as hypertensive subjects defined as having moderate obesity displayed hemodynamic and volume profiles similar to hypertensives who were non-obese (Dustan, Tarazi and Mujais, 1981; Mujais *et al.*, 1982). A careful study of hemodynamics in obese normotensive subjects confirmed the previous studies but emphasized that depression of left ventricular function was already quite striking in relatively young, obese people who were clinically free of signs of cardiomyopathy (deDivitiis *et al.*, 1981). Thus,

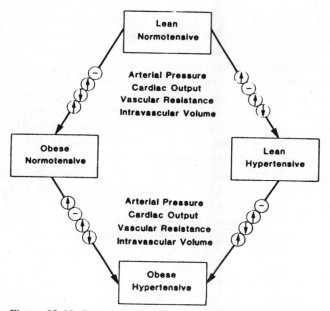

Figure 13.10 Cardiovascular effects of obesity and hypertension: disparate changes in intravascular volume and total peripheral resistance. (From Messerli, 1982, courtesy of the Publishers, *Lancet*)

even if peripheral resistance is lower in obese versus non-obese hypertensives, the impact of obesity on cardiac performance is marked.

Reisin *et al.* (1983) examined the effect of weight reduction on cardiovascular and volume profiles in obese hypertensive subjects. Reductions in blood pressure with weight loss were accompanied by decreases in circulating and cardiopulmonary blood volumes leading to a reduction in venous return. The reduction in cardiac output related directly to contracted total blood volume. In this study there was a significant decline in plasma norepinephrine concentration accompanying the hemodynamic changes suggesting that the role of adrenergic activity in contribution to the hemodynamic profile may be important. It could be proposed that the sequence of events leading to hypertension in obesity would include, as an initiating event, enhanced adrenergic activity related to excessive nutrient intake and/or the obese state. The effects of obesity on oxygen demand and the increased adrenergic activity would then lead to increases in cardiac output and intravascular volume and eventually result in increased peripheral resistance and hypertension (Messerli, 1982). The higher circulating levels of norepinephrine would contribute to the increases in peripheral resistance and perhaps maintain a higher rate of renin release and circulating angiotensin II.

TREATMENT

Guidelines for effective control of blood pressure by non-pharmacological or pharmacological means in obese hypertensive subjects are currently not well established. We have excellent examples of large-scale clinical trials that have demonstrated the lifesaving effects of pharmacological intervention therapy to normalize blood pressure in essential hypertension (Veterans Administration Cooperative Study Group on Antihypertensive Agents, 1967, 1970, 1977; Hypertension Detection and Follow-up Program Cooperative Group, 1979). The subject of obesity in these trials was given only minor consideration, although it must be presumed that a certain proportion of any essential hypertensive population would be over ideal body weight. Several studies have documented the beneficial effects of weight reduction on lowering blood pressure. However, with a few exceptions, none of these programs involved large-scale community trials with long-term efforts not only at weight reduction but also at maintenance. Additionally, only limited information is available on the comparative efficacy on non-pharmacological versus antihypertensive drugs in long-term control of hypertension in obesity. Considering the variety of antihypertensive agents used to treat hypertension, we also know very little about the consequence obesity has on their metabolism, side-effects, or efficacy.

WEIGHT REDUCTION

It is clear that weight loss in obese patients reverses several major metabolic derangements while normalizing blood pressure. More than 60 years ago Rose (1922) described the remarkable effect of weight reduction on high blood pressure. Since then several clinical trials have established that weight reduction in obese hypertensives is a very potent hypotensive modality in most but not all obese individuals (Atkinson and Kaiser, 1981; Berchtold *et al.*, 1982; Chiang, Perlman and Epstein, 1969; Dershewitz, Kahn and Solomon, 1981; Eliahou *et al.*, 1981; Fletcher, 1954; Greminger *et al.*, 1982; Kahle *et al.*, 1982; Ramsay *et al.*, 1978; Reisin *et al.*, 1978, 1983; Stamler *et al.*, 1980; Tuck *et al.*, 1981; Tyrolar, Hayden and Hames, 1975). Several aspects of these studies deserve comment. In the Evans County study, Tyrolar, Hayden and Hames (1975) pointed out that the rate of remission of hypertension was twice as great for subjects losing 4.5 kg or more over 6 years. Additionally, in a more intense weight-reducing program subjects who lost an average of 8 kg over a 1-year period had an 18 mmHg systolic and 13 mmHg diastolic reduction in blood pressure, demonstrating not only the feasibility of such a dietary approach in a general population but also the tremendous responses in blood pressure that can be attained with relatively modest weight loss. This study also revealed that white obese hypertensives had a greater depressor response per unit of weight loss than obese hypertensive blacks.

An overriding finding from most of these clinical trials is that an obese person does not need to reach ideal body weight to attain a normal blood pressure. Some studies report that as little as a 5% drop in total weight was adequate to induce major reductions in blood pressure (Greminger *et al.*, 1982; Stamler *et al.*, 1980) and that this can occur regardless of the initial severity of the obesity. Others have attempted to quantitate the rate of pressure reduction per given amount of weight loss. In the Multiple Risk Factor Intervention Trial (1976) there was a 1 mmHg fall in diastolic pressure for each 1.8 kg weight lost. A much earlier study by Fletcher (1954) in hypertensive obese females calculated that a 6.4 kg weight loss yielded a 30 mmHg fall in systolic and 19 mmHg in diastolic pressure. Reisin *et al.* (1978) reported that patients who lost 9.6 kg had a mean reduction in systolic pressure of 26 mmHg and in diastolic pressure of 20 mmHg. The Framingham study evaluated the comparative impact of a given unit of weight reduction in the general population on several risk factors including hypertension (Ashley and Kannel, 1974). The most profound effect for each 10 unit change in relative weight in men was on serum cholesterol (11.3 mg/dl decline) followed by systolic blood pressure (6.6 mmHg decline). The impact of weight loss on these risk factors was less pronounced but still significant for females. Another aspect of these observations was the projected linear response in changes in these risk parameters to changes in body weight. Somewhat similar observations in stepwise weight reductions or gains and changes in blood pressure were made in the Düsseldorf study (Berchtold *et al.*, 1981b).

The level of sodium restriction during weight reduction also seems to have little bearing on the degree or rate of blood pressure reduction (Reisin *et al.*, 1978; Tuck *et al.*, 1981). In our study employing short-term, very low calorie intake (Tuck *et al.*, 1981), hypertensive and even the normotensive obese subjects had significant reductions in blood pressure with weight loss; an observation also noted in a more long-term less severely restricted dietary and lifestyle intervention program (Stamler *et al.*, 1980). Thus, the type of dietary program employed to lower blood pressure has very little bearing on the eventual outcome of the blood pressure response and is dictated more by the degree of initial overweightness and the rate at which blood pressure should be lowered. Even the normotensive obese subject may benefit by an additional reduction in blood pressure through weight loss.

Looking at overall risk factor reductions in obese subjects it would seem that there is a differential effect on the degree of weight reduction and magnitude of change in a given risk factor. Keys *et al.* (1972) determined that high blood pressure and cholesterol levels are the leading factors in the increased cardiovascular risk in obesity. However, the effect of weight reduction on blood pressure lowering is substantially greater than on other risk factors. Berchtold *et al.* (1981a) has recently re-emphasized the fact that obese subjects may also need to lose substantial weight to achieve normal glucose tolerance. Thus, although blood pressure may be one of the easier parameters to reverse with weight loss, reversal of total risk to the obese subject may require reaching and maintaining ideal body weight.

Sims (1982) speaking for the consensus of several investigators in obesity and hypertension has emphasized that the 'stepped care' approach in drug therapy of hypertension should especially be modified in obese hypertensive subjects to include non-pharmacological modalities. The initial steps should deal with characterization of the metabolic abnormalities, reduction of energy intake, increased physical activity, education and long-term behavioral maintenance support. Surprisingly small changes in the lifestyle of the sedentary, overeating, underexercising obese hypertensive may yield satisfactory results towards attaining lower blood pressures. Our recent experience with very low calorie diets (less than 800 kcal/day) or supplemented fasting as a means of weight reduction and blood pressure control suggest that this modality should be given a more large-scale trial in obese hypertensive subjects (Tuck *et al.*, 1981) particularly in the moderate to massively obese patient. For the less obese (<20% greater than ideal body weight) a balanced hypocaloric diet may suffice to control weight and blood pressure.

EXERCISE

Björntorp (1982) has extensively examined and reviewed the role of exercise in the therapeutic approach to hypertension. Exercise in the form of physical training will cause blood pressure levels to decline in both normotensive and mildly hypertensive subjects whether they have normal and excess body weight. The reductions in blood pressure are accompanied by significant changes in sympathetic nervous system activity and in serum insulin levels (Björntorp, 1982). Exercise seems to enhance certain catecholamine-sensitive metabolic and cardiovascular functions to stimulation by adrenergic agonists. After physical training urinary catecholamine levels, which were initially high, were not reduced (Björntorp *et al*, 1977). In physical exercise studies in rats, these workers found in rat adipocytes enhanced catecholamine sensitivity (Holm *et al.*, 1980). At the beta-adrenergic receptor level this effect of physical exercise could be seen on the GTP-binding protein regulation of adenylate cyclase responses. Plasma insulin concentrations were also significantly reduced with physical training and the decline paralleled the reductions in blood pressure (Krotkiewski *et al.*, 1979). These changes in insulin levels could alter either sodium balance or sympathetic nervous system activity as part of the mechanism to explain the hypotensive effect of exercise. It is clear that these observations on physical training are important in the management of obesity hypertension, but the amount of exercise prescribed depends inversely on the severity of obesity. It is doubtful that physical exercise alone will provide the needed caloric expenditure for weight loss in the moderate to more severely obese subject. From the observed hormonal changes, however, it provides excellent and specific adjunctive therapy to any program in hypertension whether the patient is obese or not. The degree of exercise was rather extreme in these studies and it is unlikely that the more obese patient could initially adjust or perform adequately in these programs. Yet any degree of exercise in these subjects is sure to provide a better sense of satisfaction and aid in counteracting the negative influences that occur with chronic dietary programs (Sims, 1981).

ANTIHYPERTENSIVE THERAPY

Few investigations have specifically addressed the topic of antihypertensive drug therapy as it relates to the obese subject with hypertension. There are, however, theoretical considerations that obese hypertensives may exhibit differences in responses to antihypertensive agents compared to leaner patients especially regarding efficacy and side-effects. Specific cardiovascular and hormonal abnormalities in obese hypertensives such as high cardiac output, increased plasma volume, increased plasma norepinephrine and serum insulin could make certain antihypertensive agents more specific and effective based on their antihypertensive mechanism of action. The concept of employing an antihypertensive agent aimed at correction of a specific physiological abnormality in hypertension is theoretically appealing and has only been partially realized in the approach to therapy of the essential hypertensive population.

Because obese subjects may take in more salt and have expanded intravascular volume, diuretic therapy might be expected to have special efficacy in obesity hypertension. This possibility, however, has not been extensively studied; that is, no direct comparison of diuretic therapy efficacy in lean and obese hypertensive individuals has been reported. Our experience would suggest that this is not the case; obese hypertensives demonstrate only a 10–15% incidence of blood pressure normalization on diuretic therapy, a response rate identical to non-obese hypertensives. Special problems with diuretic therapy in obesity include the metabolic derangements associated with these agents, including glucose intolerance, hyperuricemia and hyperlipidemia. Obesity itself is associated with an increased incidence of glucose intolerance, hypertriglyceridemia, hypercholesterolemia and hyperuricemia. Addition of diuretics could theroretically increase the severity of these metabolic abnormalities in the obese individual. The potential long-term benefits to obese hypertensives of blood pressure reduction with diuretic agents must be weighed against the possible potentiation of these independent metabolic risk factors.

Table 13.1

	Cardiac output	Norepinephrine	Plasma renin activity	Sodium excretion	Insulin	Sodium pump
Obesity	↑	↑	↑	↑	↑	↓
Hydrochlorothiazide	±	↑	↑	↑	? ↓	↓
Propranolol	↓	↑	↓	±	↓	± ↓
Hydralazine	↑	↑	↑	↓	NA	NA
Clonidine	↓	↓	↓	↑	± ↑	NA

Vasodilator antihypertensive agents also may have limited applicability in the obese hypertensive population. The hemodynamic characteristics of obesity hypertension, including increased cardiac output with less pronounced changes in peripheral vascular resistance, make vasodilator therapy less suited for this population (*Table 13.1*). Certain cardiovascular effects of vasodilators including increased heart rate and cardiac work might not be appropriate in these subjects who already have an increased cardiac workload. Vasodilator-induced sodium retention poses a problem in this population who demonstrated increased intravascular volume. Thus, effective vasodilator therapy often requires addition of sympathetic inhibitors to attenuate cardiovascular side-effects and diuretics to offset sodium retention. This amounts to triple drug therapy in a population where in most circumstances this should not be necessary for blood pressure control.

Treatment of obese hypertensives with beta-adrenergic blocking agents may have some theoretical merit based on the hemodynamic profile in obesity as they would decrease pre-existing increased cardiac output (*see Table 13.1*). It is uncertain whether this observation has even been tested in clinical trials of beta-blockers in lean compared to obese hypertensive subjects. There is circumstantial evidence that obesity, especially with advancing age, may be accompanied by diminished antihypertensive efficacy of beta-blocking therapy. Unfortunately, none of these observations are well-founded. Since long-term beta-blocking therapy may be associated with glucose abnormalities and hyperlipidemia, these factors should be closely monitored in the treatment of obese hypertensives.

Based on the correlation between high circulating norepinephrine levels and elevated blood pressure in obese hypertensives, pharmacological methods to reduce circulating catecholamines may be the antihypertensive treatment of choice. Additionally, the high concentrations of catecholamines could stimulate renin secretion and enhance cardiac output as well as their direct effect on increasing peripheral resistance. Few antihypertensive agents specifically reduce circulating levels of catecholamines. In fact, several agents such as diuretics, vasodilators and beta-adrenergic agents are associated with elevations in plasma catecholamines compared to pretreatment levels. The antihypertensive agents alpha-methyldopa, and to a greater extent clonidine, produce significant suppression of circulating norepinephrine levels during chronic therapy. This may account for part of their antihypertensive action although other mechanisms are also important. As these agents lower sympathetic activity, lower cardiac output and reduce renin activity, they may be the therapy of choice in obese hypertensive subjects where adequate weight loss was not attainable. During a weight reduction program, patients with significant hypertension should receive antihypertensive drugs to control blood pressure until significant weight loss is attained. These dietary programs are often prolonged and, unfortunately, are not universally successful. Leaving blood pressure untreated during this period could place these individuals at increased risk. If weight reduction is successful, antihypertensive therapy can be appropriately adjusted or withdrawn.

References

AMBROSIONI, E., TARTAGNI, F., MONTEGUGNOLI, L. and MAGNANI, B. (1979) Intralymphocytic sodium in hypertensive patients: a significant correlation. *Clinical Science*, **57** (*Suppl. 5*), 325–327

ANDRES, R. and CRABBE, J. (1966) Stimulation by insulin of active sodium transport by toad skin; influence of aldosterone and vasopressin. *Archives Internationales de Physiologie et de Biochimie*, **74**, 538–540

ANDRES, R. (1980) Effect of obesity on total mortality. *International Journal of Obesity*, **4 (4)**, 381–386

ANGELIN, B. and KALMAR, K. E. (1979) Adrenal hydroxylation in genetically obese hypertensive rats. *Biochemistry and Biophysics*, **574**, 344–355

ASHLEY, F. W. and KANNEL, W. B. (1974) Relation of weight change to changes in atherogenic traits: the Framingham study. *Journal of Chronic Diseases*, **27**, 103–114

ATCHLEY, D. W., LOEB, R. F., RICHARDS, D. W., BENEDICT, E. M. JR and DRISCOLL, M. E. (1933) On diabetic acidosis. *Journal of Clinical Investigation*, **12**, 297–326

ATKINSON, R. L. and KAISER, D. L. (1981) Nonphysician supervision of a very-low-calorie diet. Results in over 200 cases. *International Journal of Obesity*, **5 (3)**, 237–241

BERCHTOLD, P., BERGER, M., JÖRGENS, V. *et al.* (1981a) Cardiovascular risk factors and HDL-cholesterol levels in obesity. *International Journal of Obesity*, **5**, 1–10

BERCHTOLD, P., JÖRGENS, V., FINKE, C. and BERGER, M. (1981b) Epidemiology of obesity and hypertension. *International Journal of Obesity*, **5**, 1–7

BERCHTOLD, P., JÖRGENS, V., KEMMER, F. W. and BERGER, M. (1982) Obesity and hypertension: cardiovascular response of weight reduction. *Hypertension*, **4** (*5 Pt 2*), III50–III55

BERCHTOLD, P., SIMS, E. A. H. and BRANDAU, K. (1981) Obesity and hypertension. *International Journal of Obesity*, **5** (*Suppl. 1*), 1

BERGLUND, G. and ANDERSON, O. (1981) Body composition, metabolism and hormonal characteristics in unselected male hypertensives. *International Journal of Obesity*, **5** (*Supp. 1*), 143–156

BERGLUND, G., LJUNGMAN, S., HARTFORD, M., WILHELMSEN, L. and BJÖRNTORP, P. (1982) Type of obesity and blood pressure. *Hypertension*, **4**, 692–696

BESARAB, A., SILVA, P. and LANDSBERG, L. (1977) Effect of catecholamines on tubular function in the isolated perfused rat kidney. *American Journal of Physiology*, **233**, F39–F45

BJÖRNTORP, P. (1982) Hypertension and exercise. *Hypertension*, **4** (*Suppl. 3*), 56–59

BJÖRNTORP, P., HOLM, G., JACOBSSON, B. *et al.* (1977) Physical training in human hyperplastic obesity. IV. Effects on the hormonal status. *Metabolism*, **26**, 319–327

BOEHRINGER, K., BERETTA-PICCOLI, C., WEIDMANN, P., MEIER, A. and ZIEGLER, W. (1982) Pressor factors and cardiovascular pressor responsiveness in lean and overweight normal or hypertensive subjects. *Hypertension*, **4** (5), 697–702

CANESSA, M., ADRANGNA, N., SOLOMON, H. S., CONNOLLY, T. M. and TOSTESON, D. C. (1980) Increased sodium–lithium countertransport in red cells of patients with essential hypertension. *New England Journal of Medicine*, **302**, 772–776

CHIANG, B. N., PERLMAN, L. V. and EPSTEIN, F. H. (1969) Overweight and hypertension. A review. *Circulation*, **39**, 403–421

CLARKE, R. P., SCHLENKER, E. D. and MERROW, S. B. (1981) Nutrient intake, adiposity, plasma total cholesterol, and blood pressure in the (Vermont) Nutrition Program for older Americans. *American Journal of Clinical Nutrition*, **34**, 1743–1751

CRYER, P. E. (1980) Physiology and pathophysiology of human sympathoadrenal neuroendocrine system. *New England Journal of Medicine*, **303**, 436

DAHL, L. K. (1972) Salt and hypertension. *American Journal of Clinical Nutrition*, **25**, 231–244

DAHL, L. K., HEINE, M. and TASSINARI, L. (1962) Effects of chronic salt ingestion: evidence that genetic factors play an important role in susceptibility to experimental hypertension. *Journal of Experimental Medicine*, **115**, 1173–1190

DAHL, L., SILVER, L. and CHRISTIE, R. (1958) Role of salt in the fall of blood pressure accompanying reduction of obesity. *New England Journal of Medicine*, **258**, 1186–1192

DANFORTH, E. J., HORTON, E. S., O'CONNELL, M. *et al.* (1979) Dietary induced alterations in thyroid hormone metabolism during overnutrition. *Journal of Clinical Investigation*, **64**, 1336–1347

DEDIVITIIS, O., FAZIO, S., PETITTO, M., MADDALENA, G., CONTALDO, F. and MANCINI, M. (1981) Obesity and cardiac function. *Circulation*, **64**, 477–482

DeFRONZO, R. A. (1981) The effect of insulin on renal handling of sodium. A review with clinical implications. *Diabetologia*, **21**, 165–178

DeFRONZO, R. A., COOKE, C. R., ANDRES, R., FALOONA, G. R. and DAVIS, P. J. (1975) The effect of insulin on renal handling of sodium, potassium, calcium, and phosphate in man. *Journal of Clinical Investigation*, **55**, 845–855

DeFRONZO, R. A., GOLDBERG, M. and AGUS, Z. (1976) The effects of glucose and insulin on renal electrolyte transport. *Journal of Clinical Investigation*, **58**, 83–90

DeFRONZO, R. A., TOBIN, J. and ANDRES, R. (1979) The glucose clamp technique. A method for the quantification of beta cell sensitivity to glucose and of tissue sensitivity to insulin. *American Journal of Physiology*, **237**, E214–E223

DeHAVEN, J., SHERWIN, R., HENDLER, R. and FELIG, R. (1980) Nitrogen and sodium balance and sympathetic nervous system activity in obese subjects treated with a low-calorie protein or mixed diet. *New England Journal of Medicine*, **302**, 477–482

DeLUISE, M., BLACKBURN, G. L. and FLIER, J. S. (1980) Reduced activity of the red-cell sodium–potassium pump in human obesity. *New England Journal of Medicine*, **303**, 1017–1022

DERSHEWITZ, R. A., KAHN, H. A. and SOLOMON, N. (1981) The relationship of weight loss to blood pressure in the obese hypertensive adolescent. *Maryland State Medical Journal*, 53–56

DeWARDENER, H. E. and MacGREGOR, G. A. (1980) Dahl's hypothesis that a saluretic substance may be responsible for a sustained rise in arterial pressure: its possible role in essential hypertension. *Kidney International*, **18**, 1–9

DiBONA, G. F. (1978) Neural control of renal tubular sodium reabsorption in the dog. *Federation Proceedings*, **37**, 1214–1217

DUNKELMAN, S. S., FAIRHURST, B., PLAGER, J. and WATERHOUSE, C. (1964) Cortisol metabolism in obesity. *Journal of Clinical Endocrinology*, **24**, 832

DUSTAN, H. P., TARAZI, R. C. and MUJAIS, S. (1981) A comparison of hemodynamic and volume characteristics of obese and non-obese hypertensive patients. *International Journal of Obesity*, **5** (*Suppl. 1*), 19–26

ELIAHOU, H. E., IAINA, A., GAON, T., SHOCHAT, J. and MODAN, M. (1981) Body weight reduction necessary to attain normotension in the overweight hypertensive patients. *International Journal of Obesity*, **5** (**1**), 157–163

ELLISON, R. C., SOSENKO, J. M., HARPER, G. P., GIBBONS, L., PRATTER, F. E. and MIETTINEN, O. S. (1980) Obesity, sodium intake, and blood pressure in adolescents. *Hypertension*, **2** (*4 Pt. 2*), 78–82

ESANU, C., OPRESCU, M., MITRACHE, L., CRISTOVEANU, A., TACHE, A. and KLEPSCH, I. (1968) A clinical form of hypercortisolism differing from Cushing's syndrome. *Revue Roumaine d'Endocrinologie*, **5**, 267–272

FADEKE-ADEROUNMU, A. and SALAKO, L. A. (1979) Abnormal cation composition and transport in erythrocytes from hypertensive patients. *European Journal of Clinical Investigation*, **9**, 369–375

FIDELMAN, M. L., MAY, J. M., BIBER, T. U. L. and WATLINGTON, D. O. (1982) Insulin stimulation of Na^+ transport and glucose metabolism in cultured kidney cells. *American Journal of Physiology*, **242**, C121–C123

FLETCHER, A. P. (1954) The effect of weight reduction upon the blood pressure of obese hypertensive women. *Quarterly Journal of Medicine*, **23**, 331–345

FRANCO-MORSELLI, R., ELGHOZI, J. L., JOLY, E., DiGRUILCO, S. and MEYER, P. (1977) Increased plasma adrenaline in benign essential hypertension. *British Medical Journal*, **2**, 1251–1254

FREIS, E. D. (1976) Salt, volume and the prevention of hypertension. *Circulation*, **53**, 589–595

GARAY, R. P., DAGHER, G., PERNOLLET, M. G., DEVYNCK, M. A. and MEYER, P. (1980a) Inherited defect in a Na^+,K^+ cotransport system in erythrocytes from essential hypertensive patients. *Nature (London)*, **284**, 281–283

GARAY, R. P., ELGHOZI, J. L., DAGHER, G. and MEYER, P. (1980b) Laboratory distinction between essential and secondary hypertension by measurement of erythrocyte cation fluxes. *New England Journal of Medicine*, **302**, 769–771

GILLUM, R. F., TAYLOR, H. L., BROZEK, J., POLANSKY, P. and BLACKBURN, H. (1982) Indices of obesity and blood pressure in young men followed 32 years. *Journal of Chronic Diseases*, **35** (3), 211–219

GOLDSTEIN, D. S. (1983) Plasma catecholamines and essential hypertension: an analytic review. *Hypertension,* **5**, 86–99

GREMINGER, P., STUDER, A., LÜSCHER, T. *et al.* (1982) Weight reduction and blood pressure. *Schweizer Medizinische Wochenschrift*, **23**, 120–123

GROSS, H. A., LAKE, C. R., EBERT, M. H., ZIEGLER, M. G. and KOPIN, I. J. (1979) Catecholamine metabolism in primary anorexia nervosa. *Journal of Clinical Endocrinology Metabolism*, **49**, 805–809

GRUBER, K. A., RUDEL, L. L. and BULLOCK, B. C. (1982) Increased circulating levels of an endogenous digoxin-like factor in hypertensive monkeys. *Hypertension*, **4**, 348–354

GRUBER, K. A., WHITAKER, J. M. and BUCKALEW, V. M. JR (1980) Endogenous digitalis-like substance in plasma of volume-expanded dogs. *Nature (London)*, **287**, 743–745

GUNBY, P. (1980) A little (body) fat may not hasten death. *Journal of the American Medical Association*, **244**, 1660

HADDY, F., PAMNANI, M. and CLOUGH, D. (1978) The sodium–potassium pump in volume expanded hypertension. *Clinical and Experimental Hypertension*, **1**, 295–311

HALLBÄCK, M. and WEISS, L. (1977) Mechanisms of spontaneous hypertension in rats. *Medical Clinics of North America*, **61**, 593–609

HAMLYN, J. M., RINGEL, R., SCHAEFFER, J. *et al.* (1982) A circulating inhibitor of (Na^+-K^+)ATPase associated with essential hypertension. *Nature (London)*, **300**, 650–652

HERRERA, F. C. (1965) Effect of insulin on short-circuit current and sodium transport across toad urinary bladder. *American Journal of Physiology*, **209**, 819–824

HERRERA, F. C., WHITTEMBURGY, G. and PLANCHART, A. (1963) Effect of insulin on short-circuit current across isolated frog skin in the presence of calcium and magnesium. *Biochimica et Biophysica Acta*, **66**, 170–172

HIRAMATSU, K., YAMADA, T., ICHIKAWA, K., IZUMIYAMA, T. and NAGATA, H. (1981) Changes in endocrine activities relative to obesity in patients with essential hypertension. *Journal of American Geriatric Society*, **29 (1)**, 25–30

HOLM, G., JACOBSSON, B., TOSS, L., SMITH, U. and BJÖRNTORP, P. (1980) The effect of physical exercise on the regulation of beta-adrenergic receptors and adenylate cyclase in rat adipocytes. Proceedings of the Third International Congress of Obesity. *Alimentazione Nutrizione Metabolismo*, **1**, 280–288

HYPERTENSIVE DETECTION AND FOLLOW-UP PROGRAM COOPERATIVE GROUP (1979) Five-year findings of the Hypertension Detection and Follow-up Program: reduction in mortality of persons with high blood pressure including mild hypertension. *Journal of the American Medical Association*, **242**, 2562–2571

JAMES, W. P., HARALDSDOTTIR, J., LIDDELL, F., JUNG, T. R. and SHETTY, P. S. (1981) Autonomic responsiveness in obesity with and without hypertension. *International Journal of Obesity*, **5 (1)**, 73–78

JUDY, W. V., WATANABE, A. M., HENRY, D. P., BESCH, H. R., MURPHY, W. R. and HOCKEL, G. M. (1976) Sympathetic nerve activity: role in regulation of blood pressure in the spontaneously hypertensive rat. *Circulation Research*, **38**, 21–29 (*Suppl*)

JUNG, R. T., SHETTY, P. S., JAMES, W. P. T., BERRAND, M. and CALLINGHAM, B. A. (1979) Reduced thermogenesis in obesity. *Nature (London)*, **279**, 322–323

JUNG, R. T., SHETTY, P. S. and JAMES, W. P. T. (1980) Nutritional effects on thyroid and catecholamine metabolism. *Clinical Science*, **58**, 183–191

KAHLE, E. B., WALKER, R. B., EISENMAN, P. A., BEHALL, K. M., HALLFRISCH, J. and REISER, S. (1982) Moderate diet control in children: the effects of metabolic indicators that predict obesity-related degenerative diseases. *American Journal of Clinical Nutrition*, **35** (5), 950–957

KANNEL, W. B., BRAND, N., SKINNER, J. J., DAWBER, T. R. and McNAMARA, P. M. (1967) The relation of adiposity to blood pressure and development of hypertension. The Framingham study. *Annals of Internal Medicine*, **67**, 48–59

KANNEL, W. B. and GORDON, T. (1979) Physiological and medical concomitants of obesity: the Framingham study. In: *Obesity in America*, edited by G. A. Bray, NIH Publication, p. 79

KAPLAN, M. L. and LEVEILLE, G. A. (1976) Calorigenic response in obese and non-obese women. *American Journal of Clinical Nutrition*, **29**, 1108–1113

KAWASAKI, T., DELEA, C. S., BARTTER, F. C. and SMITH, H. (1978) The effect of high-sodium and low-sodium intakes on blood pressure and other related variables in human subjects with idiopathic hypertension. *American Journal of Medicine*, **64**, 193–198

KEYS, A., ARAVANIS, C., BLACKBURN, H. and TAYLOR, H. L. (1972) Coronary heart disease: overweight and obesity as risk factors. *Annals of Internal Medicine*, **77**, 15–27

KLIMES, I., NAGULESPARAN, M., UNGER, R. H., ARONOFF, S. L. and MOTT, D. M. (1982) Reduced Na$^+$,K$^+$-ATPase activity in intact red cells and isolated membranes from obese man. *Journal of Endocrinology Metabolism*, **54**, 721–724

KOLANOWSKI, J. (1981) Influence of insulin and glucagon on sodium balance in obese subjects during fasting and refeeding. *International Journal of Obesity*, **5** (1), 105–114

KOLANOWSKI, J., BODSON, A., DESMECHT, P., BEMELMANS, S., STEIN, F. and CRABBE, J. (1978) On the relationship between ketonuria and natriuresis during fasting and upon refeeding in obese patients. *European Journal of Clinical Investigation*, **9**, 277–282

KOLANOWSKI, J., KETELSLEGERS, J. M. and CRABBE, J. (1980) On the role of insulin in natriuresis of fast (abstract). *16th Meeting of the European Association for the Study of Diabetes, Athens*

KOLANOWSKI, J., SALVADOR, G., DESMECHT, P., HENQUIN, J. C. and CRABBE, J. (1977) Influence of glucagon on natriuresis and glucose-induced sodium retention in the fasting obese subject. *European Journal of Clinical Investigation*, **7**, 167–175

KROTKIEWSKI, M., MANDROUKAS, K., SJÖSTRÖM, L., SULLIVAN, L., WETTERQVIST, H. and BJÖRNTORP, P. (1979) Effects of long-term physical training on body fat, metabolism and blood pressure in obesity. *Metabolism*, **28**, 650–656

LANDSBERG, L. and YOUNG, J. B. (1978a) Fasting, feeding and regulation of the sympathetic nervous system. *New England Journal of Medicine*, **298**, 1295–1300

LANDSBERG, L. and YOUNG, J. B. (1978b) Diet and the sympathetic nervous system: relationship to hypertension. *International Journal of Obesity*, **5**, 79–91

LEW, E. A. (1973) High blood pressure, other risk factors and longevity: the insurance viewpoint. In: *Hypertension Manual*, edited by J. H. Laragh, p. 43. New York: Yorke Medical Books

LIN, M. H., ROMSOS, D. R., AKARA, T. and LEVEILLE, G. A. (1978) Na$^+$-K$^+$-ATPase enzyme units in skeletal muscle from lean and obese mice. *Biochemical and Biophysical Research Communications*, **80**, 398–404

LOSSE, H., WEHMEYER, H. and WESSELS, F. (1960) The water and electrolyte content of erythrocytes in arterial hypertension. *Klinische Wochenschrift*, **38**, 393–398

LUFT, F. C., RANKIN, L. I., BLOCH, R. *et al.* (1979) Cardiovascular and humoral responses to extremes of sodium intake in normal black and white men. *Circulation*, **80**, 617–706

LUFT, F. C., WEINBERGER, M. H. and GRIM, C. E. (1982) Sodium sensitivity and resistance in normotensive humans. *American Journal of Medicine*, **72**, 726–736

LYNDS, B. G., SEYLER, S. K. and MORGAN, B. M. (1980) The relationship between elevated blood pressure and obesity. *American Journal of Public Health*, **70**, 171–173

MANN, G. V., SHAFFER, R. D., ANDERSON, R. S. and SANDSTEAD, A. H. (1964) Cardiovascular disease in the Masai. *Journal of Atherosclerotic Research*, **4**, 289–297

McCUE, C. M., MILLER, W. W. and MAUCK, H. P. (1979) Adolescent blood pressure in Richmond, Virginia schools. *Virginia Medicine*, **106**, 210–220

McGEOCH, J. E. M. (1982) Specific insulin binding to purified (Na–K)-ATPase associated with rapid activation of the enzyme. *Third International Conference on Na–K ATPase. Yale University, New Haven, Connecticut, August 17–21*

MESSERLI, F. H. (1982) Cardiovascular effects of obesity and hypertension. *Lancet*, **11**, 1165–1168

MESSERLI, F. H., CHRISTIE, B., DeCARVALHO, J. G. *et al.* (1981) Obesity and essential hypertension. Hemodynamics, intravascular volume, sodium excretion, and plasma renin activity. *Archives of Internal Medicine*, **141 (1)**, 81–85

MESSERLI, F. H., SUNDGAARD-RIISE, K., REISIN, E. *et al.* (1982) Left ventricular adaptation to obesity. *American Journal of Cardiology*, **49**, 977–1006

MILLER, J. H. and BOGDONOFF, M. D. (1954) Antidiuresis associated with administration of insulin. *Journal of Applied Physiology*, **6**, 509–512

MIR, M. A., CHARALAMBOUS, B. M., MORGAN, K. and EVANS, P. J. (1981) Erythrocyte sodium–potassium ATPase and sodium transport in obesity. *New England Journal of Medicine*, **305**, 1264–1268

MOORE, R. D. and RABOVSKY, J. L. (1979) Mechanism of insulin action on resting membrane potential of frog skeletal muscle. *American Journal of Physiology*, **236**, C249–C254

MUJAIS, S. K., TARAZI, R. C., DUSTAN, H. P., FOUAD, F. M. and BRAVO, E. L. (1982) Hypertension in obese patients: hemodynamic and volume studies. *Hypertension*, **4 (1)**, 84–92

MULTIPLE RISK FACTORS INTERVENTION TRIAL RESEARCH GROUP (1976) The multiple risk factor intervention trial (MRFIT): a national study of primary prevention of heart disease. *Journal of the American Medical Association*, **235**, 825–827

NIZET, A., LEFEBVRE, R. and CRABBE, J. (1971) Control by insulin of sodium, potassium, and water excretion by the isolated dog kidney. *Pflugers Archive, European Journal of Physiology*, **323**, 11–20

NOPPA, H., BENGTSSON, C., WEDEL, H. *et al.* (1980) Obesity in relation to morbidity and mortality from cardiovascular disease. *American Journal of Epidemiology*, **111**, 682–692

PAFFENBERGER, R. S., THORNE, M. C. and WING, A. L. (1968) Chronic disease in former college students. VIII Characteristics in youth predisposing to hypertension in later years. *American Journal of Epidemiology*, **88**, 25–34

PAGE, L. B. (1976) Epidemiologic evidence on the etiology of human hypertension and its possible prevention. *American Heart Journal*, **91**, 527–531

PATEL, Y. C., EGGEN, D. A. and STRONG, J. P. (1980) Obesity, smoking and atherosclerosis. A study of interassociations. *Atherosclerosis*, **36**, 481–490

PITTET, P. H., CHAPPUIS, K. and ACHESON, F. (1976) Thermic effect of glucose in obese subjects studied by direct and indirect calorimetry. *British Journal of Nutrition*, **35**, 281–292

RAISON, J., ACHIMASTOS, A., BOUTHIER, J., LONDON, G. and SAFAR, M. (1983) Intravascular volume, extracellular fluid volume, and total body water in obese and nonobese hypertensive patients. *American Journal of Cardiology*, **51**, 165–170

RAMIREZ, A., FLETES, L., MIZRAHI, L. and PARRA, A. (1978) Daily urinary catecholamine profile in marasmus and kwashiorkor. *American Journal of Clinical Nutrition*, **31**, 41–45

RAMSAY, L. E., RAMSAY, M. H., HETTIARACHCHI, J., DAVIES, D. L. and WINCHESTER, J. (1978) Weight reduction in a blood pressure clinic. *British Medical Journal*, **2**, 244–245

REISIN, E., ABEL, R., MODAN, M., SILVERBERG, D. S., ELIAHOU, H. E. and MODAN, B. (1978) Effect of weight loss without salt restriction on the reduction of blood pressure in overweight hypertensive patients. *New England Journal of Medicine*, **298**, 1–6

REISIN, E., FROHLICH, E. D., MESSERLI, F. H. *et al.* (1983) Cardiovascular changes after weight reduction in obesity hypertension. *Annals of Internal Medicine*, **98**, 315–319

ROBERTS, J. and MAURER, K. (1976) Blood pressure of persons 6–74 years of age in the United States. *USDHEW Advance Data No. 1.* Washington DC: US Department of Health, Education and Welfare

ROBERTSON, D., GARLAND, G. A., ROBERTSON, R. M., NIES, A. S., SHAND, D. G. and OATES, J. A. (1979) Comparative assessment of stimuli that release neuronal and adrenomedullary catecholamines in man. *Circulation*, **56**, 637 (*Suppl. 4*)

ROSE, R. H. (1922) Weight reduction and its remarkable effect on high blood pressure. *New York Medical Journal Medical Reviews*, **115**, 752–758

ROWE, J. W., YOUNG, J. B., MINAKER, K. L., STEVENS, A. L., PALLOTTA, J. and LANDSBERG, L. (1981) Effect of insulin and glucose infusion on sympathetic nervous system activity in normal man. *Diabetes*, **30**, 219–225

RUDERMAN, N. B., SCHNEIDER, S. H. and BERCHTOLD, P. (1981) The 'metabolically obese', normal-weight individual. *American Journal of Clinical Nutrition*, **34** (8), 1617–1621

SAUDEK, C. D., BOULTER, P. R., KNOPP, R. H. and ARKY, R. A. (1974) Sodium retention accompanying insulin treatment of diabetes mellitus. *Diabetes*, **23**, 240–246

SCHLOEDER, F. X. and STINEBAUGH, B. J. (1970) Renal tubular sites of natriuresis of fasting and glucose-induced sodium conservation. *Metabolism*, **19**, 1119–1128

SCHWARTZ, R. S., HALTER, J. and BIERMAN, E. L. (1980) The relation of abnormal dietary-induced thermogenesis in obesity to plasma triiodothyronine and norepinephrine. *Clinical Research*, **28**, 450A

SCHWARTZ, R. S., HALTER, J. B. and BIERMAN, E. L. (1983) Reduced thermic effect of feeding in obesity: role of norepinephrine. *Metabolism*, **35**, 114–117

SEVERS, P. S., BIRCH, M., OSIKAWSHA, B. and TUMBRIDGE, R. D. G. (1977) Plasma noradrenaline in essential hypertension. *Lancet*, **1**, 1078

SEVERS, P. S., GORDON, D., PEART, W. S. *et al.* (1980) Blood pressure and its correlates in urban and tribal Africa. *Lancet*, **2**, 60–64

SIMS, E. A. H. (1982) Mechanisms of hypertension in the overweight. *Hypertension*, **4** (*Suppl. 3*), III43–III49

SIMS, E. A. H. (1981) Hypertension and obesity: mechanisms and management. *International Journal of Obesity*, **5** (*Suppl. I*), 9–18

SOWERS, J. R., WHITFIELD, L. A., CATANIA, R. A. *et al.* (1982a) Role of the sympathetic nervous system in blood pressure maintenance in obesity. *Journal of Clinical Endocrinology and Metabolism*, **54**, 1181–1185

SOWERS, J. R., WHITFIELD, L., BECK, F. W. H., TUCK, M. L., DORNFELD, L. and MAXWELL, M. (1982b) Role of enhanced sympathetic nervous system activity and reduced Na^+-K^+-dependent adenosine triphosphatase activity in maintenance of elevated blood pressure in obesity. *Clinical Science*, **3**, 121s–124s

SOWERS, J. R., NYBY, M., STERN, N. *et al.* (1982c) Blood pressure and hormone changes associated with weight reduction in the obese. *Hypertension*, **4 (5)**, 686–691

STAMLER, J., FARINARO, E., MOHONNIER, L. M., HALL, Y., MOSS, D. and STAMLER, R. (1980) Prevention and control of hypertension by nutritional-hygenic means. Long-term experiments of the Chicago Coronary Prevention Evaluation Program. *Journal of the American Medical Association*, **243**, 1819–1823

STAMLER, R., STAMLER, J., RIEDLINGER, W. F., ALGERA, G. and ROBERTS, R. H. (1978) Weight and blood pressure. Findings in hypertension screening of 1 million Americans. *Journal of the American Medical Association*, **240**, 1607–1610

STENE, M., PANAGIOTIS, N., TUCK, M. L., SOWERS, J. R., MAYES, D. M. and BERG, G. (1980) Plasma norepinephrine levels are influenced by sodium intake, glucocorticoid administration and circadian changes in normal man. *Journal of Clinical Endocrinology and Metabolism*, **51**, 1340–1345

TOBIAN, L. (1979) The relationship of salt to hypertension. *American Journal of Clinical Nutrition*, **32**, 2739–2748

TUCK, M. L., SOWERS, J., DORNFELD, L., KLEDZIK, G. and MAXWELL, M. (1981) The effect of weight reduction on blood pressure, plasma renin activity and plasma aldosterone levels in obese patients. *New England Journal of Medicine*, **304**, 930–933

TUCK, M. L., SOWERS, J. R., DORNFELD, L., WHITFIELD, L. and MAXWELL, M. (1983) Reductions in plasma catecholamines and blood pressure during weight loss in obese subjects. *Acta Endocrinologica*, **102**, 252–257

TYROLAR, H. A., HEYDEN, S. and HAMES, C. G. (1975) Weight and hypertension: Evans County studies of blacks and whites. In: *Epidemiology and Control of Hypertension*, edited by O. Paul, pp. 177–201. New York: Stratton Intercontinental

VETERANS ADMINISTRATION COOPERATIVE STUDY GROUP ON ANTIHYPERTENSIVE AGENTS (1967) Effect of treatment on morbidity in hypertension. Results of patients with diastolic blood pressure averaging 115–129. *Journal of the American Medical Association*, **202**, 116–122

VETERANS ADMINISTRATION COOPERATIVE STUDY GROUP ON ANTIHYPERTENSIVE AGENTS (1970) Effects of treatment on morbidity in hypertension. II. Results in patients with diastolic blood pressure averaging 90–114. *Journal of the American Medical Association*, **213**, 1143–1152

VETERANS ADMINISTRATION COOPERATIVE STUDY ON ANTIHYPERTENSIVE AGENTS (1977) Propranolol in the treatment of essential hypertension. *Journal of the American Medical Association*, **237**, 2303–2310

VOORS, A. W., WEBBER, L. S., FRERICHS, R. R. and BERENSON, G. S. (1977) Body height and body mass as determinants of basal blood pressure in children – the Bogalusa Heart Study. *American Journal of Epidemiology*, **106**, 101–110

WAMBACH, G., HELBER, A., BONNER, G. and HUMMERICH, W. (1979) Natrium–kalium–adenosintriphosphatase-aktivitat in erythrozytenghosts von patienten mit essentieller hypertonie. *Klinische Wochenschrift*, **157**, 169–172

WELLE, S., LILAVIVANTHANA, U. and CAMPBELL, R. G. (1980) Effect of oral sucrose on blood pressure in the spontaneously hypertensive rat. *Metabolism*, **29**, 806–809

WELLE, S., LILAVIVANTHANA, U. and CAMPBELL, R. G. (1981) Thermic effect of feeding in man: increased plasma norepinephrine levels following glucose but not protein or fat consumption. *Metabolism*, **30**, 953–958

WEXLER, B. C. and McMURTRY, J. P. (1981) Ameliorative effects of adrenalectomy on the hyperphagia, hyperlipidaemia, hyperglycaemia and hypertension of obese, spontaneously hypertensive rats (obese/SHR). *British Journal of Experimental Pathology*, **62** (2), 146–157

WILLIAMS, L. T., LEFKOWITZ, R. J., WATANABE, A. M., HATHAWAY, D. R. and BESCH, H. R. (1977) Thyroid hormone regulation of β-adrenergic receptor number. *Journal of Biological Chemistry*, **252**, 2787–2789

WOODWARD, C. B., QUINONES, M. A. and ALEXANDER, J. K. (1978) Pathogenesis of myocardial dysfunction in extreme obesity. *Circulation*, **58** (*Suppl. 2*), 230–239

YORK, D. A., BRAY, G. A. and YUKIMURA, Y. (1978) An enzymatic defect in the obese (ob/ob) mouse: loss of thyroid-induced sodium- and potassium-dependent adenosine-triphosphatase. *Proceedings of the National Academy of Sciences of the USA*, **75**, 477–481

YOUNG, J. B. and LANDSBERG, L. (1977) Suppression of the sympathetic nervous system during fasting. *Science*, **196**, 1473–1475

YOUNG, J. B. and LANDSBERG, L. (1979) Effect of diet and cold exposure on norepinephrine turnover in pancreas and liver. *American Journal of Physiology*, **236**, E524–E533

YOUNG, J. B. and LANDSBERG, L. (1980) Impaired suppression of sympathetic activity during fasting in the gold thioglucose-treated mouse. *Journal of Clinical Investigation*, **65**, 1086–1094

YOUNG, J. B. and LANDSBERG, L. (1981) The effect of oral sucrose on blood pressure in the spontaneously hypertensive rat. *Metabolism*, **30**, 421–424

YOUNG, J. B., MULLEN, D. and LANDSBERG, L. (1978) Caloric restriction lowers blood pressure in the spontaneously hypertensive rat. *Metabolism*, **27**, 1711–1714

ZIERLER, K. and ROGUS, E. M. (1981) Effects of peptide hormones and adrenergic agents on membrane potentials of target cells. *Federation Proceedings*, **40**, 121–124

Conclusions

Christopher R. W. Edwards and Robert M. Carey

In the foregoing chapters of this book, recent developments in endocrinology important to an understanding of the pathogenesis and/or maintenance of essential hypertension have been explored in depth by a distinguished group of investigators in the field. New hormones and novel mechanisms of hormone secretion, delivery and action provide a basis for studies of physiology and pathophysiology in experimental animals and in man. The interrelationships of the various hormonal systems to each other as well as to sodium, volume and haemodynamic influences on blood pressure have been described. Although the main focus is essential hypertension, consideration of the role of hormones has been extended to the possibly related areas of hypertension in pregnancy, diabetes and obesity. The overall objective of this effort has been to consolidate present concepts of the role of endocrine factors and to emphasize their potential relevance for future research.

Over the many years since the introduction of sympathectomy for the treatment of hypertension, it has been apparent that the sympathetic nervous system and neuroendocrine factors are pivotal in the pathogenesis of essential hypertension.

In the first chapter, Ferrario and colleagues review the hormonal basis for central nervous system control of blood pressure. The important role of the brain in the regulation of peripheral autonomic nervous system function is linked to recently discovered neuroendocrine mechanisms. Monoaminergic mechanisms, vasopressin, and the renin–angiotensin system all play an important regulatory role in the central nervous system as well as serving as effector mechanisms in the control of blood pressure. The common denominators of the central nervous system in hypertension appear to be enhanced sympathetic nervous system activity as well as altered neuroendocrine function.

In the second chapter, Brown provides fascinating evidence for the hypothesis that at least one of the mechanisms leading to an increase in blood pressure in hypertensive subjects might be epinephrine released from sympathetic nerve endings after uptake from the circulation. He postulates that epinephrine is a physiological agonist at the presynaptic beta-adrenergic receptor, resulting in a positive feedback loop to enhance sympathetic nervous system activity and produce hypertension on a chronic basis.

368

Elijovich and Krakoff then summarize and evaluate the evidence that circulating vasopressin may play a role in hypertension. These authors conclude that altered smooth muscle responsiveness to vasopressin and/or buffering of the baroreceptor reflex may amplify the vascular effect of small increases in circulating vasopressin concentrations in human hypertension. With the current availability of improved methods for the measurement of blood, tissue and brain hormones and of specific hormone antagonists, the role of these neuroendocrine mechanisms should become clearer in the near future.

Sodium intake has been associated with hypertension over the 36 years since Kempner first introduced his rice diet for the treatment of hypertension. Overbeck meticulously reviews the role of sodium in hypertension from the broad perspective of clinical, *in vivo* animal and *in vitro* biochemical studies. He presents the evidence that in the early phases of hypertension depression of the vascular smooth muscle cell membrane sodium pump may be present in association with a circulating digitalis-like substance or natriuretic hormone. In this view, increased vascular wall sodium would be associated with waterlogging, causing an increase in peripheral vascular resistance.

DeWardener and MacGregor follow with a comprehensive hypothesis regarding the possible role of a natriuretic hormone. In their view there is an initial reduction in renal sodium excretion which leads to extracellular volume expansion and stimulates secretion of a hypothalamic natriuretic hormone. This then adjusts renal sodium excretion and returns sodium balance to normal. Thus sodium balance is sustained at the expense of increased circulating concentrations of this sodium transport inhibitor, which raises vascular smooth muscle reactivity and tone, elevating peripheral vascular resistance and blood pressure.

Fraser and Padfield then review the evidence in favour of a role for mineralocorticoids in the pathogenesis of essential hypertension. Important abnormalities in aldosterone secretion in the form of essential hypertension with low plasma renin activity are clearly documented, and may occur in as many as 20–30% of patients with essential hypertension. However, their specific role as well as the role of other mineralocorticoids in the pathogenesis of essential hypertension is presently unclear.

Williams and Hollenberg then present the results of their years of collaborative study which has culminated in the identification of defects in renal and adrenal responses to angiotensin II in as many as 40% of the hypertensive population. These defects include failure of modulation of renal responses during high sodium intake and a reduction in angiotensin II-induced aldosterone secretion during sodium deficiency. Recent evidence links these two important defects in the same hypertensive patient, and provides two potential explanations for the pathogenesis of hypertension. During high sodium intake, failure of renal modulation would contribute to sodium retention and volume-dependent hypertension, while an angiotensin II-dependent vasoconstrictor form of hypertension would pertain in the sodium-restricted state.

Recent evidence suggests that vasodilator substances may possibly be deficient in some forms of experimental hypertension. Peach and Singer review the role of the endothelium in the production of certain vasodilator substances such as prostanoids, purinergic substances and endothelium-dependent relaxing factors as well as importance of the endothelium in the modulation of calcium and acetylcholine-induced responses.

This is followed by a thorough discussion by Watson of the vascular and renal effects of prostaglandins, thromboxanes and leukotrienes. He relates these effects to their possible role in experimental and human hypertension.

Muirhead then details the recent discovery of the function of the renomedullary interstitial cells, and presents evidence that their secretory products, a neutral and polar lipid, fulfil Koch's postulates as possible new hormones of promising importance in the control of vascular resistance and blood pressure.

In a consideration of some selected clinical states related to hypertension, each of the last three chapters reviews the evidence for hormonal contributions to hypertension in pregnancy, diabetes mellitus and obesity. Rubin suggests that the area of pregnancy is poorly understood and a potential area for fruitful future investigation. Drury indicates the involvement of several endocrine mechanisms, including increased exchangeable sodium, inappropriately elevated angiotensin II, catecholamine and aldosterone levels and increased vascular sensitivity to pressor agents in diabetes. Tuck demonstrates a myriad of endocrine and metabolic abnormalities in obese patients with hypertension.

It will be obvious from these chapters that the field of hormones in the regulation of blood pressure is advancing at a rapid rate and that much of the important new work in hypertension centres on the primary causal role of hormonal abnormalities. Although much work needs to be done, valuable new insights into endocrine mechanisms have already contributed greatly to our understanding of the pathogenesis and treatment of this ubiquitous disease. Now, for the first time after several decades of research and with substantial assurance, we can state that essential hypertension is in a very large measure an endocrine disease.

Index